ISGE Series

Series Editor
Andrea R. Genazzani

More information about this series at http://www.springer.com/series/11871

Martin Birkhaeuser • Andrea R. Genazzani
Editors

Pre-Menopause, Menopause and Beyond

Volume 5: Frontiers in Gynecological Endocrinology

Springer

INTERNATIONAL SCHOOL OF GYNECOLOGICAL AND REPRODUCTIVE ENDOCRINOLOGY
THE EDUCATIONAL BRANCH OF ISGE

Editors
Martin Birkhaeuser
Professor emeritus for Gynaecological Endocrinology and Reproductive Medicine
University of Bern
Bern, Switzerland

Andrea R. Genazzani
International Society of Gynecological Endocrinology
Pisa, Italy

ISSN 2197-8735 ISSN 2197-8743 (electronic)
ISGE Series
ISBN 978-3-319-63539-2 ISBN 978-3-319-63540-8 (eBook)
https://doi.org/10.1007/978-3-319-63540-8

Library of Congress Control Number: 2017960823

Printed on acid-free paper

This Springer imprint is published by Springer Nature
The registered company is Springer International Publishing AG
The registered company address is: Gewerbestrasse 11, 6330 Cham, Switzerland

Preface

Proceedings of the International Society of Gynecological Endocrinology (ISGE) Winter School 2017

This volume contains the lectures presented at the 6th ISGRE 2017 Winter School, held in Madonna di Campiglio between 22 and 26 January 2017.

Important recent developments in our knowledge of premenopause and menopause, with their respective clinical implications and therapies, have encouraged the faculty to organize this Winter School. The following chapters have been selected:

- Menopause: symptoms and neuroendocrine impact: endocrine and neuroendocrine biological changes from menopause to aging—brain impact of sex steroids withdrawal of the menopause—importance and modern management of climacteric symptoms
- Intracrinology: its role in menopause
- Menopause: bone and cardiovascular impact: how to maintain healthy bones after menopause—the effect of menopause and HRT on coronary heart disease—how to prevent cardiovascular disorders: influence of gonadal steroids
- Menopause symptoms: the optimal therapies—recent changes and advances
- The breast: benign breast diseases, BRCA mutation, and breast cancer
- Infertility in late reproductive age: importance of autoimmunity—treatment after the age of 40—oocyte donation in menopausal women
- Thyroid function and pregnancy outcome after ART—what is the evidence? Thyroid disorders in climacteric women
- Polycystic ovary and metabolic syndrome: implications of cardiometabolic dysfunction—metabolic changes during menopausal transition—role of Metformin in climacteric women—weight and body composition management after menopause
- Surgical challenges after menopause: problems and solutions linked to them pelvic floor, bladder dysfunction, and urinary incontinence

On behalf of the ISGRE faculty, it is our pleasure to invite you to profit from the accumulated scientific and clinical knowledge assembled in these proceedings of our highly successful Winter School 2017.

Bern, Switzerland
Pisa, Italy

Martin Birkhaeuser
Andrea R. Genazzani

Contents

Part I

Menopause: Symptoms and Neuroendocrine Impact

Intracrinology: The New Science of Sex Steroid Physiology in Women

1

Fernand Labrie

1.1 Introduction

As example of the traditional mechanisms of endocrinology, the estrogens secreted by the ovaries are distributed by the bloodstream to all tissues of the body, thus leaving the tissue specificity to the presence or absence in each cell of various concentrations of estrogen receptors. Accordingly, in premenopausal women, the ovarian estrogens are distributed through the blood from which they control the menstrual cycle, fertility, development of the sex organs and breast, pregnancy, and lactation.

The situation, however, changes abruptly at menopause when the secretion of estradiol (E_2) by the ovaries stops and dehydroepiandrosterone (DHEA) becomes the exclusive source of sex steroids made intracellularly in each peripheral tissue independently from the ovary [1].

It is in fact remarkable that women and men, in addition to possessing a highly performant endocrine system, have largely invested in sex steroid intracrine formation in peripheral tissues, especially in women [1, 2]. In fact, while the ovaries and testes are the exclusive source of sex steroids in species below primates, the situation is very different in women and men and higher primates where the active sex steroids are in large part or wholly synthesized locally in peripheral tissues from DHEA by intracrine mechanisms, especially after menopause [1, 3–5]. In fact, all androgens in women before and after menopause are synthesized from DHEA in peripheral tissues, while, after menopause, E_2 is also exclusively synthesized from DHEA by the intracrine enzymes [1, 3, 4, 6].

Intracrinology operates in each cell in each tissue using the highly sophisticated mechanisms engineered over 500 million years and able to adjust both the

F. Labrie
Emeritus Professor, Laval University, Quebec, QC, G1V 0A6 Canada

Endoceutics Inc., Quebec, QC, Canada
e-mail: fernand.labrie@endoceutics.com

M. Birkhaeuser, A.R. Genazzani (eds.), *Pre-Menopause, Menopause and Beyond*, ISGE Series, https://doi.org/10.1007/978-3-319-63540-8_1

intracellular formation and inactivation of sex steroids to the local needs, with no biologically significant release of active estrogens or androgens in the circulation [1, 3, 6], thus avoiding systemic exposure to circulating E_2 and testosterone. This situation is very different from all animal models used in the laboratory, namely, rats, mice, guinea pigs, and all others (except monkeys) where the secretion of sex steroids takes place exclusively in the gonads with, in addition, a lack of sex steroid-inactivating enzymes [7, 8]. Such fundamental differences in sex steroid physiology between the human and the lower species markedly complicate the interpretation of data obtained in laboratory animals and very seriously limit their relevance to the human.

Long life after menopause is a recent phenomenon resulting from the impressive progress of medicine and sanitary measures which have succeeded in markedly prolonging life. In fact, life expectancy in US women has gone from 47 years in 1900 to about 79 years in 2015, for a gain of about 32 years of additional life achieved over a period of only 115 years, such a dramatic increase being equivalent to an average of 3.3 months of life added at each calendar year. In fact, women now spend one third of their lifetime after menopause. Consequently, since the menopausal symptoms and signs caused by sex steroid deficiency are a relatively recent phenomenon, evolution did not have sufficient time to develop proper control mechanisms able to increase DHEA secretion by the adrenals when the concentration of DHEA in the circulation becomes low. In fact, the secretion of ACTH which is the stimulus for both cortisol and DHEA secretion by the adrenals is exclusively controlled by the serum levels of cortisol (Fig. 1.1).

The advantage of sex steroid medicine is that accurate and reliable assays of sex steroids as well as their precursors and metabolites are available [9–17]. With the possibility of a precise knowledge about the serum levels of sex steroids, specific sex steroid replacement therapy can be prescribed with precision in response to well-quantified needs. The treatment of sex steroid deficiency is somewhat facilitated by the fact that DHEA is the unique source of both androgens and estrogens after menopause, while each target tissue makes its proper adjustments to the local requirements [5] (Fig. 1.1).

In vulvovaginal atrophy (VVA), the local replacement of the missing DHEA responsible for VVA symptoms is further facilitated by the strictly local action following intravaginal administration of low dose DHEA [18–23]. It should be remembered that the radioimmunoassays traditionally used to measure serum sex steroids had low specificity, thus giving misleading and impossible to validate values, especially at the low concentrations of serum testosterone and E_2 present in postmenopausal women [15–17, 24, 25].

The purpose of this review is to summarize the data describing the highly sophisticated, uniquely efficient, and safe mechanisms of intracrinology, which are specific to the human. This review should indicate the dramatic differences between the intracrinology of DHEA and the classical endocrinology of estrogens, which is limited to premenopause.

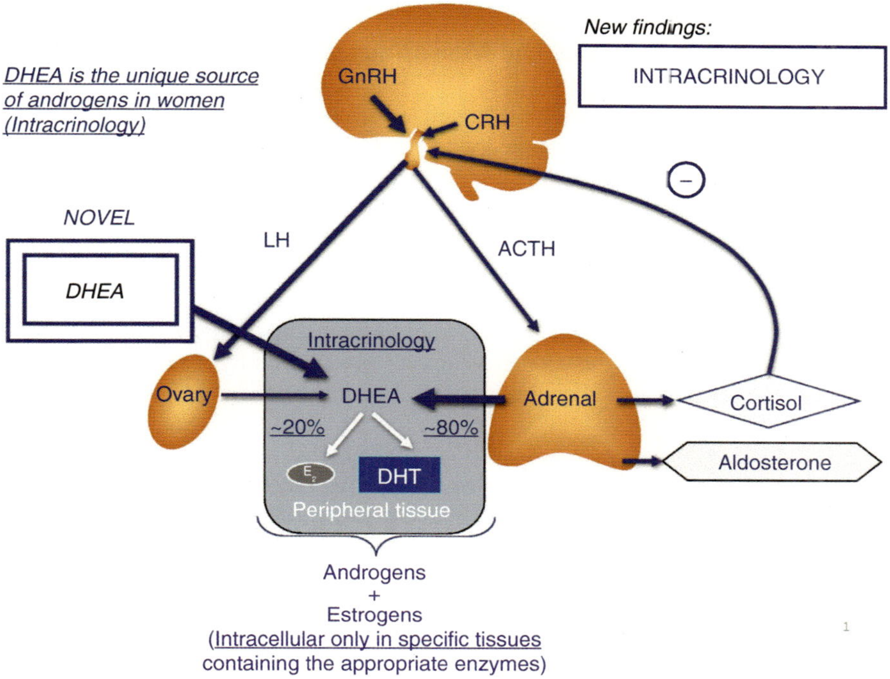

Fig. 1.1 Schematic representation of the adrenal (~80%) and ovarian (~20%) sources of DHEA in postmenopausal women. While the circulating levels of serum cortisol control the secretion of adrenocorticotropin (ACTH), ACTH stimulates the secretion of both cortisol and DHEA (dehydroepiandrosterone) by the adrenals. DHEA, however, has no influence on the secretion of ACTH. The secretion of DHEA is thus exclusively regulated by the serum levels of cortisol. *GnRH* gonadotropin-releasing hormone, E_2 estradiol, *DHT* dihydrotestosterone

1.2 Androgens Are Made Intracellularly from DHEA During the Whole Life in Women

It is important to indicate that postmenopausal women make approximately 50% as much androgens as observed in men of the same age. As mentioned above, all androgens in women are made from circulating DHEA [4]. About 80% of the serum DHEA in postmenopausal women is from adrenal origin, while approximately 20% originates from the ovary [5, 26–30] (Fig. 1.1). Since serum DHEA starts decreasing at the age of about 30 years [31, 32] with an average 60% loss already observed at time of menopause [28], women are not only missing estrogens after menopause, but they have been progressively deprived from androgens for about 20 years [4].

1.3 Serum DHEA Decreases Markedly with Age and Is the Main Cause of the Menopausal Symptoms

A problem which accompanies the relatively recent and ongoing prolongation of life is that the secretion of DHEA markedly decreases with age starting at about the age of 30 years [5, 31, 33]. Such a marked decrease in the formation of DHEA by the adrenals during aging [31, 34] results in a dramatic fall in the formation, and consequently activity, of both estrogens and androgens in peripheral target tissues. This fall in serum DHEA is the mechanism most likely responsible for the increased incidence and severity of the symptoms and signs of menopause. It is thus reasonable to believe that the loss of bone, loss of muscle mass, hot flashes, VVA, and sexual dysfunction, which often occur before the decrease in estrogen secretion by the ovaries, are secondary to the premenopausal decrease in the availability of serum DHEA [35].

1.4 At Menopause, DHEA Becomes the Exclusive Source of Both Estrogens and Androgens in Women

At menopause, or at the end of the reproductive years, the secretion of E_2 by the ovaries usually stops within a period of 6 to 12 months. Thereafter, throughout postmenopause, serum E_2 remains at biologically inactive concentrations at or below 9.3 pg/ml [3] but not 20 pg/ml as frequently used based upon inaccurate values obtained by immuno-based assays which lack specificity, thus giving approximately 100% higher values than the accurate (MS)-based assays. This difference is due to unidentified compounds other than E_2 which interfere in the assays. The maintenance of serum E_2 at low biologically inactive concentrations eliminates stimulation of the endometrium with the accompanying risk of endometrial cancer [36].

It is important to mention, at this stage, that the new understanding of the physiology of sex steroids in women [5, 37] could only become possible following the availability of the highly sensitive, precise, specific, and accurate mass spectrometry-based assays validated according to the US FDA guidelines [9, 10, 13, 14, 16, 17, 28, 33, 38]. Due to the low specificity and the inability of the radioimmunoassays traditionally used to measure low serum sex steroids adequately, the above-mentioned MS-based assays had to be developed and validated to measure with precision and accuracy the low concentrations found in postmenopausal women [16, 24, 25]. Otherwise, intracrinology would not have been developed and applied to therapeutics.

1.5 Sophisticated Battery of Sex Steroid-Synthesizing Enzymes in Peripheral Tissues: Intracrinology

Starting approximately 500 million years ago [39, 40], evolution has progressively provided the peripheral tissues with the elaborate set of enzymes able to make the DHEA-derived sex steroids intracellularly, independently from serum estrogens,

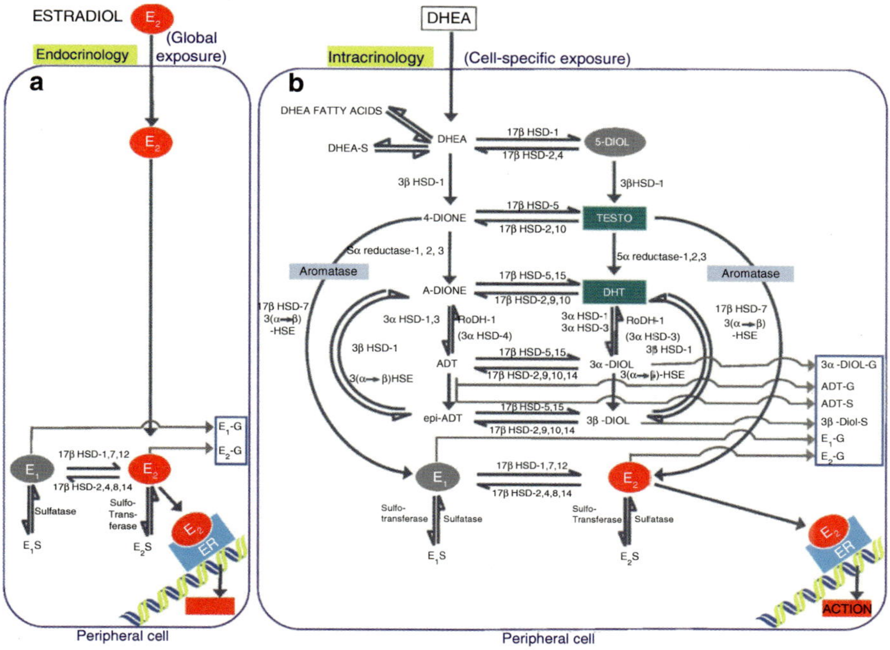

Fig. 1.2 (**a**) In the endocrine system, estradiol interacts directly with the estrogen receptors without any rate-limiting steps. (**b**) In the intracrine system, on the other hand, a much higher level of complexity is in operation with each cell controlling its level of exposure to estrogens and androgens. The inactive steroid precursor DHEA is submitted to the sophisticated enzymatic control mechanisms expressed in each cell before locally providing a minute amount of estradiol which can then exert its cell-specific activity. Evolution, though 500 million years, has succeeded in engineering more than 30 different steroidogenic and steroid-inactivating enzymes which transform DHEA, an inactive molecule by itself, into different intermediates and metabolites before ultimately making small specific amounts of estradiol and testosterone in agreement with the physiology and needs of each cell. The human steroidogenic and steroid-inactivating enzymes expressed in in peripheral intracrine tissues. *4-dione*, androstenedione, *A-dione* 5α-androstane-3,17-dione; *ADT* androsterone, *epi-ADT* epiandrosterone, E_1 estrone, E_1S estrone sulfate, E_2 17β-estradiol, E_2S estradiol sulfate, *5-diol* androst-5-ene-3α, 17β-diol, *HSD* hydroxysteroid dehydrogenase, *HSE* hydroxysteroid epimerase, *testo* testosterone, *DHT* dihydrotestosterone, *3α-DIOL* androstane-3α, 17β-diol, *3β-DIOL* androstane-3β, 17β-diol, *RoDH-1* Ro dehydrogenase 1, *ER* estrogen receptor (modified from [3])

thus avoiding a biologically significant release of active sex steroids in the circulation [17]. Since 1988, the structure/activity of more than 30 tissue-specific genes/enzymes has been elucidated (Fig. 1.2b) [2, 41–43]. A subsequent evolutionary step has been the ability of the adrenals of primates to secrete large amounts of the precursor DHEA that is used as the exclusive substrate by the steroidogenic enzymes to synthesize the required small amounts of intracellular estrogens and androgens [2, 7, 44, 45] (Fig. 1.2b). Humans, in common with other primates, are in fact unique in having adrenals that secrete large amounts of the inactive precursor steroid DHEA with some DHEA secreted by the ovaries [5] (Fig. 1.1). These extragonadal pathways of sex steroid formation are particularly essential in postmenopausal women where all estrogens and all androgens are made from DHEA at their site of action in peripheral tissues [4, 5].

1.6 The Human-Specific Intracellular Steroid-Inactivating Enzymes Avoid Significant Release of Active Sex Steroids in the Circulation

A major pathway of final sex steroid inactivation in the human is glucuronidation, which occurs by the addition of a polar glycosyl group to small hydrophilic molecules, thus facilitating their excretion [7] (Fig. 1.2b). The enzymes responsible for this transformation are members of the uridine diphosphate (UDP)-glucuronosyltransferase (UGT) family [46, 47]. In the human, UGT enzymes are expressed in the liver and most extrahepatic tissues, including the kidney, brain, skin, adipose, and reproductive tissues [48]. As expected, the glucuronides and sulfates can be measured in the circulation which is their obligatory route of elimination [49]. The extrahepatic expression and activity of the UGT enzymes are major determinants for the local inactivation of the sex steroids in the human, thus playing an essential role in the regulation of intracellular sex steroid concentration and action [7]. These enzymes permit to maintain the serum levels of sex steroids at low and biologically inactive concentrations which characterize the normal postmenopausal range, thus avoiding the risks of systemic exposure [7, 48]. The more water-soluble glucuronidated and sulfated estrogen and androgen metabolites diffuse quantitatively into the general circulation where they can be measured accurately as parameters of global sex steroid activity before their elimination by the kidneys and liver.

1.7 Serum Estradiol After Menopause and Testosterone During the Whole Life Are Not Meaningful Markers of Sex Steroid Activity

An essential characteristic of postmenopause and intracrinology is the maintenance of serum E_2 at postmenopausal or biologically inactive concentrations to avoid stimulation of the endometrium and other tissues in the absence of luteal progesterone.

In agreement with the physiology of androgens mentioned above, it is not surprising that despite long series of prospective and case-control cohort studies performed during the last 30 years, a correlation between serum testosterone and any clinical condition believed to be under androgenic control in women has remained elusive. This is somewhat expected when one considers [4, 5] that the low serum testosterone concentration in women is a consequence of the small leakage into the extracellular milieu of some testosterone made intracellularly from DHEA [4, 6]. As examples, the correlation between serum testosterone and the incidence of obesity, insulin resistance, sexual dysfunction, or other clinical problems believed to be related to androgens in women has always yielded equivocal results [28].

The recent understanding that serum DHEA but not serum testosterone is the source of intracellular testosterone in women provides an explanation for the lack of correlation reported between the serum levels of testosterone and the various tissue effects sensitive to androgens [4–6].

Due to the major role of circulating E_2 of ovarian origin before menopause for control of the menstrual cycle, pregnancy, lactation, etc., the difference in the concentration of serum E_2 between premenopause and postmenopause is very large. On the contrary, with serum testosterone, no significant change [29, 50] or a small 15% [51] or 22% difference [28, 33] has been reported between pre- and postmenopause. As mentioned above, the serum levels of testosterone in postmenopausal women are comparable to those in castrated men [33]. In intact men, on the other hand, serum testosterone is about 40-fold higher than in intact women due to the direct secretion of testosterone into the blood by the testicles [33].

Although measurement of the serum androgen metabolites is theoretically the best parameter of total androgenic activity, one would require access to the accurate assays of all the androgen metabolites. Until all such validated LC-MS/MS assays become available, it is likely that ADT-G can be used as a valid substitute [28]. It is in fact well established that the uridine glucuronosyltransferases 2 B7, 2 B15, and 2 B17 (UGT 2B7, UGT 2B15, and UGT 2B17) are the three enzymes responsible for the glucuronidation of most if not all androgens and their metabolites in the human [7, 8].

On the other hand, an example of the usefulness of serum DHEA as parameter of total androgenic activity can be provided by the serum androgen concentrations in women with female sexual dysfunction (FSD). In fact, the androgen-responsive female sexual dysfunction (FSD) has shown the best correlation with low serum DHEA-DHEA-S [52–56].

1.8 All Sex Steroids Remain Within Normal Values with Intravaginal DHEA

Following description of the mechanisms of intracrinology, it is most appropriate to examine the serum levels of DHEA, E_2, and the major estrogen metabolite estrone sulfate (E_1S) in women treated daily for 12 week with 6.5 mg prasterone DHEA who had moderate to severe dyspareunia as their most bothersome symptom of VVA [17].

From a value of 4.47 ± 0.32 ng/ml at the age of 30–35 years (n = 47), serum DHEA decreased to 1.95 ± 0.06 ng/ml in 55–65-year-old women (n = 377) [57]. Of particular interest is the observation that a value of 2.75 ± 0.07 ng/ml DHEA (n = 690 women) [17] was observed in the group of postmenopausal women treated with DHEA (Fig. 1.3a). When treating VVA, E_2 is the most interesting steroid which, as mentioned above, must remain within normal postmenopausal values to avoid systemic estrogenic stimulation [40]. In this context, it can be seen in Fig. 1.3b

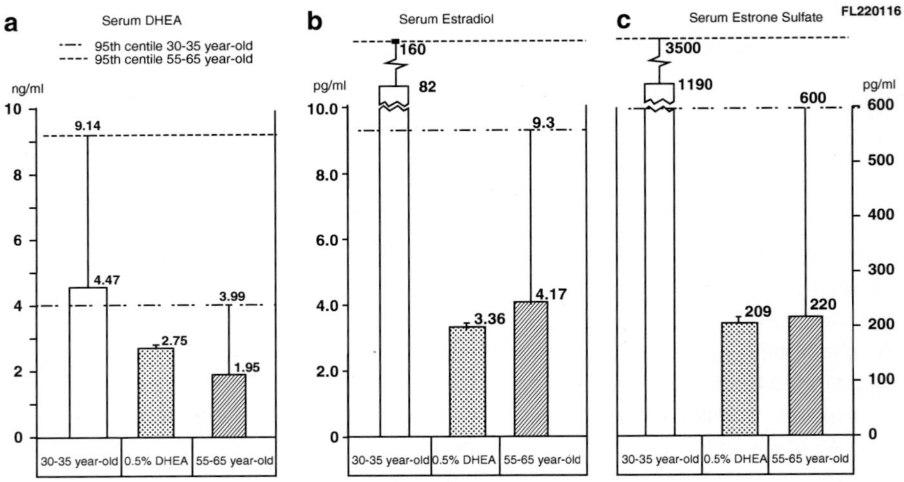

Fig. 1.3 Serum levels of DHEA (**a**), estradiol (E_2) (**b**), and estrone sulfate (E_1S) (**c**) in 30–35-year-old women (n = 47) [57], postmenopausal women treated for 12 weeks with intravaginal 0.50% (6.5 mg) DHEA (n = 690–704) [17], and in 55–65-year-old women (n = 377) [57]. After 12 weeks of daily intravaginal treatment with 6.5 mg (0.50%) prasterone (DHEA), serum E_2 was measured at 3.36 pg/ml [17] or 19% below the normal postmenopausal value of 4.17 ng/ml [57]. Similarly, estrone sulfate, the best recognized marker of global estrogenic activity, shows a serum concentration at 12 weeks of 209 pg/ml [57] or 5% below the normal average postmenopausal value of 220 pg/ml [57], in agreement with the absence of systemic exposure to estrogens after daily intravaginal 0.50% prasterone [17]

that serum E_2, after 12 weeks of daily intravaginal administration of prasterone, is measured at 3.36 ± 0.07 pg/ml (n = 694 women) [17] or 0.81 pg/ml (19.4%) below the normal serum postmenopausal value of 4.17 pg/ml [57].

Serum E_1S is recognized as the best available parameter of global estrogenic activity. This steroid is in fact considered as a “reservoir” and an important marker for assessing women’s overall estrogen exposure [58]. Whereas serum E_1S has been measured at an average of 220 pg/ml [57] in normal postmenopausal women, it can be seen in Fig. 1.3c that its concentration is somewhat lower (−5%) in women treated with DHEA at a value of 209 ± 6.47 pg/ml (n = 704 women) [17]. Since E_1S is, to our knowledge, the best marker of total estrogenic activity, the present data obtained in a particularly large cohort of women (n = 704), very strongly support the well understood local action of intravaginally administered DHEA. This data also indicates that the 6.5 mg (0.50%) of DHEA (prasterone) administered locally in the vagina is only a partial replacement for the missing DHEA. Whereas there is some increase in serum steroids reflecting the partial replacement with intravaginal DHEA, all values are well within the normal and safe postmenopausal values.

In agreement with the maintenance of serum E_2 within the normal postmenopausal values, the absence of meaningful change in serum E_1S, a well-recognized marker of total estrogenic activity, shows the absence of systemic estrogenic effect of intravaginal 0.50% (6.5 mg) DHEA [17]. These data essentially follow the mechanisms of intracrinology whereby the endometrium is protected from estrogenic stimulation [40, 59]. Such a mechanism avoids any safety concern and explains the endometrial atrophy observed in all 668 women who had endometrial biopsy after daily intravaginal administration of DHEA, including 389 women treated for 1 year [59].

1.9 Serum E_2 is Increased Above Normal with Low-Dose Intravaginal Estradiol

It is clear that the long-term consequences of increased serum E_2 concentrations with local estrogens have not been investigated to the same extent as systemic estrogens. VVA, however, unlike hot flashes, is a chronic condition, which does not tend to diminish with time. Consequently, long-term treatment is needed for the treatment of VVA since symptoms frequently recur following cessation of therapy [60]. It thus seems logical to avoid the use of intravaginal estrogen preparations which increase serum E_2 concentrations. Unfortunately, even at the lowest effective doses so far used, serum E_2 is increased [61–65]. Moreover, systemic effects on bone [66, 67] and low-density lipoprotein cholesterol [68] have been reported at the daily 7.5 μg intravaginal dose.

1.10 No Expected Safety Concern with the Exclusive Tissue-Specificity of Intracrinology Compared To Endocrinology

The control of DHEA action is completely different from that of E_2 and testosterone, as well engineered by the 500 million years of evolution which have added 30 or more intracrine enzymes controlling DHEA action in the human. In fact, the essential characteristics which differentiate the exposure to E_2 and testosterone from the exposure to DHEA, an inactive compound by itself, derive from the major differences between endocrinology and intracrinology, which can be summarized as follows:

- In the absence of control of the local formation of estrogens and androgens, the estrogen and androgen receptors are activated in all cells exposed to blood E_2 and testosterone (Fig. 1.2a): A well-known example of the relatively straightforward mechanisms of endocrinology is the ovary which synthesizes E_2 from cholesterol and secretes E_2 in the blood stream for distribution to all the tissues of the human body without discrimination. In all exposed target tissues, E_2 has direct access to all estrogen receptors with no cellular control of the amount of active sex steroid reaching its receptor (Fig. 1.2a).
- By contrast, there is a very sophisticated control of sex steroid formation from DHEA with intracrine action. In fact, with the highly sophisticated intracrine system, the exposure to estrogens and androgens is rigourously controlled in each cell of each tissue which synthesizes only small amounts of these two

steroids intracellularly according to the local physiology and needs. In fact, using the inactive DHEA as precursor, each cell synthesizes the required limited amount of estrogens and androgens required by each cell. The intracellular transformation of DHEA is thus completely dependent upon the activity of about 30 steroidogenic and steroid-inactivating enzymes expressed at various levels in each cell of each tissue (Fig. 1.2b). Consequently, the transformation of DHEA is highly variable between the different tissues, ranging from no transformation in the human endometrium, a particularly well-known tissue, to variable levels in the other tissues (Fig. 1.2b).

- It is important to remember that intracrinology is human-specific. The best illustration of the high tissue specificity achieved by intracrinology is the human endometrium where estrogens are highly stimulatory, whereas DHEA has no stimulatory effect because DHEA is not transformed into estrogens in the endometrium. In fact, it is impossible to predict the level of transformation of DHEA into E_2 and testosterone in any human tissue, except the endometrium.

References

1. Labrie F (1991) Intracrinology. Mol Cell Endocrinol 78:C113–C118
2. Labrie F, Luu-The V et al (2005) Is DHEA a hormone? Starling review. J Endocrinol 187:169–196
3. Labrie F (2015) All sex steroids are made intracellularly in peripheral tissues by the mechanisms of intracrinology after menopause. J Steroid Biochem Mol Biol 145:133–138
4. Labrie F (2015) Androgens in postmenopausal women: their practically exclusive intracrine formation and inactivation in peripheral tissues. In: Plouffe L, Rizk B (eds) Androgens in gynecological practice. Cambridge University Press, Cambridge, UK, pp 64–73
5. Labrie F, Martel C et al (2011) Wide distribution of the serum dehydroepiandrosterone and sex steroid levels in postmenopausal women: role of the ovary? Menopause 18(1):30–43
6. Labrie F, Martel C et al (2017) Androgens in women are essentially made from DHEA in each peripheral tissue according to intracrinology. J Steroid Biochem Mol Biol 168:9–18
7. Bélanger A, Pelletier G et al (2003) Inactivation of androgens by UDP-glucuronosyltransferase enzymes in humans. Trends Endocrinol Metab 14(10):473–479
8. Bélanger B, Bélanger A et al (1989) Comparison of residual C-19 steroids in plasma and prostatic tissue of human, rat and guinea pig after castration: unique importance of extratesticular androgens in men. J Steroid Biochem 32:695–698
9. Dury AY, Ke Y et al (2015) Validated LC-MS/MS simultaneous assay of five sex steroid/neurosteroid-related sulfates in human serum. J Steroid Biochem Mol Biol 149:1–10
10. Ke Y, Bertin J et al (2014) A sensitive, simple and robust LC-MS/MS method for the simultaneous quantification of seven androgen- and estrogen-related steroids in postmenopausal serum. J Steroid Biochem Mol Biol 144:523–534
11. Ke Y, Gonthier R et al (2015) A rapid and sensitive UPLC-MS/MS method for the simultaneous quantification of serum androsterone glucuronide, etiocholanolone glucuronide, and androstan-3alpha, 17beta diol 17-glucuronide in postmenopausal women. J Steroid Biochem Mol Biol 149:146–152
12. Ke Y, Gonthier R et al (2015) Serum steroids remain within the same normal postmenopausal values during 12-month intravaginal 0.50% DHEA. Horm Mol Biol Clin Investig 24(3):117–129

13. Ke Y, Labrie F (2016) The importance of optimal extraction to insure the reliable MS-based assays of endogenous compounds. Bioanalysis 8(1):39–41
14. Ke Y, Labrie F et al (2015) Serum levels of sex steroids and metabolites following 12 weeks of intravaginal 0.50% DHEA administration. J Steroid Biochem Mol Biol 154:186–196
15. Labrie F, Ke Y et al (2015) Letter to editor: superior mass spectrometry-based estrogen assays should replace immunoassays. J Clin Endocrinol Metab 100:L86–L87
16. Labrie F, Ke Y et al (2015) Why both LC-MS/MS and FDA-compliant validation are essential for accurate estrogen assays? J Steroid Biochem Mol Biol 149:89–91
17. Martel C, Labrie F et al (2016) Serum steroid concentrations remain within normal postmenopausal values in women receiving daily 6.5mg intravaginal prasterone for 12 weeks. J Steroid Biochem Mol Biol 159:142–153
18. Archer DF, Labrie F et al (2015) Treatment of pain at sexual activity (dyspareunia) with intravaginal dehydroepiandrosterone (prasterone). Menopause 22(9):950–963
19. Labrie F, Archer DF et al (2009) Intravaginal dehydroepiandrosterone (Prasterone) a physiological and highly efficient treatment of vaginal atrophy. Menopause 16:907–922
20. Labrie F, Archer DF et al (2011) Intravaginal dehydroepiandrosterone (DHEA, Prasterone), a highly efficient treatment of dyspareunia. Climacteric 14:282–288
21. Labrie F, Archer DF et al (2016) Efficacy of intravaginal dehydroepiandrosterone (DHEA) on moderate to severe dyspareunia and vaginal dryness, symptoms of vulvovaginal atrophy, and of the genitourinary syndrome of menopause. Menopause 23(3):243–256
22. Pelletier G, Ouellet J et al (2012) Effects of ovariectomy and dehydroepiandrosterone (DHEA) on vaginal wall thickness and innervation. J Sex Med 9(10):2525–2533
23. Pelletier G, Ouellet J et al (2013) Androgenic action of dehydroepiandrosterone (DHEA) on nerve density in the ovariectomized rat vagina. J Sex Med 10(8):1908–1914
24. McShane LM, Dorgan JF et al (1996) Reliability and validity of serum sex hormone measurements. Cancer Epidemiol Biomark Prev 5(11):923–928
25. Rinaldi S, Dechaud H et al (2001) Reliability and validity of commercially available, direct radioimmunoassays for measurement of blood androgens and estrogens in postmenopausal women. Cancer Epidemiol Biomark Prev 10(7):757–765
26. Cumming DC, Rebar RW et al (1982) Evidence for an influence of the ovary on circulating dehydroepiandrosterone sulfate levels. J Clin Endocrinol Metab 54(5):1069–1071
27. Labrie F (2011) Editorial: impact of circulating dehydroepiandrosterone on androgen formation in women. Menopause 18:471–473
28. Labrie F, Bélanger A et al (2006) Androgen glucuronides, instead of testosterone, as the new markers of androgenic activity in women. J Steroid Biochem Mol Biol 99(4–5):182–188
29. Longcope C, Franz C et al (1986) Steroid and gonadotropin levels in women during the perimenopausal years. Maturitas 8(3):189–196
30. Longcope C, Hunter R et al (1980) Steroid secretion by the postmenopausal ovary. Am J Obstet Gynecol 138(5):564–568
31. Labrie F, Bélanger A et al (1997) Marked decline in serum concentrations of adrenal C19 sex steroid precursors and conjugated androgen metabolites during aging. J Clin Endocrinol Metab 82(8):2396–2402
32. Orentreich N, Brind JL et al (1984) Age changes and sex differences in serum dehydroepiandrosterone sulfate concentrations throughout adulthood. J Clin Endocrinol Metab 59:551–555
33. Labrie F, Cusan L et al (2009) Comparable amounts of sex steroids are made outside the gonads in men and women: strong lesson for hormone therapy of prostate and breast cancer. J Steroid Biochem Mol Biol 113:52–56
34. Vermeulen A, Deslypene JP et al (1982) Adrenocortical function in old age: response to acute adrenocorticotropin stimulation. J Clin Endocrinol Metab 54:187–191
35. Labrie F (2007) Drug insight: breast cancer prevention and tissue-targeted hormone replacement therapy. Nat Clin Pract Endocrinol Metab 3(8):584–593
36. Hammond CB, Jelovsek FR et al (1979) Effects of long-term estrogen replacement therapy. II. Neoplasia. Am J Obstet Gynecol 133(5):537–547

37. Labrie F (2015) Intracrinology in action: importance of extragonadal sex steroid biosynthesis and inactivation in peripheral tissues in both women and men. J Steroid Biochem Mol Biol 145:131–132
38. Guidance for Industry (2013) Bioanalytical Method Validation—Revision 1. US Department of Health and Human Services, Food and Drug Administration. Center for Drug Evaluation and Research (CDER), Center for Veterinary Medicine (CVM). Division of Drug Information, September 2013 (Draft Guidance) http://www.fda.gov/Drugs/GuidanceComplianceRegulatoryInformation/Guidances/default.htm
39. Baker ME (2004) Co-evolution of steroidogenic and steroid-inactivating enzymes and adrenal and sex steroid receptors. Mol Cell Endocrinol 215(1–2):55–62
40. Labrie F, Labrie C (2013) DHEA and intracrinology at menopause, a positive choice for evolution of the human species. Climacteric 16:205–213
41. Luu-The V, Labrie F (2010) The intracrine sex steroid biosynthesis pathways. In: Martini L, Chrousos GP, Labrie F, Pacak K, Pfaff De (eds) Neuroendocrinology, pathological situations and diseases, progress in brain research, vol 181, chap 10. Elsevier. pp 177–192
42. Luu-The V, Lachance Y et al (1989) Full length cDNA structure and deduced amino acid sequence of human 3b-hydroxy-5-ene steroid dehydrogenase. Mol Endocrinol 3:1310–1312
43. Peltoketo H, Isomaa V et al (1988) Complete amino acid sequence of human placental 17b-hydroxysteroid dehydrogenase deduced from cDNA. FEBS Lett 239:73–77
44. Labrie F, Martel C et al (2013) Intravaginal prasterone (DHEA) provides local action without clinically significant changes in serum concentrations of estrogens or androgens. J Steroid Biochem Mol Biol 138:359–367
45. Luu-The V, Zhang Y et al (1995) Characteristics of human types 1, 2 and 3 17β-hydroxysteroid dehydrogenase activities: oxidation-reduction and inhibition. J Steroid Biochem Mol Biol 55:581–587
46. Mackenzie PI, Bock KW et al (2005) Nomenclature update for the mammalian UDP glycosyltransferase (UGT) gene superfamily. Pharmacogenet Genomics 15(10):677–685
47. Mackenzie PI, Owens IS et al (1997) The UDP glycosyltransferase gene superfamily: recommended nomenclature update based on evolutionary divergence. Pharmacogenetics 7(4):255–269
48. Guillemette C, Belanger A et al (2004) Metabolic inactivation of estrogens in breast tissue by UDP-glucuronosyltransferase enzymes: an overview. Breast Cancer Res 6(6):246–254
49. Bélanger A, Brochu M et al (1991) Steroid glucuronides: human circulatory levels and formation by LNCaP cells. J Steroid Biochem Mol Biol 40:593–598
50. Burger HG, Dudley EC et al (2000) A prospective longitudinal study of serum testosterone dehydroepiandrosterone sulfate and sex hormone binding globulin levels through the menopause transition. J Clin Endocrin Metab 85:2832–2838
51. Rannevik G, Jeppsson S et al (1995) A longitudinal study of the perimenopausal transition: altered profiles of steroid and pituitary hormones, SHBG and bone mineral density. Maturitas 21(2):103–113
52. Basson R (2010) Is it time to move on from "hypoactive sexual desire disorder?". Menopause 17(6):1097–1098
53. Basson R, Young A et al (2015) RE: is there a correlation between androgens and sexual desire in women? J Sex Med 12(7):1654–1655
54. Davis SR, Davison SL et al (2005) Circulating androgen levels and self-reported sexual function in women. JAMA 294(1):91–96
55. Guay AT, Jacobson J (2002) Decreased free testosterone and dehydroepiandrosterone-sulfate (DHEA-S) levels in women with decreased libido. J Sex Marital Ther 28(Suppl 1):129–142
56. Wahlin-Jacobsen S, Pedersen AT et al (2015) Is there a correlation between androgens and sexual desire in women? J Sex Med 12(2):358–373
57. Labrie F, Cusan L et al (2008) Effect of intravaginal DHEA on serum DHEA and eleven of its metabolites in postmenopausal women. J Steroid Biochem Mol Biol 111(3–5):178–194
58. Corona G, Elia C et al (2010) Liquid chromatography tandem mass spectrometry assay for fast and sensitive quantification of estrone-sulfate. Clin Chim Acta 411(7–8):574–580

59. Portman DJ, Labrie F et al (2015) Lack of effect of intravaginal dehydroepiandrosterone (DHEA, prasterone) on the endometrium in postmenopausal women. Menopause 22(12):1289–1295
60. Skouby SO, Al-Azzawi F et al (2005) Climacteric medicine: European Menopause and Andropause Society (EMAS) 2004/2005 position statements on peri- and postmenopausal hormone replacement therapy. Maturitas 51(1):8–14
61. Eugster-Hausmann M, Waitzinger J et al (2010) Minimized estradiol absorption with ultra-low-dose 10 microg 17beta-estradiol vaginal tablets. Climacteric 13(3):219–227
62. Holmgren PA, Lindskog M et al (1989) Vaginal rings for continuous low-dose release of oestradiol in the treatment of urogenital atrophy. Maturitas 11(1):55–63
63. Nilsson K, Heimer G (1992) Low-dose oestradiol in the treatment of urogenital oestrogen deficiency—a pharmacokinetic and pharmacodynamic study. Maturitas 15(2):121–127
64. Notelovitz M, Funk S et al (2002) Estradiol absorption from vaginal tablets in postmenopausal women. Obstet Gynecol 99(4):556–562
65. Pickar JH, Amadio JM et al (2016) Pharmacokinetic studies of solubilized estradiol given vaginally in a novel softgel capsule. Climacteric 19(2):181–187
66. Naessen T, Berglund L et al (1997) Bone loss in elderly women prevented by ultralow doses of parenteral 17beta-estradiol. Am J Obstet Gynecol 177(1):115–119
67. Salminen HS, Saaf ME et al (2007) The effect of transvaginal estradiol on bone in aged women: a randomised controlled trial. Maturitas 57(4):370–381
68. Naessen T, Rodriguez-Macias K et al (2001) Serum lipid profile improved by ultra-low doses of 17 beta-estradiol in elderly women. J Clin Endocrinol Metab 86(6):2757–2762

From Menopause to Aging: Endocrine and Neuroendocrine Biological Changes

2

Alessandro D. Genazzani, Andrea Giannini, and Antonella Napolitano

2.1 Introduction

Aging is strongly related to the female hormonal status; indeed it is well known how relevant the impact of the hormonal deficiency in the postmenopause is on the general health of the woman. Aging and in particular the menopause transition are associated with the occurrence of the typical symptoms related to estrogen deficiency such as vasomotor, genitourinary, and musculoskeletal symptoms [1–3]. In this period women become markedly vulnerable to cardiovascular diseases and neurodegenerative disorders that, at this moment of women's life, occur more frequently than in men [4]. With the increase of life expectancy, in 2025 it is expected that there will be more than 1.1 billion in postmenopausal women and most of them will suffer from eating disorders and menopausal-related symptoms (Fig. 2.1).

This issue has a significant economic impact since it has been shown that the menopausal symptoms determine a 10–15% lower working efficiency, a 23% increase in terms of days of absence from work due to illness, and a 40% increase of health-related costs.

A.D. Genazzani (✉) • A. Napolitano
Department of Obstetrics and Gynecology, Gynecological Endocrinology Center, University of Modena and Reggio Emilia, Modena, Italy
e-mail: algen@unimo.it

A. Giannini
Department of Experimental and Clinical Medicine, Division of Obstetrics and Gynecology, University of Pisa, Pisa, Italy

M. Birkhaeuser, A.R. Genazzani (eds.), *Pre-Menopause, Menopause and Beyond*, ISGE Series, https://doi.org/10.1007/978-3-319-63540-8_2

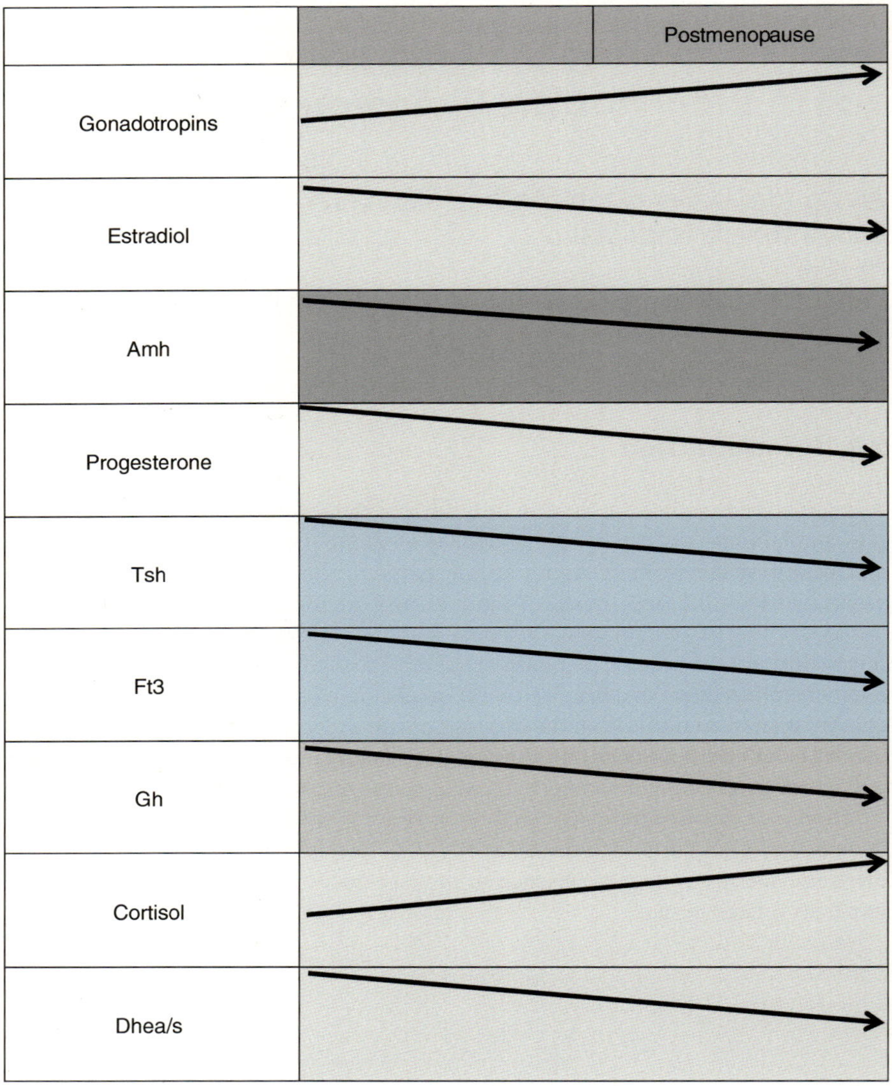

Fig. 2.1 Schematic representation of the main endocrine changes from perimenopause to menopause

2.2 Neuroendocrine Aging

The onset of menopause is mainly related to the biological delay of the ovaries and of the follicles. The number of follicles is determined before birth, when the oocytes are 6–7 million during mid-gestational development. Afterward, their number quickly reduces due to the mechanism of apoptosis, remaining approximately 700,000 during infancy and 300,000 at puberty.

The continuation of the mechanism of apoptosis, with the loss of 400–500 eggs during each follicular recruitment cycle in reproductive life (sometimes involving multiple follicles in a single cycle), determines the functional breakdown of these cells close to the 45–50 years of age, thus inducing the onset of menopause. The time of ovarian function with few ovulations is mainly determined by the entity and rapidity of the mechanisms of apoptosis; it remains still unknown what triggers this process. The granulosa and theca cells determine, with their steroid synthesis, the process of the menstrual cycle, even in the presence of a highly reduced oocyte number that takes place at the beginning of the menopause.

Follicular cell function is regulated by the pituitary gonadotropins and by the hormones produced locally. Probably the reduced sensitivity of the follicular cells to stimulating factors can play a role in the decline of ovarian function. According to this hypothesis, the progressive reduction of both the anti-Müllerian hormone (AMH) and inhibin B levels is the most reproducible and consistent endocrine change observed during the menopausal transition, and this change is related to the decrease of the mass and/or follicular functionality and explains the reduction of the fertility before any changes in menstrual cycle take place.

During aging and particularly during menopausal transition, the hypothalamic-pituitary-ovarian axis shows relevant changes that depend partially on ovarian function declines, but also on several functional changes at the CNS level, that are induced by the aging process [5]. According to this hypothesis, menopause similar to puberty may be affected by specific hypothalamic processes triggering and modulating the reproductive axis [5].

During perimenopause (i.e., 4–6 years before menopause), FSH increase can be identified in middle-aged women long before the evidence of the decrease of estrogen levels and/or the occurrence of menstrual irregularities. Similarly, luteinizing hormone (LH) secretion pattern changes during the menopausal transition with higher pulse amplitude and lower pulse frequency. Experimental studies on rats have suggested that age-related desynchronization in neurochemical signals, which are involved in the activation of GnRH neurons, may occur before the onset of the modifications of the estrous cycle.

Many neuropeptides and neurochemical molecules, i.e., glutamate, noradrenaline, and vasoactive intestinal peptide that determine the estrogen-mediated GnRH and LH peaks, decrease with aging or modify the precise temporal correlation that is required for the specific GnRH secretory pattern. These changes at the hypothalamic level could lead to the progressive modification of the LH pulsatile release and to a reduced ovarian responsiveness typical of this stage of female reproductive life. Therefore, as explained earlier, during the menopausal transition, many complex endocrine modifications take place, typical of the last years of reproductive life and related to the hypothalamus and ovarian dysfunction. In general the menopausal transition is characterized by the reduction of duration of the follicular phase and the concomitant increase in FSH levels. This explains the shorter intervals between cycles that most of women have in this period of life. Cohort studies have demonstrated that the shortening of the follicular phases is associated with an acceleration toward ovulation of many small follicles. The most appropriate explanation of this phenomenon seems to be the reduced or complete loss of production of inhibin B, which would lead to an increase of the release of FSH and, as a result, a sort of "hyperstimulation" inducing a relatively high production of estrogens. This should facilitate (and accelerate) the achievement of LH peak. Over time, age-related hypothalamic changes result in a reduction in sensitivity for estrogens and LH peak becomes increasingly erratic and unpredictable [6]. In addition, follicles become less sensitive to gonadotropins, determining luteal phase deficiency due to anovulatory cycles and triggering the first menstrual irregularities. At this moment of the menopausal transition, the inadequate hypothalamic sensitivity to estrogen causes menopausal symptoms, such as hot flashes and night sweats, though women still have relatively high estrogen levels [7, 8]. This situation explains why exogenous estrogen administration blunts most of the symptoms.

Natural menopause is the consequence of the loss of ovarian function. This is the result of a long cascade of events that occur in the ovaries and in the brain. In menopause, estrogen secretion ends and sex steroids, necessary for the organism, continue to be produced locally.

Menopausal symptoms and related symptoms would be more intense, significantly reducing quality of life and life expectancy, as soon as there is the reduction also of the action of estrogens and androgens produced specifically with the mechanisms of "intracrinology" such as adrenal DHEA (80%) and ovarian DHEA (20%) [9, 10]. In other words, while menopause estradiol serum levels should remain below normal levels and with biologically inactive concentrations, the function of peripheral tissues (except the endometrium) requires physiological intracellular concentrations of estrogen and/or androgens. Indeed, clinical research focused almost exclusively on the blockade of the secretion of estradiol and progesterone by the ovary and consequently on the replacement of ovarian estrogens. The endogenous decrease at very low levels of ovarian estradiol secretion at the time of menopause is positive since it decreases and avoids the risk of endometrial hyperplasia and carcinoma, so we cannot consider it a complete negative event that requires estrogen therapy.

Several years ago Baulieu et al. [11, 12] demonstrated that brain cells can synthesize numerous steroids, and after this study, many clinical and experimental studies have been performed showing interesting results. Baulieu [11], in the initial observations, measured the levels of dehydroepiandrosterone (DHEA) in the central nervous system (CNS) showing that DHEA levels were higher in the CNS than in serum and remained high even after removal of the adrenal glands. Later it was shown that the brain is responsible for the synthesis of DHEA. This type of steroids has been called "neurosteroids" to differentiate them from those steroids produced in the peripheral tissue. The main neurosteroids are DHEA and pregnenolone, DHEA sulfate (DHEAS), progesterone, deoxycorticosterone sulfate, and their 5 α-reduced metabolites especially allopregnanolone (ALLO). They mediate their actions not through interaction with steroid hormone nuclear receptors, but with membrane receptors [13].

Although the role of neurosteroids is not yet well defined, many studies showed their main roles. In some neurodegenerative conditions (Alzheimer's disease and Parkinson's disease or multiple sclerosis) or other CNS pathologies (depression, schizophrenia) or cerebral trauma pathologies, neurosteroid levels decrease; moreover it has been demonstrated that they can play an important role in the modulation of glia and neuronal cells during intrauterine life, puberty, and adolescence or in response to emotional/cognitive stimulations. These data clearly means that the central neurosteroidogenesis might influence or can be influenced by endogenous or exogenous circulating steroid levels [14].

Therefore, it is difficult to understand the functional significance of neurosteroids and to recognize, quantify, and diversify their central and peripheral endocrine glandular secretion. There is evidence that local paracrine/autocrine effects and biosynthesis of neurosteroids can quickly modify the neuronal function in a manner not achievable with other steroids. During menopause, the ovarian estrogen secretion blunts in all women, but not all of them suffer the typical climacteric symptoms and signs (75% of menopausal women show menopausal symptoms and signs of various entities), and this event can be explained only considering other sources of alternative sex steroids. All tissues, except the endometrium, have specific enzymes that transform the DHEA into androgens and/or estrogens.

Humans and other primates are the only animals to have adrenal glands that can secrete amounts of inactive precursor of steroids, such as DHEA that as a prohormone is converted into androgens and/or estrogens that are active on specific peripheral tissues in accordance with so-called intracrinology [9]. Our evaluation permitted the expression of steroidogenic enzymes, cellular specific, that in combination with a high secretion of DHEA can permit the production of amounts of intracellular androgens and/or estrogens.

During aging and the menopausal transition, neurotransmitters, neuropeptides, and neurosteroids undergo major changes as a result of reduced gonadal hormone production. Many activities of central nervous system deteriorate, particularly those associated with hippocampal functions like memory, attention, logic, and control of the autonomic nervous system.

Recently it has been proposed a relevant role of neurotransmitters on triggering menopausal symptoms. In fact, the menopausal transition is associated with a reduction in the levels of ALLO, mainly due to reduced ovarian progesterone synthesis, and such event is the possible cause of the pathophysiology of mood disorders during menopause. In addition, the synthesis of neurosteroids is critical for brain aging processes and related cognitive diseases. Neurosteroid concentrations were significantly reduced in the human brain affected by Alzheimer's disease, and this reduction was correlated with the severity of the disease. According to these results on humans, a low basal level of ALLO was found in cerebral cortex of the transgenic rats' brain with Alzheimer's disease (3 TgAD), thus suggesting either an alteration of the production as well as an accelerated catabolism of allopregnanolone. Data derived from a comparative analysis of the allopregnanolone levels in the plasma and in the cerebral cortex of these mouse models have strongly suggested that the low levels of ALLO in the cerebral cortex represent a specific problem of CNS, since systemic levels of ALLO are normal.

The reduction of ALLO levels in the cerebral cortex of mice model with Alzheimer was evident even in animals treated with the ALLO; this probably could be ascribed to the mitochondrial catabolism of neurosteroids. Inside the CNS, ALLO acts as a proliferative factor for the nerve stem cells and for the precursors of oligodendrocytes. ALLO reduces proliferation of the peripheral nervous system (PNS), where it promotes the proliferation of Schwann cells, the recovery of spinal cord damages, and regeneration of axons of the peripheral nerves. ALLO induces mitosis in the hippocampus and in vitro cultured neurons. The cell proliferation induced by ALLO on undifferentiated cells derived from embryonic and adult rat neurons is between 20 and 30%, while the proliferation observed on undifferentiated human nerve cells is about 37–49%.

Brinton [15] has recently assessed the potential treatment with ALLO to promote the regeneration of brain cells. ALLO seems to be able to reduce the impact of CNS diseases and to activate some mechanisms to repair and to regenerate CNS neurons. Moreover, the regenerative processes of neurogenesis and synaptogenesis reduce also the inflammation, and all these events support the potential use of the ALLO as a therapeutic agent to repair and regenerate.

In conclusion, during neuroendocrine aging the reduced levels of sex steroids induce greater changes in the production and clearance of several neurotransmitters and neuromodulators, implicated in the modulation of the hypothalamic-pituitary-ovary as well as of hippocampal areas. After the failure of the ovarian activity, expression of steroid receptors, which are ubiquitous in the brain, is no longer being sustained, and consequently the equilibrium of CNS mechanisms that dominated throughout the fertile life is severely impaired [5, 16].

2.3 Adrenal Axis Aging

With menopause the ovarian activity and functionality progressively reduce, but also thyroid function and the levels of GH decrease, but the most relevant changes occur at the adrenal gland level. The aging process that begins in the third decade gradually leads to a reduction up to 50% of the adrenal androgen levels, in about 20 years, due to the reduction of the function of the adrenal gland, even if in the presence of an adequate amount of estrogen.

Glucocorticoids, the final products of the hypothalamic-pituitary-adrenal axis, regulate many of our physiological functions by playing important roles on regulating the mechanisms. Experimental studies on human model and on primates have demonstrated that the concentrations of DHEAS significantly reduce during senescence, while the circulating levels of cortisol increase with aging. The concentrations of DHEAS reduce during chronic stress and diseases, while plasma concentrations of cortisol generally grow or remain stable, resulting in a reduction in DHEAS to cortisol ratio. DHEA/cortisol ratio is important and any reduction may indicate abnormal physiological processes, and this can induce impairment of mechanisms of learning and memory. Indeed low DHEA/cortisol ratio is associated with a greater cognitive impairment.

During aging across menopausal transition and postmenopause, plasma androgen concentration changes and becomes lower, particularly the level of DHEA/DHEAS, while cortisol levels progressively increase over the years [17]. This leads to a relative hypercortisolism at the higher levels of normality, typical of the elderly that represents a biological mechanism defensive, although this event represents a metabolic and neurological imbalances trigger since hypercortisolism induces neurotoxicity over the years. This gradual increase of cortisol level, together with a reduction in the levels of DHEA and other adrenal androgens, causes significant changes.

The main effects of androgen deficiency in women are the sexual impairment, namely, to reduce the motivation, imagination, fun, and sexual excitement but also quality of life due to alterations of mood, irritability, and the reduction of energy. The lack of ovarian androgens, both the low DHEAS and adrenal androgen levels, induces functional changes and disorders to the limbic system, such as anxiety and insomnia, mood disorders, migraine and cefalea, depression, fatigue, decreased libido, and progressive loss of memory up to real dementia of the Alzheimer's type [13]. It is well worth mentioning that in a recent study on patients with Alzheimer's disease, a significant lower level of allopregnanolone was observed in the temporal cortex, than healthy controls, and another study already [18] showed a positive correlation between DHEAS levels and the integrity of executive functions, the ability to concentrate, and working memory.

The changes that occur in the hypothalamus are responsible for vasomotor symptoms, associated with profuse sweating, hypertension, and obesity. Analyzing the biosynthetic pathway of adrenal steroid hormones, it has been observed that the onset of aging induces a progressive DHEA level decline, probably due to reduced expression and/or enzyme functions, while cortisol increases. As mentioned above, high plasma levels of cortisol are neurotoxic and in addition are also responsible for the increase of gluconeogenic processes as well as of hyperinsulinemia. There is also the increase of all anabolic processes and the reduction of the release of fatty acids from adipose tissue, a condition that affects the overall metabolism.

2.4 Thyroid Axis Aging

Thyroid function and the gonadal axes are related throughout the woman's fertile period and their relationship is mutual [19, 20]. Thyroid hormones increase the synthesis of sex hormone-binding globulin (SHBG), testosterone, and androstenedione, reduce the clearance of estradiol and androgens, and increase the peripheral conversion of androgens to estrone [19]. In oocytes there are receptors for thyroid hormones that act synergically with follicle-stimulating hormone (FSH) for the production of progesterone.

Estrogens induce the increase of the serum concentration of thyroxine-binding globulin (TBG), through higher liver synthesis, and this activity decreases soon after menopause onset.

Normal aging is accompanied by a slight decrease in pituitary TSH release and a reduction of thyroid iodine uptake, so there is reduction of peripheral degradation of T4, which results in a gradual age-dependent reduction in serum triiodothyronine (T3) concentration but with minimal changes of serum T4 levels. Dysfunction of the thyroid axis is common in the general population and even more prevalent in the elderly, with an increased incidence of overt thyroid under- or overactivity [21]. This means that there are a significant number of patients with subclinical thyroid pathology, which is found in more than 10% of patients aged over 80 years [21].

In the "Colorado thyroid disease prevalence study," it was demonstrated that there is a higher rate of elevated TSH plasma levels with age, ranging from below 5% at 18–24 years to about 20% in women aged 74 and older. This occurs more frequently in women than in men [22].

Studies on relationship between menopause and thyroid function are few and do not allow to demonstrate whether menopause has any effects on thyroid regardless of aging.

In the Women's Health Across the Nation study, a community-based multiethnic study of the natural history of the menopausal transition, it was observed that there was a 9.6% prevalence of TSH values outside the euthyroid range [23]. Although TSH was associated with abnormal menstrual bleeding and self-reported fearfulness, it was not associated with indicators of the menopausal transition, such as menopausal blockade of menstrual bleeding, menopausal symptoms, or reproductive hormone concentration.

Menopause is not strictly related to an increased or decreased risk of thyroid dysfunctions, and thyroid function is not directly involved in the pathogenesis of any complications of menopause with the exception for cardiovascular risk and bone metabolism that may be aggravated when hyperthyroidism or hypothyroidism occurs [24, 25].

Oral et al. [26] demonstrated that, in a population of climacteric women, clinical thyroid disease was found in 2.4% and subclinical disease in 23.2%, and in this group subclinical disease hypothyroidism (73.8%) is more frequent than hyperthyroidism (26.2%).

Another study reported that about 70% of the patients with hypothyroidism were over the age of 50 years at the time of diagnosis [27]. Primary hypothyroidism, the most common pathological hormone deficiency, occurs more often in women than in men and increases in incidence with age [28]. Like hyperthyroidism, the occurrence of hypothyroidism may be overt or subclinical (high TSH with normal free T4 and free T3 concentrations). The symptoms of hypothyroidism and the effects on central nervous system and neuromuscular abnormalities such as depression, memory loss, cognitive impairment, general slowness, sensitivity to cold, and a variety of neuromuscular complaints are well known. Other symptoms of hypothyroidism similar to those that start in postmenopause are cardiopulmonary dysfunction, increased total cholesterol, and low-density lipoprotein (LDL) as well as reduced high-density lipoprotein (HDL) inducing increase of cardiovascular risk. Subclinical hypothyroidism occurs in 10% and more in women after the age of 60 [24, 25].

It is evident from what the above described that there are an unfavorable serum lipid profile, impaired heart function, an increase in systemic vascular resistance, and arterial stiffness, and due to changes of endothelial function, there is a higher risk of atherosclerosis and coronary artery disease as well as a higher risk to develop major depressive disorders.

Similarly, the prevalence of hyperthyroidism increases with age up to 10%. Subclinical hyperthyroidism in iodine-replete areas changes from 3.9% in all ages to 5.9% in those aged 60 years and older. The prevalence was thought to be even higher than average in areas of iodine deficiency [27–29].

Common manifestations of hyperthyroidism may be confused with perimenopausal symptoms including palpitations, nervousness, insomnia, easy fatiguability, excessive sweating, and intolerance to heat but also weight loss, systolic hypertension, tremor, and muscle weakness. Women with subclinical hyperthyroidism may have mild symptoms or signs. These dysfunctions favor resorption and bone formation and progressive bone demineralization.

Menopause may modify the clinical expression of some thyroid diseases, in particular the autoimmune ones. Indeed thyroid autoimmunity is more common in females than in males, probably for the direct effects of estrogens and androgens on the immune system. Serum thyroid autoantibodies are detectable in up to 25% of women over the age of 60 years, and autoimmune hyperthyroidism is eight to nine times more common in women than in men and increases with age [30]. It is clear that serum TSH investigation has to be checked at least once every 1–2 years in perimenopausal and postmenopausal women. Estrogen replacement therapy is useful in particular to postmenopausal women with subclinical or clinical hyperthyroidism, since bone loss is positively influenced by estrogens. In older age the need for iodine and L-thyroxine is reduced. Therefore, therapy needs to be controlled and adapted to the symptoms, and women with overt thyroid dysfunction should be treated.

2.5 Somatotropic Axis Aging

The growth hormone (GH)/insulin-like growth factor-1 (IGF-1) axis is an important regulator of growth and development during childhood and adolescence and controls the nutritional status through the complex family of growth factors. Indeed chronic malnutrition, in particular lack of carbohydrates and amino acids, causes a marked reduction of IGF-1 plasma levels [31]. Catabolic conditions, such as hepatic failure, renal failure, inflammatory bowel disease, and malabsorption syndromes, are associated with low or very low plasma IGF-1 concentrations [32]. This axis also regulates body composition, metabolism, and aerobic capacity throughout life, increasing fat mobilization and decreasing body fat, adipocyte size, and lipid content. GH synthesis, assessed by measurement of serum IGF-1, the most sensitive marker of GH action, and its pulsatile release are regulated by the hypothalamic neuropeptides GH-releasing hormone (GHRH) and somatotropin release-inhibiting factor (somatostatin) and by gastric hormone ghrelin [33].

IGF-1 inhibits GH synthesis and release [34, 35], but also multiple negative feedback loops autoregulate the GH axis and a number of central neurotransmitter and neuropeptides are involved in GH regulation (a-adrenergic mechanisms, dopaminergic pathways, cholinergic pathways, stimulatory role of histamine and serotonin, endogenous opioids).

Androgens and estrogens may play different roles in the regulation of somatotropic axis, because there is important gender dimorphism of GH secretion. Young women have 24-h integrated serum GH concentrations 50% higher than young men, due to higher incremental and maximal GH peak amplitudes, but there is no significant difference in GH half-life, interpulse times, or pulse frequency between male and female [36, 37]. Human data suggest that GHRH is tonically secreted during the daytime in women but not in men. Levels of both GH and IGF-1 decrease during aging, in particular during the third decade, and reach a plateau during the seventh decade [38, 39]; however, endogenous GH status showed considerable variability [36, 40]. GH secretion shows a reduction of the nocturnal peaks of serum GH during adulthood, and these peaks are reduced in amplitude. Some individuals over the age of 40 release little GH during sleep [41].

This process of GH delay is termed "somatopause" and indicates the potential link between age-related decline in GH and frailty in older subjects.

Little is known concerning the biological effects of somatopause. Given that a number of factors are known to differentially stimulate GH/IGF-1 action and activity, it is perhaps unsurprising that the clinical impact of altered GH/IGF-1 levels in older age remains unclear [41]. The age-dependent decline in GH secretion is paralleled by changes in body composition, with a decrease in lean body mass and an increase in total body fat (especially intra-abdominal fat) [41].

GH secretory patterns differ between sexes; the spontaneous GH secretion decreases with aging, and it is less pronounced in premenopausal women (remaining relatively stable), until after the menopause, when GH levels significantly fall [38, 42]. Estrogens are involved in the determination of body fat distribution, with greater accumulation of subcutaneous fat in the gluteofemoral region and less visceral fat mass than in men. With the menopause, estrogen deficiency may contribute, together with the aging-related GH decline, under estrogen modulation, to increase visceral fat deposition. Due to this, women tend to accumulate visceral fat. Body mass index is a major negative determinant of GH secretory burst amplitude [43].

Following the fifth decade, a reduction of sleep-related GH secretion has been observed. This is probably related to changes in sleep pattern associated with increasing age [44]. The negative impact of aging on GH secretion is twofold more evident in men than in premenopausal women of similar age [45]. Twenty-four-hour mean serum GH concentrations in premenopausal women remain relatively stable until the menopause, when these gender differences tend to disappear. The age-related decline of GH secretion is coupled with a reduction of both IGF-1 and its binding protein IGFBP-3 [46].

The mechanisms underlying the reduced GH secretion are not clear, although an unbalanced secretion of hypothalamic GHRH and somatostatin into the portal circulation might be the cause. The pituitary remains responsive to direct stimulation by secretagogues, although some authors found a reduction in GH response to GHRH with increasing age [47, 48].

In studies where some inhibitory influences on GH secretion were removed, the acute GH response to GHRH is well maintained in old age. Co-administration of compounds that are believed to suppress somatostatin, such as arginine, can restore the GH response in elderly subjects to levels similar to those observed in young adults [49].

Thus, the available data suggest that the effect of age upon spontaneous and stimulated GH secretion probably includes an increase in somatostatinergic tone, although a decline in GHRH (or other stimulating factors) may participate to this process. The former could be due to the hypothalamic cholinergic hypoactivity that has been described in aging [50].

Conclusions

The functional life of human ovaries is determined by a complex and yet largely unidentified set of genetic, hormonal, and environmental factors. Women undergo menopause when follicles in their ovaries are exhausted. However, the clinical manifestations experienced by women approaching menopause are the result of a dynamic interaction between neuroendocrine changes that take place in the brain with the reproductive endocrine axis governing the function of ovaries. Although menopause is ultimately defined by ovarian follicular exhaustion, several lines of scientific evidence in humans and animals now suggest that dysregulation of estradiol feedback mechanisms and hypothalamic-pituitary dysfunction contributes to the onset and progression of reproductive senescence, independently from the ovarian failure [16, 51].

The understanding of the mechanisms that make women enter into the menopausal transition may offer opportunities for interventions that delay menopause-related increase of disease morbidity and thus might improve the overall quality of life for aging women.

Results from epidemiologic studies give a median age of natural menopause (ANM) of 48–52 years among women in wealthy nations [52]. In a more recent meta-analysis of 36 studies spanning 35 countries, the overall mean ANM was estimated at 48.8 years (95% CI: 48.3, 49.2), with significant variation by geographical region. ANM was generally occurring earlier among women in African, Latin American, and Middle Eastern countries (regional means for ANM: 47.2–48.4 years), while in Europe and Australia, ANM occurs later (ANM 50.5–51.2 years) and tends to be even later in women living in western countries over the twentieth century; however the connections of biological and environmental factors, regional differences, and historical trends on the timing of menopause remain far from being clear [53–56].

The timing of the ANM reflects a lot of endocrine, genetic, and epigenetic factors, other than socioeconomic and lifestyle factors. Heritability in menopausal age is estimated to range between 30 and 85% [57, 58]. Women whose mothers or other first-degree relatives were known to have early menopause have been found to be 6- to 12-fold more likely to undergo early menopause themselves [59, 60].

Linkage analysis studies pinpoint areas in chromosome X (Xp21.3 region) that is associated with early (<45 years) or premature (<40 years) menopause. A region in chromosome 9 (9q21.3) contains a gene which encodes for a protein of the B-cell lymphoma 2 (BCL2) family; BCL2 is involved in apoptosis and may thus be relevant in determining menopause through follicular depletion [61]. Other linkage analysis studies have identified a region in chromosome 8 that is associated with age at menopause. Interestingly, near this identified DNA sequence is the gene encoding for gonadotropin-releasing hormone (GnRH) [62]. Other genes specific to ovarian function such as the follicle-stimulating hormone (FSH) and inhibin receptors have been shown to be associated with early and premature menopause [63]. Women who are carriers for the fragile X mutation and have an intermediate number of CGG repeats in their fragile X mental retardation 1 (FMR1) gene on their X chromosome have been observed to undergo premature and early menopause [64].

Candidate gene association studies, looking at possible association between genes encoding with factors involved in reproductive pathophysiology and menopause, failed to identify clear associations. The beginning of the abnormal HPO axis function is the reduction of the ovarian gametes which are the key players in determining the start of menopause, but it is not the unique determinant of female reproductive senescence.

The number of follicular cells before birth is very high; oocytes expand to a maximum of 6–7 million at mid-gestation. Afterward, a rapid loss of oocytes starts because of apoptosis, leading to a population of 700,000 at birth and of 300,000 at puberty. The ongoing of apoptotic loss, along with the use of oocytes during the 400–500 cycles of follicular recruitment taking place in a normal reproductive life, combined with the recruitment of multiple follicles per cycle, leads to final exhaustion of these cells at midlife, determining menopause occurrence around 45 and 55 years [1].

In this view, life span of the ovaries is only marginally influenced by ovulation, while it mostly depends on the extent and rapidity of the apoptotic process of its oocytes, and molecular mechanisms regulating this process are still unknown.

The finding from previous studies supports the hypothesis that the specialized steroid-secreting cells of granulosa and theca drive the menstrual cycle. Follicular cells are regulated by pituitary gonadotropins as well as by locally produced hormones. Loss of sensitivity of follicular cells to stimulating factors has a key role in the decline of ovarian function [2].

According to this, the most relevant endocrine modification throughout the menopausal transition is the progressive decline of both inhibin B and anti-Müllerian hormone (AMH), thus inducing the decrease of the number of follicles and/or their functionality. This explains why fertility is impaired in women before any kind of dysregulation in menstrual cyclicity occurs [3]. During the menopausal transition, the HPO axis undergoes significant modifications which are in part due to the decline of the ovarian function and in part due to functional modifications induced by the onset of reproductive senescence [5]. According to this hypothesis, menopause may have some similarity with puberty, since specific hypothalamic processes of both these events might have genetic triggers. To this extent the increase of FSH concentrations can be detected in middle-aged women before estrogen declines or cycle irregularities occur. Similarly, in this period LH pulses secretion patterns show some modifications.

Findings from experimental studies in rat models suggest that an age-related desynchronization of the neurochemical signals involved in activating GnRH neurons takes place before modifications in estrous cyclicity show up several hypothalamic neuropeptides and neurochemical agents (glutamate, norepinephrine, vasoactive intestinal peptide) that regulate the estrogen-mediated GnRH/LH surge that seems to diminish with age or lose the precise temporal coupling with GnRH secretion [6]. Disruption of this hypothalamic biological clock would lead to progressive impairment in the timing of the preovulatory LH surge, which would add to the poor ovarian response typical of this moment of women's life.

Thus, it becomes clear that the endocrine modifications of perimenopausal period depend on the combination of both dysfunction of the ovaries and of the hypothalamus. A shortened follicular phase associated with elevation of FSH plasmatic concentrations is common of the early menopausal transition during which patients typically have a shorter intermenstrual interval and frequent anovulation.

Several experimental studies demonstrated that shortened follicular phases are associated with abnormal ovulation, involving follicles with smaller size. The most plausible explanation of this phenomenon is the loss of inhibin B production, leading to higher FSH release and therefore to a higher estrogen production. This would facilitate and accelerate the achievement of the LH surge but not to a good ovulation.

Throughout years of menopausal transition, the age-related hypothalamic modifications lead to a reduction in estrogen sensitivity and the LH surge becomes more erratic. Follicles also become less sensitive to gonadotropins, thus leading to luteal phase defect (LPD) and anovulatory cycles, as a consequence to menstrual irregularities. Hypothalamic insensitivity to estrogens and the lowering of estradiol levels explain why menopausal symptoms, such as hot flushes and night sweats, commonly show up at this moment and why hormone replacement with estrogens are effective in reducing the symptoms [8].

The impairment of the basic symptoms is related to any abnormal triggers in that minimal changes of core temperature produce excessive vasodilation, sweating, or shivering. Declining of estrogens and of inhibin and the increasing FSH explain only in part the impaired thermoregulation, which is associated with changes of neurotransmitters (noradrenaline, beta-endorphin, dopamine, serotonin, NPY) in different brain areas and in peripheral vascular reactivity [65]. These impairments are at the basis also of the onset of sleep disturbances. Mood disorders, such as depression and anxiety, are not caused only by menopausal changes, but predisposed women, however, may have their first episodes just before or during perimenopausal transition. Muscle and joint pain is also typical during menopause, and it is closely related with hot flushes, thermoregulation, and the depressed mood. Moreover, the metabolic changes lead to an increase of body fat which tends to locate at the trunk level resulting in the development of visceral adiposity. Considering all of these events, the decline of HPO axis has a key role in determining several symptoms that affect women's life and reduce quality of life [66–68].

During menopausal transition also, androgen levels decrease resulting in lack of energy, sexual arousal, and satisfaction and long-term development of cognitive, metabolic, and mood disorders. Hypothalamic–pituitary–adrenal axis (HPA) hyperactivity has been demonstrated in chronic diseases affecting nervous system disorders like depression [9]. The end products of HPA axis, glucocorticoids (GCs), regulate many physiological functions and play an important role in affective regulation and dysregulation. Despite DHEAS levels which markedly decrease throughout adulthood, an increase in circulating cortisol with advanced age has been observed in human and nonhuman primates [10]. In addition, unlike DHEAS concentrations that decline under conditions of chronic stress and medical illness, cortisol concentrations generally either rise or do not change, resulting in a decrease in DHEAS to cortisol ratio [11–14]. Therefore, it may be important to consider the ratio of both steroids in addition to their absolute concentrations. The resulting decrease in the DHEA/cortisol ratio may have drastic implications for many physiological processes, including learning and memory, a view that is supported by the finding that lower DHEA/cortisol ratio area associated with greater cognitive impairment [69]. However, the relationship between steroidal concentrations and cognitive impairment is still debated.

In summary, the natural evolution of menopause is the consequence of gradual loss of ovarian function. This is the final step in a long and irregular cascade of events taking place both in the CNS and at the ovarian level. Genetic factors influence the timing of these processes, but the key molecular pathways involved are yet unclear. Identifications of such factors would be important to set new strategies to treat reproductive dysfunction and menopause-related diseases.

References

1. Nejat EJ, Chervenak JL (2010) The continuum of ovarian aging and clinicopathologies associated with the menopausal transition. Maturitas 66(2):187–190
2. Broekmans FJ, Soules MR, Fauser BC (2009) Ovarian aging: mechanisms and clinical consequences. Endocr Rev 30(5):465–493
3. Burger HG, Hale GE, Robertson DM, Dennerstein L (2007) A review of hormonal changes during the menopausal transition: focus on findings from the Melbourne Women's Midlife Health Project. Hum Reprod Update 13(6):559–565
4. de Kat AC, Dam V, Onland-Moret NC, Eijkemans MJ, Broekmans FJ, van der Schouw YT (2017) Unraveling the associations of age and menopause with cardiovascular risk factors in a large population-based study. BMC Med 15(1):2
5. Wise PM (1999) Neuroendocrine modulation of the "menopause": insights into the aging brain. Am J Phys 277:E965–E970
6. Downs JL, Wise PM (2009) The role of the brain in female reproductive aging. Mol Cell Endocrinol 299:32–38
7. Butler L, Santoro N (2011) The reproductive endocrinology of the menopausal transition. Steroids 76:627–635
8. Santoro N et al (2003) Impaired folliculogenesis and ovulation in older reproductive aged women. J Clin Endocrinol Metab 88:5502–5509
9. Labrie F (2004) Adrenal androgens and intracrinology. Semin Reprod Med 22(4):299–309

10. Chalbot S, Morfin R (2006) Dehydroepiandrosterone metabolites and their interactions in humans. Drug Metabol Drug Interact 2:21–23
11. Baulieu EE (1997) Neurosteroids: of the nervous system, by the nervous system, for the nervous system. Recent Prog Horm Res 5:21–32
12. Baulieu EE, Robel P, Schumacher M (2001) Neurosteroids: beginning of the story. Int Rev Neurobiol 46:1–32. Review
13. Dong Y, Zheng P (2012) Dehydroepiandrosterone sulphate: action and mechanism in the brain. J Neuroendocrinol 24(1):215–224
14. Compagnone NA, Mellon SH (2000) Neurosteroids: biosynthesis and function of these novel neuromodulators. Front Neuroendocrinol 21:1–56
15. Brinton RD (2013) Neurosteroids as regenerative agents in the brain: therapeutic implications. Nat Rev Endocrinol 9(4):241–250. Review
16. Brann DW, Mahesh VB (2005) The aging reproductive neuroendocrine axis. Steroids 70(4):273–283
17. McConnell DS, Stanczyk FZ, Sowers MR, Randolph JF Jr, Lasley BL (2012) Menopausal transition stage-specific changes in circulating adrenal androgens. Menopause 19(6):658–663
18. Davis SR, Shah SM, McKenzie DP, Kulkarni J, Davison SL, Bell RJ (2008) Dehydroepiandrosterone sulfate levels are associated with more favorable cognitive function in women. J Clin Endocrinol Metab 93(3):801–808
19. Krassas GE, Poppe K, Glinoer D (2010) Thyroid function and human reproductive health. Endocr Rev 31(5):702–755
20. Krassas GE (2000) Thyroid disease and female reproduction. Fertil Steril 74(6):1063–1070
21. Boelaert K (2013) Thyroid dysfunction in the elderly. Nat Rev Endocrinol 9:194–204
22. Canaris GJ, Manowitz NR, Major G et al (2000) The Colorado thyroid disease prevalence study. Arch Intern Med 160:526–534
23. Sowers M, Luborsky J, Perdue C, Araujo KL, Goldman MB, Harlow SD, SWAN (2003) Thyroid stimulating hormone (TSH) concentrations and menopausal status in women at the mid-life: SWAN. Clin Endocrinol 58(3):340–347
24. Danzi S, Klein I (2012) Thyroid hormone and the cardiovascular system. Med Clin North Am 96(2):257–268
25. Kahaly GJ (2000) Cardiovascularand atherogenic aspects of subclinical hypothyroidism. Thyroid 10(8):665–679. Review
26. Oral E, Senturk LM, Hallac M et al (2002) Screening for thyroid disease at the menopause clinic. Climateric 5(Suppl 1):162
27. Davis PJ, Davis FM (1984) Hypothyroidism in the elderly. Compr Ther 10:17–23
28. Faughnan M, Lepage R, Fugere P et al (1995) Screening for thyroid disease at the menopausal clinic. Clin Invest Med 18:11–18
29. Parle JV, Maisonneuve P, Sheppard MC et al (2001) Prediction of all-cause and cardiovascular mortality in elderly people from one low serum thyrotropin result: a 10-year cohort study. Lancet 358:861–865
30. Laurberg P, Cerqueira C, Ovesen L, Rasmussen LB, Perrild H, Andersen S, Pedersen IB, Carlé A (2010) Iodine intake as a determinant of thyroid disorders in populations. Best Pract Res Clin Endocrinol Metab 24(1):13–27
31. Phillips LS, Unterman TG (1984) Somatomedin activity in disorders of nutrition and metabolism. Clin Endocrinol Metab 13:145–189
32. Mock DM (1986) Growth retardation in chronic inflammatory bowel disease. Gastroenterology 91:1019–1021
33. Smith RG, Jiang H, Sun Y (2005) Developments in ghrelin biology and potential clinical relevance. Trends Endocrinol Metab 16:436–442
34. Yamashita S, Melmed S (1986) Insulin-like growth factor I action on rat anterior pituitary cells: suppression of growth hormone secretion and messenger ribonucleic acid levels. Endocrinology 118:176–182
35. Hartman ML et al (1993) A low dose euglycemic infusion of recombinant human insulin-like growth factor I rapidly suppresses fasting-enhanced pulsatile growth hormone secretion in humans. J Clin Invest 91:2453–2462

36. Zadik Z, Chalew SA, McCarter RJ Jr, Meistas M, Kowarski AA (1985) The influence of age on the 24-hour integrated concentration of growth hormone in normal individuals. J Clin Endocrinol Metab 60:513–516
37. Van den Berg G, Veldhuis JD, Frölich M, Roelfsema F (1996) An amplitude-specific divergence in the pulsatile mode of growth hormone (GH) secretion underlies the gender difference in mean GH concentrations in men and premenopausal women. J Clin Endocrinol Metab 81:2460–2467
38. Ho KY et al (1987) Effects of sex and age on the 24-hour profile of growth hormone secretion in man: importance of endogenous estradiol concentrations. J Clin Endocrinol Metab 64:51–58
39. Hoffman DM, O'sullivan AJ, Baxter RC, Ho KK (1994) Diagnosis of growth-hormone deficiency in adults. Lancet 344:482–483
40. Finkelstein JW, Roffwarg HP, Boyar RM, Kream J, Hellman L (1972) Age-related change in the twenty-four-hour spontaneous secretion of growth hormone. J Clin Endocrinol Metab 35:665–670
41. Rudman D et al (1990) Effects of human growth hormone in men over 60 years old. N Engl J Med 323:1–6
42. Winer LM, Shaw MA, Baumann G (1990) Basal plasma growth hormone levels in man: new evidence for rhythmicity of growth hormone secretion. J Clin Endocrinol Metab 70:1678–1686
43. Giustina A, Veldhuis JD (1998) Pathophysiology of the neuroregulation of growth hormone secretion in experimental animals and the human. Endocr Rev 19:717–797
44. Kamel NS, Gammack JK (2006) Insomnia in the elderly: cause, approach, and treatment. Am J Med 119:463–469
45. Weltman A et al (1994) Relationship between age, percentage body fat, fitness, and 24-hour growth hormone release in healthy young adults: effects of gender. J Clin Endocrinol Metab 78:543–548
46. Corpas E, Harman SM, Blackman MR (1993) Human growth hormone and human aging. Endocr Rev 14:20–39
47. Lang I, Schernthaner G, Pietschmann P, Kurz R, Stephenson JM, Templ H (1987) Effects of sex and age on growth hormone response to growth hormone-releasing hormone in healthy individuals. J Clin Endocrinol Metab 65:535–540
48. Russell-Aulet M, Dimaraki EV, Jaffe CA, DeMott-Friberg R, Barkan AL (2001) Aging-related growth hormone (GH) decrease is a selective hypothalamic GH-releasing hormone pulse amplitude mediated phenomenon. J Gerontol A Biol Sci Med Sci 56:M124–M129
49. Ghigo E et al (1990) Growth hormone (GH) responsiveness to combined administration of arginine and GH-releasing hormone does not vary with age in man. J Clin Endocrinol Metab 71:1481–1485
50. Gibson GE, Peterson C, Jenden DJ (1981) Brain acetylcholine synthesis declines with senescence. Science 213:674–676
51. Klein NA et al (1996) Reproductive aging: accelerated ovarian follicular development associated with a monotropic folliclestimulating hormone rise in normal older women. J Clin Endocrinol Metab 81(3):1038–1045
52. Tom SE, Mishra GD (2013) A life course approach to reproductive aging. In: Dvornyk V (ed) Current topics in menopause. Bentham Science Publishers Sharjah, Oak Park, IL, pp 3–19
53. Schoenaker DA et al (2014) Socioeconomic position, lifestyle factors and age at natural menopause: a systematic review and meta-analyses of studies across six continents. Int J Epidemiol 43:1542–1562
54. Nichols HB et al (2006) From menarche to menopause: trends among US Women born from 1912 to 1969. Am J Epidemiol 164:1003–1011
55. Dratva J et al (2009) Is age at menopause increasing across Europe? Results on age at menopause and determinants from two population-based studies. Menopause 16:385–394
56. Flint MP (1997) Secular trends in menopause age. J Psychosom Obstet Gynaecol 18:65–72
57. Kok HS, van Asselt KM, van der Schouw YT et al (2005) Genetic studies to identify genes underlying menopausal age. Hum Reprod Update 11:483–493

58. van Asselt KM et al (2004) Heritability of menopausal age in mothers and daughters. Fertil Steril 82:1348–1351
59. Torgerson DJ, Thomas RE, Reid DM (1997) Mothers and daughters menopausal ages: is there a link? Eur J Obstet Gynecol Reprod Biol 74:63–66
60. Crame DW, Xu H, Harlow BL (1995) Family history as a predictor of early menopause. Fertil Steril 64:740–745
61. Van Asselt KM et al (2004) Linkage analysis of extremely discordant and concordant sibling pairs identifies quantitative trait loci influencing variation in human menopausal age. Am J Hum Genet 74:444–453
62. Murabito JM et al (2005) Genome-wide linkage analysis to age at natural menopause in a community-based sample: the Framingham Heart Study. Fertil Steril 84:1674–1679
63. Ferrarini E et al (2013) Clinical characteristics and genetic analysis in women with premature ovarian insufficiency. Maturitas 74:61–67
64. Nelson LM (2009) Clinical practice. Primary ovarian insufficiency. N Engl J Med 360:606–614
65. Archer DF et al (2011) Menopausal hot flushes and night sweats: where are we now? Climacteric 14:515–528
66. Al-Safi ZA, Santoro N (2014) Menopausal hormone therapy and menopausal symptoms. Fertil Steril 101:905–915
67. Vivian-Taylor J, Hickey M (2014) Menopause and depression: is there a link? Maturitas 79:142–146
68. Bay-Jensen AC et al (2013) Role of hormones in cartilage and joint metabolism: understanding an unhealthy metabolic phenotype in osteoarthritis. Menopause 20:578–586
69. Maurice T, Gregoire C, Espallergues J (2006) Neuro (active) steroids actions at theneuromodulatory sigma1 (sigma1) receptor: biochemical and physiologicalevidences, consequences in neuroprotection. Pharmacol Biochem Behav 84(4):581–597

3 Brain Impact of Sex Steroid Withdrawal at Menopause

Nicola Pluchino and Andrea R. Genazzani

3.1 Introduction

In the last century, longer female life expectancy has implied that women now live a third of their lives beyond the end of their ovarian function, increasing the need for new therapeutic strategies to facilitate successful aging (defined as low probability of disease), high cognitive and physical abilities, and active engagement in life. The incidence of hypertension, diabetes mellitus, and psychiatric and degenerative brain diseases, especially stroke and dementia, is more frequently seen in older people. Each of these conditions can, separately or in combination, results in similar signs and symptoms of cognition, memory, mood, and motor function disorders.

Adrenal and ovarian steroids play pivotal neuroactive and brain region-specific roles. Their protective effects are multifaceted and brain regions dependent. They encompass a system that ranges from chemical to biochemical and genomic mechanisms, protecting against a wide range of neurotoxic insults. Consequently, adrenal and ovarian steroid withdrawal, during the reproductive senescence, impacts negatively the brain function at neuronal, vascular, and metabolic levels.

Convergent evidence for the effects of estrogen on cognitive function comes from studies that have examined cognition in relation to menstrual cycle phase, biomarkers of lifelong estrogen exposure, estrogen receptor polymorphisms, neuroimaging studies, and circulating hormone levels. The menopausal transition and aging process represent the main objective of hormone intervention in female life in terms of brain function and cognitive vitality, and several experimental and clinical evidences support this theory. In this chapter, we critically review the evidence on

N. Pluchino
Obstetrics and Gynecology, University Hospital of Geneva, Geneva, Switzerland

A.R. Genazzani (✉)
International Society of Gynecological Endocrinology, Pisa, Italy
e-mail: argenazzani@gmail.com

M. Birkhaeuser, A.R. Genazzani (eds.), *Pre-Menopause, Menopause and Beyond*, ISGE Series, https://doi.org/10.1007/978-3-319-63540-8_3

the intriguing hypothesis that the early female brain senescence is a highly responsive period to estrogen treatment for cognitive vitality.

3.2 Menopause and Mood Disorders: Depression and Anxiety

Epidemiologic data suggest an increased incidence and prevalence of depressive symptoms in women in their mid-40s and again between the ages of 55 and 64 years. Estrogen deficiency has been suggested as a cause of this increased prevalence of depressive disorders in women, and the menopausal transition appears to be a period of vulnerability to depressive symptoms with or without a history of depression [1–4]. It has demonstrated that psychological distress appears to increase in early perimenopause compared with premenopause, and vasomotor symptoms further increase the risk of psychological distress [5]. The Study of Women's Health Across the Nation (SWAN) reported that more than 40% of participants had increased irritability, nervousness, mood changes, and dysphoric mood in the previous 2 weeks in early perimenopause compared with premenopause [6]. Additionally, 14.3% reported feeling depressed 6 or greater days within the past 2 weeks [7]. Considering that the perimenopause can last up to some years, the risk of developing depression during the perimenopause can be as high as 14 times that of premenopausal women [8]. Depression is the second leading cause of disability in developed countries [9], and the potential burden of illness experienced by depressed perimenopausal women is significant. In particular, women experiencing long transitions to menopause were at greater risk of depression than those having short transitions [10, 11]. The association between a long perimenopause and depression appeared to be explained by increased menopausal symptoms rather than by the menopause status. The presence of vasomotor symptoms appears to be associated with a higher prevalence of depressed mood, and anxiety is a significant predictor of hot flashes among women in the late reproductive years [12, 13].

Additionally, Brown et al., in a population-based cross-sectional study of 639 women, found significant links between depressive symptoms and several menopausal symptoms including hot flashes, sleep disturbance, and irritability (the Harvard Study of Moods and Cycles). In particular, Brown et al. found a twofold increase in the risk of developing depressive symptoms during perimenopause among women who experience nocturnal hot flashes without a history of depression [14], and experience of hot flashes at baseline was marginally significantly more frequent among women who reported severe depressive symptoms during an 8-year follow-up as compared to women who did not exhibit mood symptoms during the follow-up period. Additionally, participants with severe mood symptoms during follow-up were 2.16 times more likely to report hot flashes at the same visit.

The effect of the menopausal transition and sex hormones on anxiety disorders is much less studied than depression, despite the finding that nearly half of the women during the climacterium experience anxiety and stress symptoms. Data from the Penn Ovarian Aging Study (POAS) strongly support that anxiety was associated with hot flashes in a community-based cohort of African-American and white women. The most anxious women had the most severe and most frequent vasomotor symptoms [15]. The relationship between hot flashes and anxiety persisted after adjusting for menopause transition stage, depressed mood symptoms, smoking, body mass index, estradiol, age, race, and time since the baseline measures in the study.

Interesting data on the relationship between sex steroids, menopause, and mood disorders come from the Mayo Clinic Cohort Study of Oophorectomy and Aging by Rocca et al [16]. The study involves a population-based cohort of women residing in Olmsted County, MN, who underwent oophorectomy before the onset of menopause for a noncancer indication from 1950 to 1987. For a median follow-up period of 24 years, the risk of anxiety symptoms increased significantly in women who underwent bilateral oophorectomy compared with referent women (adjusted HR, 2.29; 95% CI, 1.33–3.95). The increased risk of anxiety symptoms was particularly evident among women who underwent surgery before the age of 48 years (adjusted HR, 2.66; 95% CI, 1.39–5.09). Bilateral oophorectomy was also a risk factor for depression diagnosed by a physician (adjusted HR, 1.54; 95% CI, 1.04–2.26).

Neurobiologically, both vasomotor symptoms and mood disorders are regulated by the monoamine neurotransmitters serotonin, norepinephrine, and dopamine. Dysregulation of these systems can lead to depression when that deregulation occurs within brain areas deputed to mood control (prefontal cortex, limbic system) and can lead to vasomotor symptoms when the deregulation involves the hypothalamic centers deputed to thermoregulation.

Treating vasomotor symptoms using estrogens can likely prevent depressive symptoms in vulnerable women. Moreover remission from symptoms of mood disorders such as anxiety, depression, and sleep disturbance without a full reduction of vasomotor symptoms is a risk factor for mood disorder relapse [17].

A role for neurosteroids in central menopausal symptoms has been also recently hypothesized. Menopause transition is associated with decreased allopregnanolone levels, mainly due to reduced ovarian synthesis of progesterone, supporting its role in the mood disorder physiology during the climacterium. Low circulating allopregnanolone levels are associated with the onset of depression and anxiety during the reproductive aging.

In postmenopausal women, HRT is able to modify circulating levels of neurosteroids, determining an increase in allopregnanolone levels and a decrease in DHEA. These data indicate a main role for these compounds as neuroendocrine mediators of the effects of estrogens on the CNS, and the effect exerted by HRT on allopregnanolone levels might be related to the anxiolytic and sedative effects of HRT in menopausal women. However, synthetic progestins available in the clinical setting have different effects on central neurosteroidogenis supporting the concept that synthetic progestins may show differential activity on brain biology. This feature involves the synthesis of brain allopregnanolone and the specific activity on GABA-A receptor of progestins, rather than the activation of PRs [18].

Neurosteroid biology in menopausal-related mood changes offers several new perspectives to understand the brain pathophysiology during the climacterium and aging process. Allopregnanolone replacement therapy serves as proof of concept for therapeutics that target endogenous brain regeneration, windows of therapeutic opportunity for regeneration, and critical system biology factors that will determine the efficacy of regeneration.

3.3 Menopause and Cognitive Decline: Early Symptoms for an Early Treatment

The detection of early neural markers of brain aging and cognitive dysfunction is one of the main challenges during the climacterium, and the early postmenopause and the degree of cognitive vitality during the aging process could depend on early clinical interventions.

The evidence that estrogen has several neuroprotective effects brings new meaning to the potential impact of the prolonged postmenopausal hypoestrogenic state on learning and memory and the potential increased vulnerability of aging women to brain injury and neurodegenerative diseases.

Although the apparent dichotomy between the beneficial actions of E2 on the brain of experimental animals (see previous paragraphs) and report from randomized controlled trials in women (mainly WHI) could be a great conundrum, a critical analysis of clinical data robustly supports the neurotrophic effect of estrogen.

Results from the Mayo Clinic Cohort Study of Oophorectomy and Aging provide the degree of the long-term influence that sex steroid deprivation has on cognitive vitality. In particular women who underwent either unilateral or bilateral oophorectomy had an increased risk of cognitive impairment or dementia compared with women with natural menopause (adjusted HR, 1.46; 95% CI, 1.13–1.90) [16]. In another study, the risk of Parkinson disease was higher in women who underwent either unilateral or bilateral oophorectomy (adjusted HR, 1.68; 95% CI, 1.06–2.67) [19]. In both studies, a younger age at menopause was associated with increased risk of neurological impairment. In particular, Rocca et al. observed significant linear trends of increasing risk for either outcome with younger age at oophorectomy. Estrogen deficiency is the initial step in a chain of causality that determined the increased risk of cognitive impairment or dementia. In support of a neuroprotective effect of estrogen, women who underwent bilateral oophorectomy before age of 49 years but were given estrogen treatment until at least age 50 years had no increased risk.

Epidemiological surveys prospectively monitoring women as they progress through the menopause transition have suggested that self-reports of decreased concentration and poor memory are frequent accompaniments of this phase of life and the postmenopause. In the Study of Women's Health Across the Nation (SWAN), more than 40% of perimenopausal and postmenopausal women endorsed forgetfulness on a symptom inventory compared with 31% of premenopausal women [20]. In the Seattle Midlife Women's Health Study, approximately 62% of midlife women reported an undesirable change in memory [21].

Maki et al. investigated the relationship between objective measures of hot flashes and one particular domain, verbal episodic memory, in a sample of midlife women.

In particular, the presence of objective hot flashes is a negative predictor of verbal memory in midlife women with moderate to severe vasomotor symptoms. This relationship appears to be primarily due to nighttime rather than daytime hot flashes supporting the concept that hot flashes and sleep disturbances are signs of brain vulnerability to sex steroid withdrawal with a negative impact of cognition [22]. Hypothalamic and HPG axis senescence induces vasomotor symptoms and hypogonadism that could trigger menopause-related mental decline in other brain areas years before deficits in learning and cognition would normally start to become evident. The epidemiological data on the neuroprotective effects of estrogen-base therapy were reviewed by Leblanc and colleagues: women who were symptomatic from menopause had improvement in verbal memory, vigilance, reasoning, and motor speed when given HRT. The same meta-analysis of observational studies examining HRT and cognitive function also suggests a significant reduction in the risk of AD among women who have ever used HRT [23]. In particular, the strongest evidence for an association between HRT and Alzheimer disease comes from two cohort studies: the Manhattan Study of Aging [24] and The Baltimore Longitudinal Study of Aging [25]. The two prospective cohort studies that reported a significantly reduced risk of AD in estrogen users are particularly compelling because they avoid both recalling and prescribing practice bias. In the Italian Longitudinal Study on Aging, ERT was associated with a reduced prevalence of AD in 2816 women (OR, 0.24; 95% CI, 0.07–0.77) [26]. Analysis of observational data from the Cache County Study suggested a reduction in the risk of AD for past HRT users for 3–10 years. In the same study, the "excess" risk of AD when compared with age-equivalent men disappeared among women who received HRT for more than 10 years [27].

In conclusion, the majority of studies and meta-analyses evidencing cognitive benefits during HRT analyze young symptomatic postmenopausal women, supporting the concept of the "window of opportunity" for estrogen neurotrophic effects.

3.4 Evidences and Perspectives in the Post-WHIMS Era

The overall analysis of studies on estrogens and cognitive function from basic science to clinical applications provides some answers for their discrepant findings and suggests new research directions.

Compared to observational and longitudinal studies, randomized controlled trials (RCTs) provide stronger evidence of an estrogen effect on cognition; while the preponderance of findings shows that estrogen users performed better on cognitive tests and experienced less deterioration in aspects of cognition with increasing age than the never-users, findings from longitudinal and observational studies are much more inconsistent that those from the RCTs. Different hypotheses have been argued to explain these differences—the selection bias, since the observational and longitudinal studies encompass self-selected women, and usually women taking HRT have better education and higher socioeconomic status. Thus, it is difficult to sort out, in these studies, the effects of genetics and environment from the effects of estrogen.

Another point of reflection should be the methodological approach to evaluate cognitive function and brain aging throughout different trials. For the majority of studies, the cognition does not represent the primary endpoint, and many used the 3MSE as the sole measure of cognitive functioning. The 3MSE is an omnibus test of cognitive functioning, which is generally used as a screening instrument to detect cognitive decline, and it is unable to distinguish performance between specific cognitive domains. It is possible that the real effects of estrogen on cognitive protection even with samples of elderly women may have been underestimated due to the lack of precision and specificity of the measuring instrument. Therefore, assessments of specific cognitive functions, such as memory, attention, executive functions (judgment, planning, organization, and cognitive flexibility), language, and spatial ability, are critical for tests of hypotheses regarding effects of estrogens on cognitive function.

Data from the WHI Study of Cognitive Aging (WHISCA), an ancillary study to the WHI and WHIMS, report that the effect of CEE + MPA on cognitive function varies across cognitive domains in older women, reflecting both possible beneficial and detrimental actions of ovarian steroids on the aged brain, suggesting directions for future research [28].

In conclusion, convergent evidences suggest that estrogen treatment has positive effects on aspects of memory and cognition when it is administered to naturally menopausal women shortly after the cessation of their menstrual cycles or immediately following surgical menopause. Data from literature suggest that estrogen treatment to older women have scant beneficial or even detrimental effects on cognitive aging. A "critical period" shortly after menopause, when HT needs to be prescribed to protect cognitive function, has been suggested.

To test the "critical period" hypothesis directly, two recent intervention studies were conducted examining the effects of HT initiation soon after menopause on cognitive function. Firstly, the WHIMS-Young (WHIMS-Y) study investigated 1326 women who had taken part in the WHI CEE-based randomized controlled trials when aged 50–55 years. In an average of 14.2 years after randomization to treatment and 7.2 years after treatment discontinuation, when the women were approximately 67.2 years of age, a battery of cognitive tests was administered via a telephone interview [29]. This study addressed the critically important question of whether cognition is impacted years later when women undergo HT during early menopause. Contrary to the initial WHI results, these data indicated neither harm nor benefit to cognitive ability in women initiating HT early in menopause.

An ancillary study of KEEPS, the National Institutes of Health's National Institute on Aging (NIH-NIA), called the KEEPS Cognitive and Affective study (KEEPS Cog), evaluated the differential efficacy of transdermal estradiol and oral CEE on measures of cognitive function and mood in women enrolled in the parent KEEPS study. The collection of baseline cognitive data from over 700 women enrolled in the KEEPS Cog study was recently completed. The KEEPS Cog study is the first multisite, randomized, placebo-controlled, double-blind, parallel-group design clinical study that will address major HT-related issues raised by WHI and WHIMS. Specifically, the KEEPS Cog study compares the differential efficacy of CEE and transdermal estradiol on a comprehensive battery of cognition and mood measures, sensitive to cognition changes associated with HT in perimenopausal and recently postmenopausal women. The hypothesis of the KEEPS Cog study is that, compared to CEE, treatment with transdermal estradiol will enhance cognitive function of healthy peri- and early menopausal women (i.e., decreased rate of cognitive decline or enhanced rate of cognitive improvement compared to placebo-treated group).

Given the adverse findings of WHIMS in postmenopausal women and the fact that HT is still approved for the treatment of menopausal symptoms commonly experienced by younger perimenopausal women, it is critical that the potential cognitive effects of HT, both beneficial and adverse, be identified in women undergoing menopausal transition. The KEEPS Cog study is the first clinical study to characterize the differential effects of oral CEE and transdermal estradiol on cognitive function of perimenopausal women. As with the WHIMS-Y results, there were neither advantageous nor harmful effects of HT on measures of memory or other cognitive functions. Interestingly, the KEEPS investigators did find an improvement in symptoms of depression and anxiety in women randomized to oral CEE. The major limit of KEEPS Cog is the short follow-up; 4 years might be not sufficient to demonstrate cognitive differences in healthy, well-educated, early postmenopausal women [30].

Results of the KEEPS Cog study will provide a pivotal data and an exclusive opportunity for future studies to follow the KEEPS cohort over an extended period of 20–25 years to determine whether HT initiated during the perimenopausal period could delay or preferably prevent future development of neurodegenerative diseases like mild cognitive impairment (MCI) and AD.

References

1. Bromberger JT, Meyer PM, Kravitz HM et al (2001) Psychologic distress and natural menopause: a multiethnic community study. Am J Public Health 91:1435–1442
2. North American Menopause Society (2006) Menopause guidebook, 6th edn. North American Menopause Society, Cleveland, OH
3. Gallicchio L, Schilling C, Miller SR, Zacur H, Flaws JF (2007) Correlates of depressive symptoms among women undergoing the menopausal transition. J Psychosom Res 63:263–268
4. Moline ML, Broch L, Zak RZ (2004) Sleep in women across the life cycle from adulthood through menopause. Med Clin N Am 88:705–736
5. McKinley JB, McKinley SM, Brambilla D (1987) The relative contributions of endocrine changes and social circumstances to depression in mid-aged women. J Health Soc Behav 28:345–363
6. Avis NE, Stellato R, Crawford S et al (2001) Is there a menopausal syndrome? Menopausal status and symptoms across racial/ethnic groups. Soc Sci Med 52:345–356
7. Bromberger JT, Assmann SF, Avis NE, Schocken M, Kravitz HM, Cordal A (2003) Persistent mood symptoms in a multiethnic community cohort of pre- and perimenopausal women. Am J Epidemiol 15:347–356
8. Schmidt PJ, Haq N, Rubinow DR (2004) A longitudinal evaluation of the relationship between reproductive status and mood in perimenopausal women. Am J Psychiatry 161:2238–2244
9. Murray CJL, Lopez AD (eds) (1996) The global burden of disease. A comprehensive assessment of mortality and disability from diseases, injuries and risk factors in 1990 and projected to 2020. Harvard School of Public Health, Cambridge, MA

10. Richards M, Rubinow D, Daly R, Schmidt P (2006) Premenstrual symptoms and perimenopausal depression. Am J Psychiatry 163(1):133–137
11. Bromberger JT, Matthews KA (1996) A longitudinal study of the effects of pessimism, trait anxiety, and life stress on depressive symptoms in middle-aged women. Psychol Aging 11(2):207–213
12. Avis NE, Brambilla D, McKinlay SM, Vass K (1994) A longitudinal analysis of the association between menopause and depression. Results from the Massachusetts Women's Health Study. Ann Epidemiol 4(3):214–220
13. Freeman EW, Sammel MD, Grisso JA et al (2001) Hot flashes in the late reproductive years: risk factors for Africa American and Caucasian women. J Womens Health Gend Based Med 10(1):67–76
14. Cohen LS, Soares CN, Vitonis AF, Otto MW, Harlow BL (2006) Risk for new onset depression during the menopausal transition. Arch Gen Psychiatry 63:385–390
15. Freeman EW, Sammel MD, Lin H, Gracia CR, Pien GW, Nelson DB, Sheng L (2007) Symptoms associated with menopausal transition and reproductive hormones in midlife women. Obstet Gynecol 110(2 Pt 1):230–240
16. Rocca WA, Shuster LT, Grossardt BR et al (2009) Long-term effects of bilateral oophorectomy on brain aging: unanswered questions from the Mayo Clinic Cohort Study of Oophorectomy and Aging. Women's Health (Lond Engl) 5(1):39–48
17. Morgan ML, Cook IA, Rapkin AJ, Leuchter AF (2007) Neurophysiologic changes during estrogen augmentation in perimenopausal depression. Maturitas 56(1):54–60
18. Bernardi F, Pieri M, Stomati M et al (2003) Effect of different hormonal replacement therapies on circulating allopregnanolone and dehydroepiandrosterone levels in postmenopausal women. Gynecol Endocrinol 17(1):65–77
19. Rivera CM, Grossardt BR, Rhodes DJ, Rocca WA (2009) Increased mortality for neurological and mental diseases following early bilateral oophorectomy. Neuroepidemiology 33(1):32–40
20. Gold EB, Sternfeld B, Kelsey JL et al (2000) Relation of demographic and lifestyle factors to symptoms in a multi-racial/ethnic population of women 40-55 years of age. Am J Epidemiol 152(5):463–473
21. Woods NF, Mitchell ES, Adams C (2000) Memory functioning among midlife women: observations from the Seattle Midlife Women's Health Study. Menopause 7(4):257–265
22. Maki PM, Drogos LL, Rubin LH, Banuvar S, Shulman LP, Geller SE (2008) Objective hot flashes are negatively related to verbal memory performance in midlife women. Menopause 15(5):848–856
23. LeBlanc ES, Janowsky J, Chan BK, Nelson HD (2001) Hormone replacement therapy and cognition: systematic review and meta-analysis. JAMA 285(11):1489–1499
24. Tang MX, Jacobs D, Stern Y et al (1996) Effect of oestrogen during menopause on risk and age at onset of Alzheimer's disease. Lancet 348:429–432
25. Kawas C, Resnick S, Morrison A et al (1997) A prospective study of estrogen replacement therapy and the risk of developing Alzheimer's disease: the Baltimore Longitudinal Study of Aging [published correction appears in Neurology. 51:654]. Neurology 48:1517–1152
26. Baldereschi M, Di Carlo A, Lepore V et al (1998) Estrogen-replacement therapy and Alzheimer's disease in the Italian Longitudinal Study on Aging. Neurology 50(4):996–1002
27. Zandi PP, Carlson MC, Plassman BL et al (2002) Hormone replacement therapy and incidence of Alzheimer disease in older women: the Cache County Study. JAMA 288(17):2123–2129
28. Resnick SM et al (2006) Effects of combination estrogen plus progestin hormone treatment on cognition and affect. J Clin Endocrinol Metab 91(5):1802–1810
29. Espeland MA, Shumaker SA, Leng I, Manson JE, Brown CM, LeBlanc ES et al (2013) Long-term effects on cognitive function of postmenopausal hormone therapy prescribed to women aged 50 to 55 years. JAMA Intern Med 173(15):1429
30. Gleason CE, Dowling NM, Wharton W, Manson JE, Miller VM, Atwood CS, Brinton EA, Cedars MI, Lobo RA, Merriam GR, Neal-Perry G, Santoro NF, Taylor HS, Black DM, Budoff MJ, Hodis HN, Naftolin F, Harman SM, Asthana S (2015) Effects of hormone therapy on cognition and mood in recently postmenopausal women: findings from the randomized, controlled KEEPS-cognitive and affective study. PLoS Med 12(6):e1001833

4 Climacteric Symptoms: Importance and Management

Martin Birkhaeuser

4.1 Introduction

Most middle-aged women suffer from climacteric symptoms such as hot flushes, sweating, insomnia, mood changes, muscle pain, joint and back pain, vaginal dryness, urological symptoms and sexual disorders. In industrialized countries, up to 75–85% of climacteric women experience at least one of these symptoms.

Climacteric symptoms may vary across cultures and different regions of the world. For instance, in western countries, vasomotor symptoms (VMS) are the cardinal symptom of menopause [1–7]. In other regions such as South America [8–10], Asia [9–11], Hong Kong [12], India [10, 13, 14] or Japan [15–17] the leading symptoms are pains in joints and muscles and backache.

Climacteric complaints have to be assessed in relation to the cultural background, the economic and educational level and the social and familiar situation [1, 2, 5, 7]. All menopausal symptoms depend on women's perception, self-awareness and attitude towards the menopause [18–20]. For a substantial minority of women, climacteric symptoms persist into the late postmenopausal years [21].

To objectivize an intended therapeutic effect on climacteric symptoms, validated rating scales [22] should be used (Table 4.1). The Menopause Rating Scale II (MRS II, Table 4.2) is a short standardized questionnaire for clinical use. Three important dimensions of this scale were characterized by cluster and factor analysis: (1) somatic, (2) psychological and (3) urogenital symptoms. MRS II has been validated in many languages, including several non-European languages, and used for intercultural studies.

M. Birkhaeuser
Professor emeritus for Gynaecological Endocrinology and Reproductive Medicine, University of Bern, Bern, Switzerland

Postal correspondence/address: Gartenstrasse 67, CH-4052, Basel, Switzerland
e-mail: martin.birkhaeuser@balcab.ch

M. Birkhaeuser, A.R. Genazzani (eds.), *Pre-Menopause, Menopause and Beyond*, ISGE Series, https://doi.org/10.1007/978-3-319-63540-8_4

Table 4.1 Most used scales for the evaluation of climacteric symptoms and Quality of Life after menopause

Scale	Reference
Greene Climacteric Scale	Greene [23], Greene (1976, cited in [23])
Women's Health Questionnaire (WHQ)	Hunter [24], Girod et al. [25]
Qualifemme	Le Floch [26]
The Menopause-Specific QOL Questionnaire (MENQOL)	Hilditch [27]
Menopause Rating Scale (MRS)	Schneider and Doeren [28], Potthoff et al. [29]
Menopausal Symptom List (MSL)	Perz [30]
Menopausal Quality of Life Scale (MQOL)	Jacobs et al. [31]
Utian Quality of Life Scale (UQOL)	Utian et al. [32]

From: Schneider and Birkhaeuser [22]

Table 4.2 Menopause rating scale

Menopause Rating Scale (MRS II)

Which of the following symptoms apply to you at this time? Please, mark the appropriate box for each symptom. For symptoms that do not apply, please mark 'none'.

Symptoms:	none	mild	moderate	severe	very severe
Score	= 0	1	2	3	4
1. Hot flushes, sweating (episoded of sweating)	☐	☐	☐	☐	☐
2. Heart discomfort (unusual awareness of heart beat, heart skipping, heart racing, tightness)	☐	☐	☐	☐	☐
3. Sleep problems (difficulty in falling asleep,) difficulty in sleeping through, waking up early)	☐	☐	☐	☐	☐
4. Depressive mood (feeling down, sad, on the verge of tears, lack of drive, mood swings)	☐	☐	☐	☐	☐
5. Irritability (feeling nervous, inner tension, feeling aggressive)	☐	☐	☐	☐	☐
6. Anxiety (inner restlessness, feeling panicky)	☐	☐	☐	☐	☐
7. Physical and mental exhaustion (general decrease in performance, impaired memory, decrease in concentration, forgetfulness)	☐	☐	☐	☐	☐
8. Sexual problems (change in sexual desire, in sexual activity and satisfaction)	☐	☐	☐	☐	☐
9. Bladder problems (difficulty in urinating, increased need to urinate bladder incontinence)	☐	☐	☐	☐	☐
10. Dryness of vagina (sensation of dryness or burning in the vagine, difficulty with sexual intercourese)	☐	☐	☐	☐	☐
11. Joint and muscular discomfort (pain in the joints, rheumatoid complaints)	☐	☐	☐	☐	☐

The Menopause Rating Scale II is a short standardized questionnaire for clinical use. The MRS has the benefit of being a self-administrative tool for the assessment of climacteric complaints with convenient applicability, and representative reference data. Three important dimensions of this scale were characterized by cluster and factor analysis: (1) somatic, (2) psychological and (3) urogenital symptoms MRS II has been validated in many languages, including several non-European languages, and used for intercultural studies (see [22])

It has to be stressed that climacteric complaints have always to be assessed in relation to the cultural background, the economic and educational level and the social and familiar situation

4.2 The Climacteric Syndrome

4.2.1 Vasomotor Symptoms and Sleep Disorders

4.2.1.1 Vasomotor Symptoms

Hot flushes may occur at any time of day or night. They are spontaneous or triggered by common situations such as sudden ambient temperature change, embarrassment, client contact, stress, any warm drink, caffeine or alcohol [1]. Alimentation, socio-economic factors and exercise may have an impact on frequency and severity of VMS [2, 33–35]. Prevalence peaks at the age 52–54 years. The median total VMS duration is over 7 years [5, 6]. About 25% of all women suffer at the age of 65 years still from hot flushes. VMS may last far into the ages of 80–90 years [5, 21, 36]. Among a group of women aged 85 years, about 16% experienced hot flushes during the day and/or during the night and 6.5% were currently using MHT, and almost 10% were very to moderately distressed by their hot flushes [36].

In Western countries, the overall incidence of hot flashes may reach 88%, but it has been found to be as low as 9.5% in Japan (Fig. 4.1) [1–7, 14–17]. In addition, huge differences in the experience of VMS (hot flushes, night sweats) are identified among women within the same culture [4, 5, 34, 35]. Figure 4.1 presents the highest and the lowest estimates reported within some regions.

Hot flushes may interfere with work and daily activities. They have an impact on family life as well as sexual function, partner relationships, the socio-economic

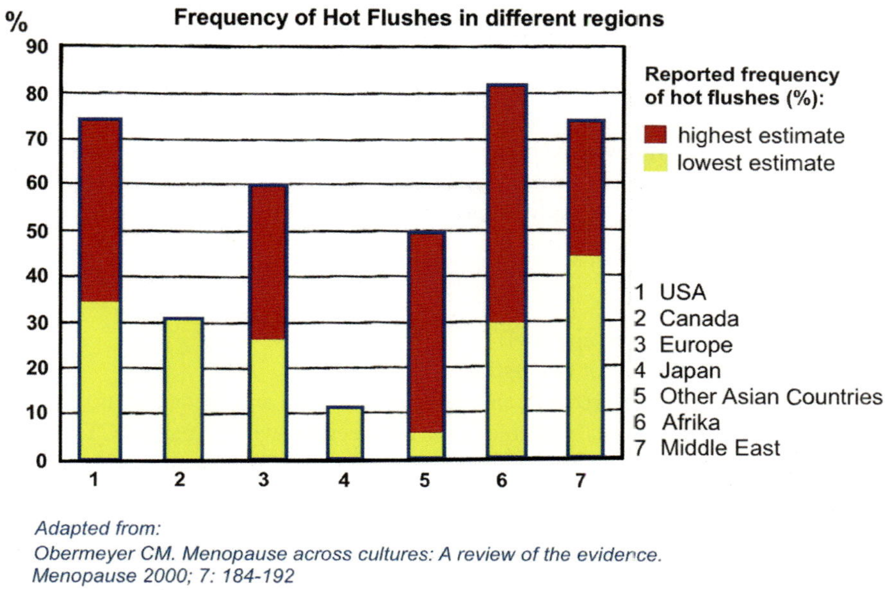

Fig. 4.1 Menopause across cultures: Frequency of hot flushes in different regions. This figure presents for all countries except Canada and Japan (highest estimate not available) the highest and the lowest estimates reported within some countries and regions (modified from [9])

position and health-related quality of life [5, 22, 37]. VMS impair sleep, causing subsequent fatigue, loss of concentration and symptoms of depression [1, 3, 22, 33, 34, 37, 38]. Risk factors for severe and burdensome hot flushes include surgical menopause, obesity, childhood neglect or abuse, smoking, lower levels of education, low socio-economic status, and prior anxiety and depression [1, 2, 5, 10, 39].

Menopause itself does not influence quality of life, but the impact of VMS on quality of life may be considerable and is often underestimated [1, 5, 22, 34, 37]. The impact of climacteric symptoms depends also on the attitude against menopause. In women with natural menopause a negative feeling has been reported in 35.3% and a positive feeling against menopause in 33.3%. 27.5% were indifferent whereas relief and indifference have been indicated by 3.9% [20]. Negative beliefs and depressed mood are associated with a high problem-rating. This may lead to a vicious circle. Women having experienced surgical menopause perceive menopause more negatively than women with natural menopause [19]. Women with VMS have an increased risk for cardiovascular diseases (CVD) [40, 41].

Some diseases may simulate VMS. The differential diagnosis includes hyperthyroidism, carcinoid syndrome (excessive serotonin secretion), mastocytosis (secretion of histamine and prostaglandins), pheochromocytoma (catecholamines), medullary thyroid cancer (calcitonin secretion), VIPomas (in 90%, pancreas), and other rare causes (such as dumping syndrome, renal cell carcinoma, sarcoidosis, bronchogenic lung cancers).

Treatment of VMS

General Measures

In women complaining of low and medium intensity symptoms, changes in lifestyle is the first measure to take, such as regular exercise, weight loss and avoiding hot drinks and alcohol [1, 42]. Behavioural intervention techniques include paced respiration (slow, deep breathing), muscle relaxation and bio-feedback. Psychological interventions aim at relieving symptoms through their effects on behaviour, understanding, cognitive processes (memory, beliefs) or emotions. There is no evidence showing that yoga or homeopathic therapy [42] is effective intervention for menopausal symptoms.

Hormonal Treatments

Menopausal Hormone Therapy (MHT)

Oestrogens (With or Without Progestins)

In women suffering from frequent and severe hot flushes and night sweats, MHT is the most efficient treatment available, as it has been shown by many RCTs, meta-analyses, reviews [1, 3, 42–56] and by a Cochrane analysis published in 2004 [45]. A systematic review and meta-analysis of 14 RCTs [47] calculated that the pooled mean difference in the number of hot flushes per week was identical for the three main forms of MHT used today: oral CEE, oral 17β-oestradiol, and transdermal 17β-oestradiol. Compared to placebo, the decrease in hot flushes was −16.8 (CI −23.4 to −10.2) for oral 17β-oestradiol, −22.4 (CI, −35.9 to −10.4) for transdermal 17β-oestradiol and −19.1 (CI, −33 to −5.1) for peroral CEE [47]. The significant improvement of VMS occurred in all groups within the first treatment month. Although in this meta-analysis, not all the dosages used in the RCTs included have been strictly comparable, there was no statistical difference between the three groups.

Oral and transdermal 17β-oestradiol are equally efficient in treating VMS [45–47]. The oestrogen dose recommended to treat climacteric symptoms should be the lowest needed to relieve symptoms effectively in order to minimize side effects and risks [55–57]. However, this same low dose proven effective to treat VMS might be insufficient for fracture prevention.

The risks of MHT outweigh clearly the risks [44, 56, 58]. If indicated, there is no mandatory limit to oestrogen use [44, 58].

The specific risks and benefits of MHT are discussed elsewhere in this volume.

Tibolone

Tibolone, a synthetic tissue-specific sexual steroid, is efficient in reducing VMS and urogenital symptoms due to mucosal atrophy [49, 50, 52, 58]. It is a good alternative to MHT in women suffering from climacteric symptoms. Tibolone, used at the daily dose of 2.5 mg, has been slightly less effective than combined MHT in some trials in alleviating menopausal symptoms, in others it has been equal or superior. Tibolone has a low to inexistent incidence of vaginal bleeding if started at least 12 months after menopause. However, if tibolone is administered in the perimenopause, it may increase spotting and bleeding as does the continuous administration of combined MHT, in the opposite to sequential MHT. Tibolone prevents fragility fractures [50]. In younger women not affected by breast cancer, there was no increased breast cancer or stroke risk. However, in women who had already suffered from breast cancer and whose mean age was over 60 years, both risks have been increased [53].

Treatment in the Perimenopause

Menopausal transition is a slowly progressive process. Climacteric symptoms may start before menopause, together with the appearance of an abnormal cyclic pattern including luteal insufficiency, anovulation, irregular frequency, decreased or increased flow and dysfunctional bleeding. Symptoms that may occur before menopause are hot flushes, atrophic changes (urogenital, mucosae), pains in joints and muscles and mood changes. If symptoms are limited to the luteal phase, the cyclic administration of a progestagen alone for 12–14 days is appropriate, preferably a neutral one, such as dydrogesterone or micronized progesterone. In presence of constant symptoms sequential MHT is indicated.

Often, safe contraception is still needed. Combined hormonal contraceptives (CHC) should not be initiated after the age of 35 years. The continuation of a former well-tolerated use of a CHC has to be evaluated at least yearly based on the existing national guidelines and the WHO Medical eligibility criteria for contraceptive use [43]. An elegant alternative to CHC and to the often disliked non-hormonal methods is the insertion of a levonorgestrel (LNG)-releasing IUD containing 52 mg LNG. The initial release of LNG is 20 μg/day. This is sufficient for endometrial safety if an oestrogen has to be added because of VMS, or if heavy bleeding has to be treated.

Non-hormonal Pharmacological Treatments

SSRIs/SNRIs

The second best choice to improve VMS are SSRIs and SNRIs [42, 59–61]. Venlafaxine 75 mg, desvenlafaxine 50–100 mg, paroxetine 20 mg, citalopram 10–20 mg, escitalopram 20 mg and some other products have been used effectively to reduce the frequency and severity of VMS in short-term, randomized trials [1, 60, 61]. In general, these preparations reduce the frequency and severity of HF by 50–60%. However, placebo has been shown to be nearly as effective in some other trials. Desvenlafaxine 100 mg/day may cause nausea and vomiting within the first week of treatment. Titration was found to reduce these side effects. SSRIs and SNRIs may increase the risk of falls and therefore of fragility fractures.

Women with a history of breast cancer and taking tamoxifen should avoid SSRIs, which have been shown to interfere with tamoxifen metabolism. For these patients, administration of SNRIs is the safest treatment; the drugs of first choice are venlafaxine or desvenlafaxine.

Gabapentin

Gabapentin is a centrally acting anti-epileptic agent. In one trial, Gabapentin (300 mg three times a day) was as effective as low-dose oestrogen (0.5 mg Premarin or 25 μg estradiol patch) in reducing the frequency and severity of VMS, but it has several disagreeable side effects, mainly somnolence, unsteadiness and drowsiness [1, 42, 59–61]. Because of its side effects, Gabapentin is very rarely used to treat VMS. Pregabalin, like gabapentin, binds to the alpha-2-delta subunit of voltage-dependent calcium channels and has been tested successfully in Phase III as an option to treat menopausal hot flushes [42].

Clonidine

Clonidine, an α-2-adrenergic agonist, reduces in doses of 50 μg 2–3 times daily VMS to a modest extent compared to placebo. Its side effects include constipation, dryness of the mouth and drowsiness [1, 42].

Veralipride

Veralipride, a benzamide neuroleptic drug, is used in some countries to control menopausal vasomotor symptoms and seems to be a safe option [42].

Stellate Ganglion Blockade

The stellate ganglion (SG) is a sympathetic ganglion located just below the subclavian artery. SG block with local anaesthetic should be reserved for cancer patients having severe VMS with a contraindication against oestrogens where all alternative treatments have failed [42, 60].

Phytoestrogens, Black Cohosh, Other Herbal Products

Phytoestrogens

Phytoestrogens such as isoflavones, coumestans and lignans are found in soybeans (isoflavones), hops (*Humulus lupulus*), flaxseed (lignans), fruits, vegetables, whole grains and legumes. Although the efficacy of extracted or synthesized soy isoflavones has been demonstrated in clinical trials, and confirmed in meta-analyses and reviews [42, 60–62], the only substance recommended in the key results of the COCHRAN analysis from 2013 has been Genistein [62]. The effect of Isoflavones is obviously independent of the dietary source: positive results have been obtained with soy food, soy or red clover extracts and with isolated isoflavones [63].

Black Cohosh

Black cohosh (*Cimicifuga racemosa*) has been shown in short-term RCTs to be an effective therapy [64–66] for relieving menopausal symptoms, primarily hot flushes, if a standardized extract is used. Long-term data are not available. The standardized preparations of *C. racemosa* using well-defined extracts (such as CR BNO 1055, Ze 450) are an efficient alternative to the Menopausal Hormone Therapy (MHT) in moderate to medium VMS. Because *C. racemosa* does not contain phytoestrogens, it may be prescribed in women presenting a contraindication against oestrogens [59, 64, 67]. In vitro, black cohosh inhibits breast cancer cells [65, 68]. In an observational study (18,861 breast cancer patients; 1102 in the *C. racemosa* group, 17,759 controls;. mean age at diagnosis 61.4 years; mean observational time 4.6 years), the *verum* group showed a significantly lower cancer relapse rate compared to the placebo group (HR 0.83, 95% CI 0.69–0.99) [69]. Confirmations by RCTs are still missing. Other Cimicifuga species than *C. racemosa* and perhaps *Cryptocarya foetida* used in China are ineffective but still contained in several preparations on the US market explaining largely the negative image of Black Cohosh in the US.

Other Herbal Products

For herbs such as St. John's wort, gingseng, *Gingko biloba* and dong quai, *Rheum rhaponticum* and French maritime pine bark evidence of efficacy and safety is conflicting [42, 60, 67]. There is insufficient evidence regarding the efficacy of so-called Chinese herbs [42, 60, 70].

Acupuncture

Although the literature is controversial some RCTs have given positive results [71–73]. Acupuncture treatment for relieving menopausal symptoms may be effective for decreasing hot flushes in postmenopausal women where MHT is not indicated or not accepted by the patient.

4.2.1.2 Sleep Disorders

Sleep disorders and insomnia affect 12–57% of all peri- and postmenopausal women. They belong to the most troublesome climacteric symptoms [74, 75] and are strongly related to VMS, to depressive mood and to anxiety [76, 77]. Persisting sleep disorders should be screened for underlying causes, such as chronic stress, pain, socio-economic factors, family or partner problems, drug abuse or nycturia.

Treatment

If VMS are the main cause of the sleep disorder, the same therapeutic possibilities can be used as mentioned above for the treatment of VMS. Again, the first-line treatment is MHT. Oestrogens improve REM sleep [42, 58, 78]. Progesterone (but not synthetic progestins) and particularly its metabolite pregnanolone possess a strong sedative effect, increasing NREM-sleep. Pregnenolone, a precursor of progesterone, also improves several components of sleep quality [78]. Oestradiol combined with oral micronized progesterone is a potent hormonal combination to induce sleep.

If MHT is not indicated or not accepted by the patient, high-intensity exercise has been recommended [78]. Valerian root was shown to improve sleep in a cohort of 100 perimenopausal women with chronic insomnia. Valerian root is suggested because of its low risk of side effects [78].

As a next step, antidepressants (SSRIs/SNRIs, in particular paroxetine, venlafaxine, desvenlafaxine and citalopram) may be used. SSRIs/SNRIs may reduce simultaneously VMS [78]. Compared to soporifics, the global risks of antidepressants are lower. Low-dose trimipramine (5–10 mg in the evening; drops 4%, 1 drop = 1 mg) has been shown to be effective in climacteric sleep disorders. If needed, the dosage can be slowly increased, and tapered off as soon as possible.

It has to be stressed that it is a mistake to use sleeping pills in menopause-induced sleep disorders in the peri- and early postmenopause as a first-line treatment. The dangers of sleeping pills, including the risk of falls resulting in fractures, are largely underestimated [79]. Compared to MHT, sleeping pills possess independent of age an increased risk of morbidity and mortality [79–81]. In a study with 23,676 paired untreated controls and 10,529 patients (63% women) with sleep disorders treated with >132 doses of sleeping pills/year for a mean duration of 2.5 years, the Hazard Ratio (95% CI) for an increased mortality was 5.3 (4.5–6.3), and the one for an increased cancer incidence 1.35 (1.2–1.5) [81].

Frequency and severity of HFs have an approximately linear relationship with quality of life and sleep parameters. Improvements in hot flushes are associated with improvements in quality of life and sleep. This correlation may allow to predict the changes in sleep and quality of life expected from different VMS treatments [82].

4.2.2 Symptoms Caused by Connective Tissue Degeneration

The physio-pathological degenerative mechanisms leading to climacteric symptoms of the connective tissues in the *musculo-skeletal system, the ligaments, the skin* and in the height loss of the *intervertebral disks* are similar. Recent studies have found oestrogen receptors in chondrocytes, synoviocytes and in many skin elements such as keratinocytes, melanocytes, fibroblasts, hair follicles and sebaceous glands. Animal and preclinical studies have evidenced a decrease of cartilage, connective tissue, and skin degradation when oestrogens and SERMs are administered [83, 84].

4.2.2.1 Musculo-skeletal Symptoms

Importance

At the time of menopausal transition, diffuse chronic pains of joints and limbs and backache are significantly more frequent in women than in men of the same age [85, 86]. Chronic musculo-skeletal pain is mostly linked to a decrease of muscular strength and increases therefore the risk of falls. They possess a negative impact on quality of life [87].

Despite the practical importance of musculo-skeletal symptoms after menopause, and despite the fact that these symptoms are listed in all modern rating scales, such as the MRS II, too many menopause specialists largely neglect this fact. A recent review on "Menopausal Symptoms and Their Management" written for endocrinologists does not even mention these for many women bothersome non-specific pains [3], although generalized muscle and joint aches as well as backache are among the commonest symptoms experienced by women at menopause. In a Finnish study, the incidence of backache was 20% in peri- and 17.1% in postmenopausal women, the one of muscular pain 20.3% and 22.1%, respectively. The difference to premenopausal controls was significant for backache ($p < 0.001$ in the peri- and <0.01 in the postmenopause, respectively) and for muscular pain ($p < 0.05$ both groups) [88].

Musculo-skeletal pain and backache around menopause are mostly a consequence of oestrogen deficiency and not of osteoarthritis. However, in climacteric women a clear association has been found between lifetime oestrogen exposure and the risk of osteoarthritis. The increase of prevalence and incidence of osteoarthritis is greater in middle-aged women when compared to men, and arthritis is more likely to be progressive and symptomatic in post- than in premenopausal women.

In contrast to western countries, musculo-skeletal pain is the dominant climacteric symptom in South America, in India and in some Asian countries. In Latin American [8, 89], 77% of 300 climacteric women suffered from musculo-skeletal pain, 74.6% from depressive mood, 69.6% from sexual disorders, 65.5% from VMS and 45.6% from sleep disorders. A study from Northern India found musculo-skeletal pain in 55.8 of the climacteric women tested followed by fatigue and loss of energy in 51.9%, eye problems in 49.6% and headaches in 43.4% [14]. In Japan, symptoms linked to musculo-skeletal pain and backache rank far before VMS [9, 15–17]. Furthermore, the incidence of pains of joints, limbs and shoulder (the Japanese "stiff shoulder") and of backache depends on emotional, socio-economic and mental factors as well as on the attitude against menopause [85, 86, 90].

Treatment

Effect of Oestrogens

Menopausal symptoms are taken often for rheumatism, and they are wrongly treated by non-steroidal anti-inflammatory drugs or painkiller. Wrong treatment might also be linked to the old misbelief that back pain is *eo ipso* caused by osteoporosis. However, osteoporosis remains a differential diagnosis.

In the WISDOM Trial, MHT users complained significantly less about aching joints and muscles ($p = 0.001$) than non-users [87]. In both arms of the WHI trial, the users of CEE combined with MPA [91] as well as of CEE alone [92] indicated a significant amelioration of their initial musculo-skeletal symptoms. In the CEE + MPA arm, the basal incidence of musculo-skeletal symptoms and joint pain was the same in the MHT- ($n = 8506$) and in the placebo-group ($n = 8102$). After a follow-up of 5.6 years, significantly more MHT-users compared to placebo indicated a decrease of joint pain or stiffness (47.1 versus 38.4%; 1.43; 1.24–1.64) and general aches or pains (49.3 versus 43.7%; 1.25; 1.08–1.44) [91]. In the 10,739 postmenopausal women participating at the CEE alone trial, joint pain frequency was significantly lower after 7.1 years of mean follow-up in the CEE compared to the placebo group (76.3 vs 79.2%, $P = 0.001$) as was the severity of joint pain (1.16 ± 0.87 (CEE) vs 1.22 ± 0.88 (placebo), mean ± SD; $P < 0.001$, respectively). In contrast, joint swelling frequency was higher in the CEE alone group (42.1 vs 39.7%, $P = 0.02$) [92]. After the end of MHT use, the WHI investigators observed a significant increase of bodily pain and stiffness of joints (Odds Ratio (OR) 2.16; 95% CI 1.95–2.40), particularly in women suffering initially from these symptoms (OR 3.21; 95% CI 2.90–3.56) [93]. Last but not least, the WHI has demonstrated a 45% reduction in total joint surgery among women using MHT compared to the placebo group [94].

In a prospective study over 12 months in 367 symptomatic postmenopausal women, we have demonstrated that transdermal MHT is also effective in treating climacteric backache and pains in joints and limbs due to oestrogen deficiency [95]. Transdermal MHT consisted in the sequential administration of an E2-alone patch for 2 weeks (50 μg/day), followed by a combined E2/NETA-patch (E2 50 μg/day + NETA 250 μg/day) for the next 2 weeks over 12 months. All musculo-skeletal symptoms decreased significantly at month three and stayed significantly lower until the end of the treatment compared to baseline ($p < 0.001$) (Fig. 4.2; [95]).

In a RCT (78 women aged 49–55 years), not only backache but also reduced mobility of the spine decreased significantly in the MHT group compared to placebo ($p < 0.05$) [96].

It has been demonstrated that about 50% of climacteric women suffering from bodily pain react well to MHT. It is therefore recommended to administer oestrogens as a first-line treatment to women where the appearance of these symptoms shows a temporal relationship to the menopausal transition, and not to prescribe automatically non-steroidal anti-inflammatory drugs.

4.2.2.2 Skin, Mucosae, Eye

Importance and Treatment

As a consequence of normal ageing, skin becomes thinner and wrinkled. Elasticity decreases. This degenerative ageing process is accelerated by menopause. Skin and mucosae thin more rapidly after menopause, and there is a loss of viscoelasticity. Oestrogen receptors in the skin suggest that oestrogen deficiency will have a negative impact on skin health [97].

It has been demonstrated that the negative effect of menopausal oestrogen loss can be slowed down or partly reversed by the systemic administration of oestrogens [97, 98]. The oestrogenic mechanisms involved in skin reparation are comparable to the ones observed at the intervertebral disks and the carotid [97]. Non-confirmed data suggest that a topical oestrogen administration might also improve the quality of the skin surface [99]. However, it is evident that a skin permanently damaged by heavy smoking or excessive sun exposition cannot be positively influenced by oestrogens [98].

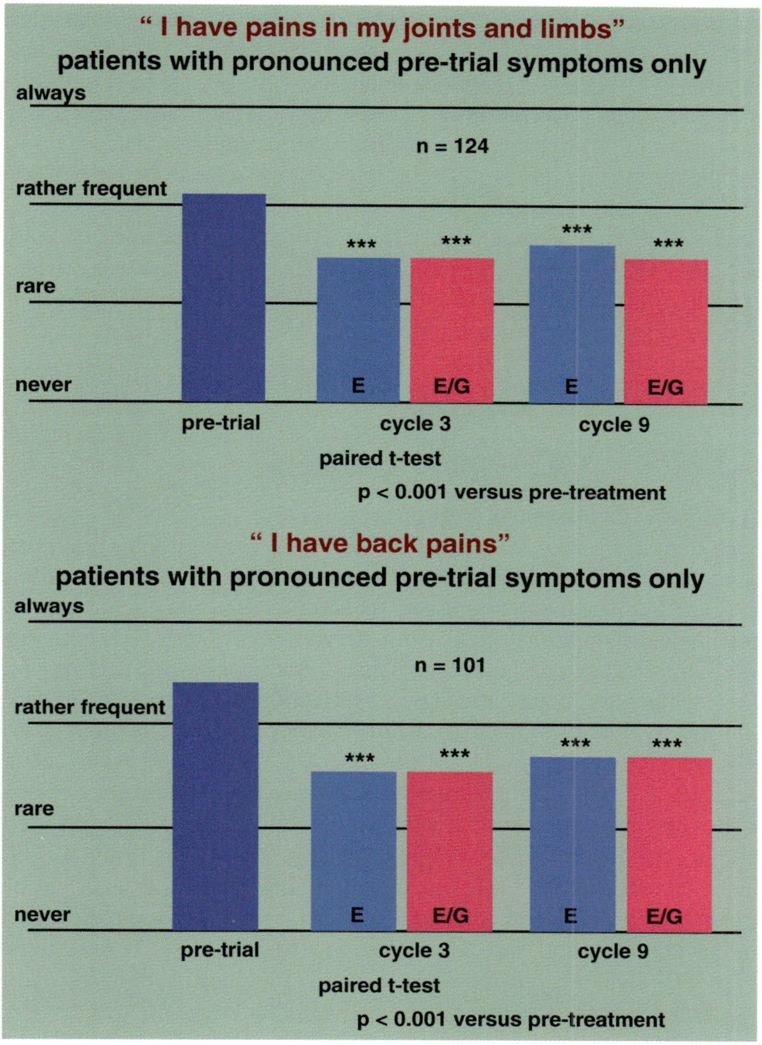

Fig. 4.2 Efficacy of transdermal MHT for the treatment of musculo-skeletal pain. A prospective study over 12 months in 367 symptomatic postmenopausal women has demonstrated that transdermal MHT is also effective in treating climacteric backache and pains in joints and limbs [95]. Transdermal MHT consisted in the sequential administration of an E2-alone patch for 2 weeks (50 µg/day), followed by a combined E2/NETA-patch (E2 50 µg/day + NETA 250 µg/day) for the next 2 weeks over 12 months. The two questions presented on this figure have been: "I have pains in my joints and limbs", and "I have back pains". All musculo-skeletal symptoms decreased significantly at month three and stayed significantly lower until the end of the treatment compared to baseline (paired t-test; $p < 0.001$) (from [95])

The phenomenon of thinning, loss of elasticity, and a decrease of the physiological secretion is also observed at the mucosae. It is particularly bothersome at the eye. The dry eye syndrome (keratoconjunctivitis sicca) may be due to oestrogen loss, but other somatic causes, such as allergies, smoking, local infections, or the Sjögren syndrome [100], have to be excluded. Furthermore, the dry eye syndrome might be the leading symptom of a depression expressed mainly through somatizations, or reflect a drug side effect.

Systemic MHT may worsen ocular dryness (probably depending on the progestin used) [101, 102], whereas the combination of oestradiol and testosterone might have a positive effect [101]. In contrast, local administration of oestrogen drops improves the dry eye symptoms significantly [103]. Other ocular hormonal effects have been recently reviewed [104].

4.2.3 Mental Changes, Mood

4.2.3.1 Clinical Expression, Prevalence

Oestrogen deficiency may lead to mental changes. Through their brain receptors, oestrogens modulate the metabolism of serotonin and noradrenalin, as do antidepressants, and influence therefore mood, mental function, and cognition [105, 106].

Psychological symptoms reach from nervousness, aggressiveness, irritability and agitation to instable and depressive mood. Menopausal women may feel controlled by an inner tension. Psychological symptoms such as anxiety and depression are significantly more frequent in women suffering from medium and severe VMS. There is a clear correlation between VMS and depression and anxiety (Fig. 4.3) [40, 42, 105–108]. Depressive symptoms are more likely to precede hot flushes in women who report both symptoms [109]. Chronic lack of sleep due to frequent hot flushes and sweats at night correlates with mental symptoms in symptomatic climacteric women [77]. This condition may end in a state of physical and mental exhaustion with a general decrease in performance, an impaired memory, a decrease in concentration and an augmenting forgetfulness. If not treated adequately, mental changes may generate serious difficulties at the working place as well as at home (partner, children) and may end in social isolation.

It is well known that women suffer in their lifetime twice as much from depression than men. Overall, the risk for major depression is approximately 1.5 to 3 times higher in women than in men. The estimated lifetime prevalence in women is 21.3% [104–106]. Endocrine unstable life periods such as puberty, pregnancy, postpartum and menopause are "windows of increased vulnerability" for depressive states. In particularly vulnerable women, the menopausal transition might trigger a depressive disorder [105, 106, 109–112]. The incidence of depressive mood (feeling down, sad, on the verge of tears, lack of drive, mood swings) and anxiety (inner restlessness, feeling panicky) is significantly increased in women with early and precocious menopause [113]. In a longitudinal study, a concordant restoration of ovarian function, characterized by an increase of serum oestradiol and a decrease of serum FSH, and a spontaneous amelioration of mood in perimenopausal

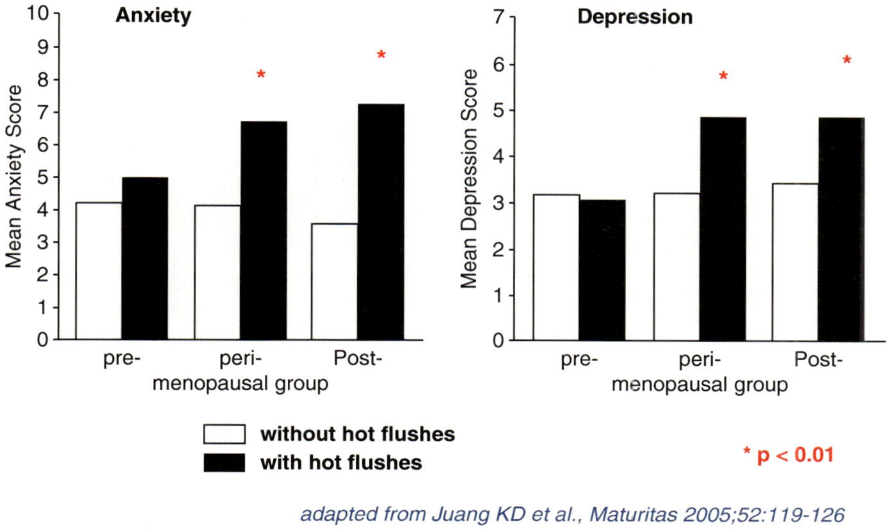

Fig. 4.3 Anxiety and depression scores in women with and without hot flushes in the pre-, peri- and postmenopause. There is a clear correlation between VMS and depression and anxiety. Both symptoms are significantly more frequent in women suffering from medium and severe VMS (modified from [107])

depression has been observed [114]. In the prospective Melbourne Women's Midlife Health Project a large increase in FSH levels over this period was associated with depressive symptoms (OR: 2.6; 95%CI: 1.0–6.7) [115]. Both longitudinal studies confirmed the hypothesis of the "window of increased vulnerability" in peri- and early postmenopausal women, as do the data in early menopause. Hormone levels and menopausal status are predictors of depression in women in transition to menopause [116].

4.2.3.2 Treatment

Twenty years ago, a meta-analysis [117] came to the conclusion that oestrogens improved depressive mood significantly (mean $d = 0.69$; $p = 0.0001$), and that androgens plus oestrogens combined had been even more effective than oestrogens alone (mean $d = 1.37$; $p = 0.003$). The effect size (d-value) used on this meta-analysis is a scale-free measure of the strength of research findings and a measure of the differences between two means. It is expressed in standard deviation units (d-value of 0.00 = no treatment effect). Newer data are consistent in demonstrating that oestrogen therapy decreases aggressiveness and improves affective disorders, mood, depressive symptoms and anxiety in climacteric women with VMS in the peri- and early postmenopause [117–130]. The KEEPS trial, a large recent 4-year RCT, reported that CEE (0.45 mg/day, with cyclic progesterone) but not transdermal estradiol (0.05 mg/day, with cyclic progesterone) improved depressive symptoms and anxiety compared to placebo [131]. However, observational studies and other RCTs (including our own data, Fig. 4.4; [93, 104]) had shown that efficacy of

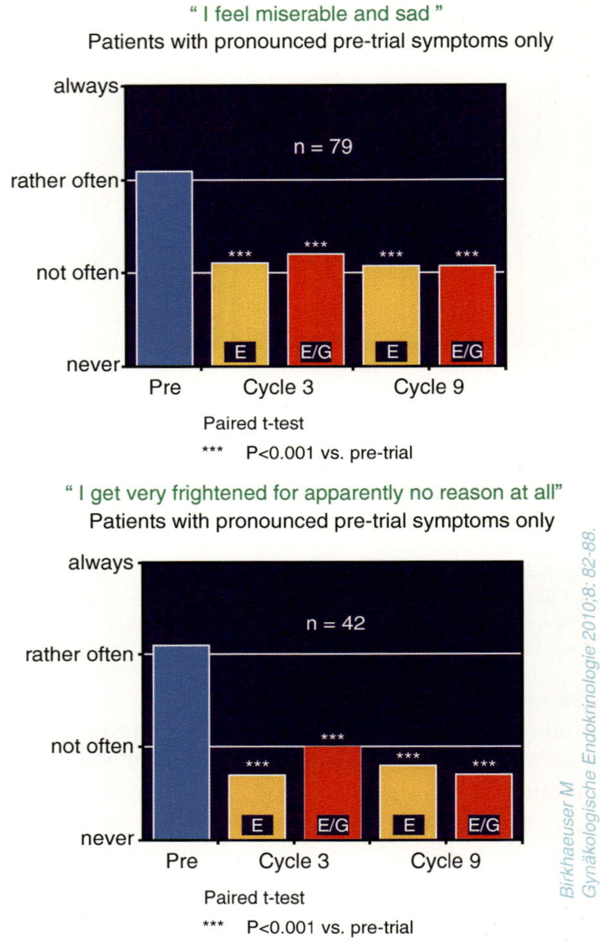

Fig. 4.4 Efficacy of transdermal MHT for the treatment of depressive symptoms. A prospective study over 12 months, 367 symptomatic postmenopausal women have been given transdermal MHT [95, 105]. Transdermal MHT consisted in the sequential administration of an E2-alone patch for 2 weeks (50 µg/day), followed by a combined E2/NETA-patch (E2 50 µg/day + NETA 250 µg/day) for the next 2 weeks over 12 months. The answers to the following two questions, representative for depression and anxiety, are presented in this figure: "I feel miserable and sad", and "I get very frightened for apparently no reason at all". The symptoms of depression and anxiety decreased significantly at month three and stayed significantly lower until the end of the treatment compared to baseline (paired t-test; $p < 0.001$ vs pre-trial) (adapted from [105])

transdermal oestradiol was at least equal to the one of peroral oestrogens [104, 118, 121, 124, 126, 129]. Inversely, current use of oestrogens decreases the risk for the occurrence of depressive symptoms significantly compared to non-users (OR 0.7; CI 0.5–0.9; $p = 0.01$) [132].

In contrast to these positive results, a 4-month pilot study, a RCT, found no effect on mood for MHT (CEE 0.625 mg/day + continuous medroxyprogesterone acetate = MPA) in women aged 45–55 years [133]. These data are congruent with an earlier observation showing in a placebo-controlled trial that MPA neutralizes the positive effect of CEE alone on depressive symptoms in postmenopausal women [134]. Already in the nineties, it has been pointed out that some progestins such as MPA block the favourable mental-tonic effect of oestrogens on mood [117, 135]. No such negative impact is known for micronized progesterone, dydrogesterone or NETA.

The combination of oestrogens with androgens is increasing the effect on mood of oestrogens alone [117, 119]. The combination of oestrogens and androgens may be helpful in women suffering from depressive symptoms together with a loss of libido.

No positive effect on depressive mood has been observed in trials where climacteric women being otherwise asymptomatic had been included in their late postmenopause [123, 136, 137].

Oestrogens may potentiate the effect of antidepressants [127, 138–140]. Oestrogens modulate the metabolism of noradrenaline and serotonin in a similar way to many antidepressants, resulting in an increase of the adrenergic and serotonergic activity. In a double-blind RCT in 358 depressed postmenopausal women, 72 received fluoxetine (20 mg/day) plus CEE, 286 received CEE alone, fluoxetine alone or placebo. Patients on ERT plus fluoxetine had a substantially greater mean Ham-D percentage improvement than patients on ERT plus placebo (40.1% vs. 17.0%, respectively; $p = 0.015$); fluoxetine-treated patients not on ERT did not show benefit significantly greater than placebo-treated patients not on ERT [139].

Oestrogens may improve cognition [108, 133, 141], but the data are still controversial although a correlation has been shown between low endogenous oestradiol levels and the decrease in cognitive ability [142]. As for cardiovascular diseases, there might be a window of opportunity for oestrogen use [143, 144].

In peri- and early postmenopausal women with climacteric vasomotor symptoms, oestrogens might be considered as a first-line treatment for depressive symptoms. Elderly depressed patients may profit from the combined administration of oestrogens and fluoxetine. However, SSRIs or antidepressants remain the first-line treatment of depressive mood in asymptomatic women in their late postmenopause.

4.2.4 Uro-Genital Disorders and Low Sexual Desire

4.2.4.1 Urogenital Symptoms

Unlike hot flushes and night sweats which mostly decrease with time, atrophic symptoms affecting the vagina and lower urinary tract are often progressive. Frequently, atrophic symptomatic vulvo-vaginal atrophy (VVA) requires treatment up to the old age. However, symptomatic VVA may be present before menopause. Vaginal dryness causes itching, burning and dyspareunia. Prevalence increases from 15% in the perimenopause to 59% in the postmenopause (≥4 years after menopause). Taken together, 25–50% of all women will suffer once in their life from urogenital symptoms [145]. In contrast to surveys including women who were known to have symptomatic VVA, a study of 98,705 postmenopausal women aged 50–79 years who were not specifically recruited for a survey on VVA or sexual function found lower rates of vaginal symptoms. Only 19–27% reported dryness, irritation or itching [146].

As VMS, the symptomatology of VVA depends hugely on cultural, religious and socio-economic factors [147]. The reported incidence of symptomatic VVA and the acceptance of medical help is linked to the taboo represented by female sexual organs still today in many countries and in some religious or social groups (recommended reading: IMS recommendations for the management of postmenopausal vaginal atrophy [147]).

There is an association between vaginal dryness and painful intercourse. Sexual activity is often compromised. Inadequate lubrication is a common cause of dyspareunia, defined as a recurrent or persistent pain with sexual activity that causes marked distress. In an online survey conducted in six countries, an estimated 45% of postmenopausal women reported experiencing vaginal symptoms [148], but only 4% could identify the symptoms of VVA related to menopause. For US women, the following opinions have been expressed in relation to vaginal discomfort (VIVA study; [148]): 80% considered symptomatic VVA to negatively affect their lives, 75% reported negative consequences on sex life, 68% that it makes them feel less sexual and 36% that it makes them feel old. Thirty-three percent reported negative consequences on marriage/relationship, 26% a negative effect on self-esteem and still 25% that it lowers QOL. The largest US survey (REVIVE; 3046 women with symptoms of VVA; [149]) added the following information: 85% of women with a partner felt “some loss of intimacy”, 59% indicated that VVA symptoms detracted from enjoyment of sex and 47% of partnered women that VVA interfered with their relationship. Then, 29% reported that VVA had a negative effect on sleep and 27% that it had a negative effect on their general enjoyment of life.

A total of 749 postmenopausal women from five European countries (150 in the UK, 150 in France, 150 in Spain, 150 in Germany and 149 in Italy) participated in an analytical study [150]. The attitudes and behaviours of postmenopausal women towards their VVA allow for the clear definition of different profiles of women, with varying representation among countries. This study identified several profiles of postmenopausal women. Forty nine percent of the study participants belonged to the 4 of the 8 profiles where speaking about urogenital problem (particularly to a doctor) was difficult to nearly impossible and where the opinion prevailed that symptomatic VVA should not be medicated (even if it has had a great impact on sex and quality of life), but that you have to cope with it [150]. These nearly 50% of climacteric women require clearly more effort in communication by their health care provider to diagnose and treat their condition in routine clinical practice. This status quo is nothing to be proud of.

The VIVA study done in five countries, including the United States and Canada, showed that less than half (37–42%) were satisfied with the existing information [148]. In the same study, in contrast to these five countries, Finland reached a degree of satisfaction of 76% with the available information about VVA, pointing to huge cultural and educational differences. Mirroring these figures, only 63% out of 500 US women associated vaginal symptoms with menopause. And only 41% of respondents believed that enough information about vaginal discomfort is available to them [148]. All these surveys prove that much more frequently than expected the discussion about vaginal health has to be opened by the gynaecologist because too many women still feel ashamed to do it. Unfortunately, reality is completely different: in a US survey, only 7% reported that their healthcare practitioner initiated a conversation about VVA [151].

Non-Hormonal First-Line Therapies for Women with Symptomatic VVA

Despite the various effective options available today, only a minority (about 25% in the Western world and probably considerably less in other areas) will seek medical help [147].

Non-Hormonal Treatments

In some women, non-hormonal local measures might be sufficient. Vaginal dryness can be helped by simple lubricants and moisturizers [145, 150]. This is safe, effective and with few contraindications. Lubricants and moisturizers are relieving effectively discomfort and pain during sexual intercourse for women with mild to moderate vaginal dryness. It is the best option for women who prefer not to use oestrogens, or who have a genuine contraindication to oestrogens [147, 150].

There is a distinction between lubricants and moisturizers and notable differences between commercially available products. Women should be advised to choose a product that is optimally balanced in terms of both osmolality and pH, and is physiologically most similar to natural vaginal secretions. Suitable products are listed in a recent review. In general, oil-in-water creams seem to be superior to vaginal gels [145, 147, 152].

Hormonal Treatments

For symptomatic women with moderate to severe VVA and for those with milder VVA who do not respond to lubricants and moisturizers, oestrogen remains the therapeutic standard. Although systemic MHT is efficient in 75% of vaginal complaints, local administration of oestrogens is superior and should be preferred. Local oestrogen therapy is also effective for the treatment of dyspareunia caused by vulvovaginal atrophy.

Studies support the use of local (but not systemic) oestrogen therapy for the treatment of urge urinary incontinence, overactive bladder and to reduce the number of urinary tract infections. But the current evidence does not favour a beneficial effect on stress urinary incontinence [58].

Although endometrial safety data are not available for use longer than 1 year, it is agreed upon that the addition of a progestagen is generally not indicated when low-dose or ultra-low-dose vaginal oestradiol is administered for symptomatic VVA [58].

For women treated for non-hormone-dependent cancer, management of VVA is similar to that for women without a cancer history. The new recommendations for the local vaginal state that ultra-low-dose vaginal tablets of oestradiol and low-dose administration of oestriol may be prescribed to women after treatment of an ER-positive breast cancer [153, 154]. Data do not show an increased risk of cancer recurrence among women currently undergoing treatment for breast cancer or those with a personal history of breast cancer who use vaginal oestrogens to relieve urogenital symptoms. The decision to use vaginal oestrogen may be made in coordination with a woman's oncologist. An informed decision-making and consent process in which the woman has the information and resources to consider the benefits and potential risks of low-dose vaginal oestrogen should precede the start of the treatment [153, 154].

The intravaginal administration of DHEA (=Prasterone) for treating symptomatic VVA has been approved in November 2016 by the US FDA, but not EMA. The daily intravaginal administration of 0.50% (6.5 mg) DHEA has shown highly significant beneficial effects on symptomatic VVA [155]. The observed strictly local action of DHEA is in line with the absence of significant drug-related adverse events and with the actual understanding of the physiology of sex steroids in women.

A novel intravaginally administered SERM, ospemifene, demonstrated in Phase III studies efficacy in treating vaginal dryness and dyspareunia, regenerating vaginal cells, improving lubrication, and reducing pain during sexual intercourse. Symptoms improved in the first 4 weeks and endured for up to 1 year. It had a good endometrial, cardiovascular system and breast safety profile [156]. Ospemifene has been approved by the FDA (but not EMA) for treatment of dyspareunia caused by VVA.

4.2.4.2 Low Sexual Desire

Introduction

Human sexual desire and sexual enjoyment are enabled through highly complex mechanisms where hormonal and non-hormonal factors are involved, including all senses, such as olfactory (e.g., individual odour, pheromones, perfumes), tactile (skin), auditory, visual and psychological. Low or absent sexual desire is the most common sexual dysfunction in women, but it is not one frequently volunteered by women [147]. Although oestradiol and testosterone are indispensable for normal sex life, the responsibility of decreasing sexual steroids for low sexual desire is usually overestimated in healthy women with an intact uterus and both ovaries. In healthy women, there are no data correlating androgen levels with specific signs or symptoms, therefore there is no androgen deficiency syndrome [157, 158].

Prevalence of Dypareunia

Dyspareunia increases and libido decreases over the menopausal transition. The prevalence of low or absent sexual desire peaks during midlife, and it varies in function of regional, cultural and religious conditions. In a RCT including 1749 US women aged 18–59 years, 33% of the women surveyed reported reduced sexual interest. Out of these 33%, 87% reported sexual dissatisfaction and 43% considered this to be a problem [159]. Another study revealed that more than 50% of women wanted professional help for the sexual problems self-disclosed in 41% of them [160]. In most older studies, prevalence reached ≥30% [159–163]. A more recent study in 2207 women aged 30–70 years reported a prevalence of low sexual desire ranging from 26.7% among premenopausal women to 52.4% among naturally menopausal women. The prevalence of hypoactive sexual desire distress (HSDD) was highest among surgically menopausal (12.5%) and lowest among naturally menopausal women (6.6%). Among premenopausal women, HSDD reached 7.7% [164]. Therefore, only a small percentage of women with a low sexual desire are distressed by it, and there is no increase from premenopausal to naturally postmenopausal women.

In the SWAN study, a large US study of 3302 women of 42–52 years at inclusion, the most important variable related to sexual functioning was importance of sex, followed by psychological status, physical health, relationship status and emotional satisfaction with partner, sexual arousal, frequency of sexual intercourse, and physical pleasure [165]. These findings confirm the earlier data from the Melbourne Women's Midlife Health Project [166]. In both longitudinal studies, relationship variables and dissatisfaction with partner relationship, attitudes toward sex and aging, vaginal dryness, and cultural background have a greater impact on most aspects of sexual function than the transition to early perimenopause and hormonal factors. Major risk factors for sexual dysfunction include poor health status, depression, certain medications, history of physical abuse, sexual abuse, or both. A recent publication from the WHI Observational Study demonstrated an association of sexual disorders with sleep disturbances, maintained after corrections for confounders [167]. Sexual dysfunction may be associated with medical disease or neurological conditions affecting the autonomic nervous system (e.g. in diabetes mellitus), with pharmacological treatment, e.g. serotonergic antidepressants, with medical therapies, with pelvic radiation, or with surgical procedures. Dysfunction may also be associated with past or current psychological factors that may have influenced psychosexual development [156].

Clinical evaluation should include medical history, sexual history, and a physical examination. Laboratory data are of limited value, except when warranted by history or physical examination.

Endocrine Changes

Oestrogens: The endocrine changes, which underlie menopausal transition, are predominantly the consequence of a marked decline in ovarian follicle numbers [168]. In the perimenopause, the increase in FSH appears to be an important factor in the maintenance of estradiol (E2) concentrations until late in reproductive life until it drops in the postmenopause. Endogenous E2 levels may be important predictors of change in sexual function in elderly women who are sexually active [169].

Androgens: In women, levels of testosterone, androstenedione, DHEA and DHEAS peak in the third to fourth decade of life and then decline with age. Concentrations of testosterone fall by about 50% during reproductive life, between the ages of 20 and 40. Levels of total testosterone and DHEAS are unchanged by the menopausal transition, but bioavailable free testosterone may rise [168, 170–173]. In the Melbourne study, DHEA and DHEAS decline with age, without any specific influence of the menopause [171, 172]. In contrast, the SWAN study observed in most women an increase of four adrenal androgens (DHEA, DHEAS, androstenedione, and androstenediol [Adiol]) during the menopausal transition [174].

Treatment

Sexual dysfunction should only be treated if it reduces sexual satisfaction and causes distress. At high risk for distress are women with pathological causes of low testosterone including hysterectomy with and without bilateral oophorectomy at any age, primary ovarian insufficiency, hypopituitarism, adrenal insufficiency and iatrogenic ovarian suppression.

Non-Pharmacologic Interventions

Non-pharmacologic interventions include education, office-based counselling, psychotherapy, cognitive-behavioural therapy (CBT) and couple therapy. CBT adds attention to cognitive restructuring of distortions and myths that may be related to the sexual difficulty, and places a heavy emphasis on "in session" and homework assignments. In a RCT, only 26% of women with HSDD randomized to the CBT condition met diagnostic criteria for this disorder at post-treatment, stabilizing at 36% at one-year follow-up. Compared to the control group, CBT also led to significant improvements in the quality of the sexual and marital life, sexual satisfaction and pleasure, perception of sexual arousal and several other related factors [156]. Couple therapy is commonly a component of, or adjunct to sex therapy. It focuses on interpersonal issues such as communication training that affect the sexual relationship.

Non-Hormonal Pharmacological Treatment

Bupropion

Although there are no approved non-hormonal treatments for low sexual desire, Bupropion has been used for this purpose. Bupropion is an antidepressant approved for treating nicotine dependency. It has been shown to improve desire in some women with and without depression (off-label use) [175]. Of a group of non-depressed women diagnosed with hypoactive sexual desire receiving bupropion hydrochloride in single-blinded manner, 29% responded. None had responded to an initial four-week placebo phase [156]. Further studies are needed.

Flibanserin Treatment with flibanserin, on average, resulted in one-half additional satisfying sexual event per month while statistically and clinically significantly increasing the risk of dizziness, somnolence, nausea and fatigue [176]. The actual evidence is graded as very low and does not allow to recommend its use.

Hormonal Treatment

MHT (Including Tibolone)

Systemic MHT is not recommended for sexual dysfunction in the absence of vasomotor symptoms, if sexual dysfunction is not directly associated with desire, or in the absence of a feeling of distress. A Cochrane analysis concluded that MHT with oestrogens alone or in combination with progestogens is associated with an improvement in sexual function when used specifically in women with menopausal symptoms or who were in early postmenopause, but not when used for any postmenopausal woman [177]. On the other hand, MHT and tibolone are the first-line treatment for women with spontaneous or iatrogenic (e.g. chemotherapy, irradiation) premature menopause suffering from decreased or absent libido [58, 177]. Figure 4.5 demonstrates the efficacy of an individualized MHT on sexual satisfaction in women previously exposed to bone marrow transplantation after whole body irradiation [178].

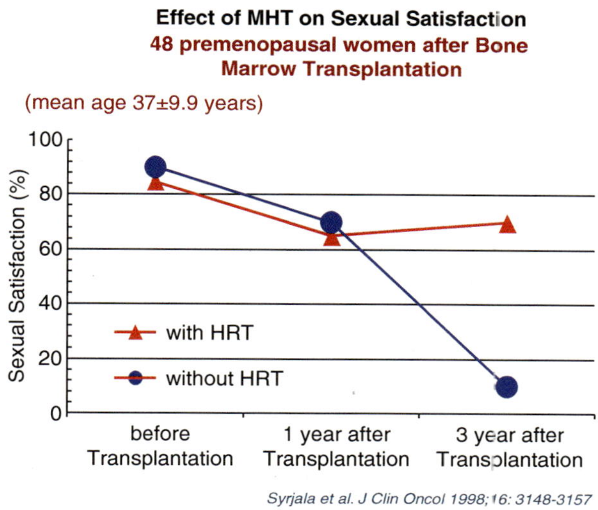

Fig. 4.5 Efficacy of Menopausal Hormone Therapy (MHT, HRT) on low sexual desire. Efficacy of an individualized MHT on sexual satisfaction in 102 women previously exposed to bone marrow transplantation after whole body irradiation (modified from [178])

Evidence regarding raloxifene and bazedoxifene does not suggest an important effect on sexuality.

Vaginal oestrogen may be needed in addition to systemic MHT in patients presenting with concomitant vaginal atrophy and dyspareunia.

Testosterone (T) Therapy Exogenous T has demonstrated efficacy in treating loss of desire in subgroups of postmenopausal women [58, 179–185]. It is not clear from any human data if sexual benefit from T is via the androgen receptor or solely via the oestrogen receptor from aromatization of T to E2. Women with complete androgen insensitivity syndrome mostly report healthy desire and response [122].

There is no indication for the general prescription of androgens for sexual dysfunction other than hypoactive sexual desire disorder. T therapy in otherwise healthy women with low sexual desire is very rarely indicated, and only justified after the exclusion of all known general risk factors, in particular a partnership problem [180–184]. Endogenous T levels do not predict the response to androgen therapy. Both hysterectomy alone or with bilateral oophorectomy result in a significant loss of androgen production [186, 187] (Fig. 4.6). MHT combined with androgen substitution should not be withheld to these women.

Unfortunately, since the withdrawal of the T-patch approved for the treatment of women with distressing low sexual desire, other physiological T preparations have not been approved for use in women. The remaining practical solution is to

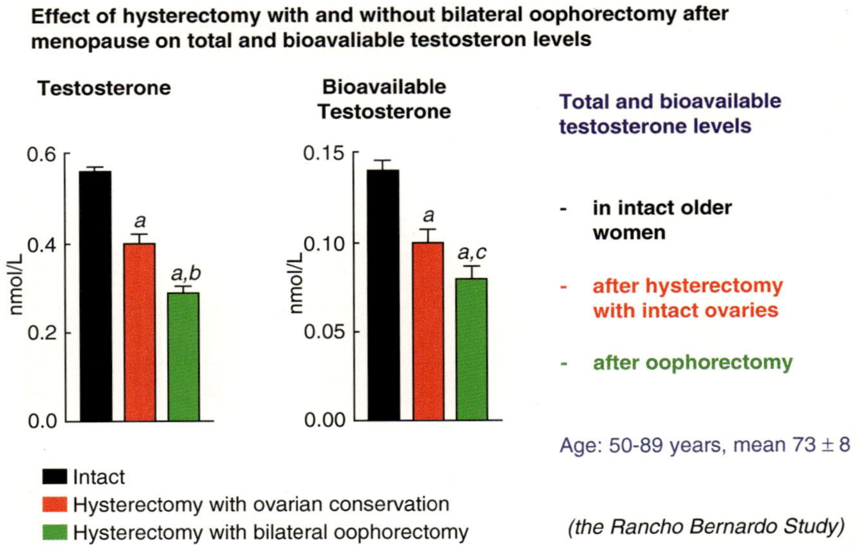

Fig. 4.6 Both hysterectomy alone or with bilateral oophorectomy result in a significant loss of androgen production. In the Rancho Bernardo Study. 684 women, aged 50–89 years, were surveyed for hysterectomy and oophorectomy status and had plasma samples obtained between 1984–1987. Of these, 438 (67%) had not undergone hysterectomy or oophorectomy (intact), 123 (18%) reported hysterectomy with bilateral oophorectomy, and 123 (18%) reported hysterectomy with conservation of 1 or both ovaries. After adjustment for age and body mass index, both total and bioavailable testosterone levels were reduced by more than 40% ($P < 0.001$) in hysterectomized women with bilateral oophorectomy compared to those in intact women, with intermediate levels observed in hysterectomized women with ovarian conservation. (a, $P < 0.001$ vs. intact. b, $P < 0.001$; c, $P < 0.01$ vs. hysterectomy with ovarian conservation). (modified from [187])

prescribe, as an off-label-use, an androgen preparation approved for males. Some suggestions are presented in Table 4.3. These off-label treatments have to be adapted to each individual patient. Because short- and long-term safety data are lacking in women, these patients should be supervised closely to avoid unwanted hyperandrogenic side effects.

DHEA Administration

A recent systematic review concluded that DHEA improved aspects such as sexual interest, lubrication, pain, arousal, orgasm and sexual frequency [188, 189]. DHEA was efficient in populations with sexual dysfunction where other causes of HSDD have been excluded, especially in perimenopausal and postmenopausal women, and in women suffering from adrenal insufficiency or hypopituitarism. The doses successfully used have been 25–50/day, ≥100 mg/day should not be used routinely. DHEA treatment has to be supervised closely due to limited data concerning its safety.

Table 4.3 Remaining approved androgen preparations for female use and practical suggestions for off-label androgen treatment in women

ANDROGEN THERAPY IN WOMEN

Androgen preparations: only a few old ones are approved.
But: you may prescribe Androgens individually and off-label

Approved	
Gynodian Dep. Ampoules (EU)	4 mg Estradiol valerate/ml + 200 mg Prasterone enantate=DHEA/ml
Primodian Dep. Ampoules (SA)	4 mg Estradiol valerate/ml + 90.3 mg Testosteron enantate/ml
Individual prescription	
Testosterone cristals	Estradiol 50 mg+Testosterone 50 mg per implant (1 implant every 3 months, UK)
Testosterone supp.	20 mg Testosterone/suppository (pharmacists)
DHEA-caps.	10-25 (-50) mg DHEA/capsule (pharmacists)
Testosterone Cream	T 1% (AndroFeme Cream (AUS)) (Start: 0.5ml/day, supervision by T-determinations!)
Products for men (off-label for women)	
Andractim Gel (man, France)	2,5% andostranolone (=DHT)*
Testogel (man, EU)	5 g Gel/Tag (=1 sachet=50mg testosterone =recommended dose for males)*

*Doses for women: start with ¼ of the male dose, increase if needed.

® *Martin Birkhaeuser, 2017*

All these off-label treatments have to be adapted meticulously to each individual patient. Because short- and long-term safety data are lacking, these women should be supervised closely to avoid unwanted hyperandrogenic side effects

4.3 Quality of Life

Changes of Health related quality of life (HRQL) in climacteric women are integrating all the negative and positive factors a woman lives in her menopausal transition due to the physiologic changes occurring in this period [190] and secondary to the treatments that may be used [22, 44, 46, 48, 49, 58]. Symptoms experienced during menopause as well as socio-demographic characteristics affect HRQL in climacteric women. HRQL is the only global criterion that is decisive for their daily well-being. In symptomatic climacteric women, HRQL may decrease seriously: the more and the heavier the symptoms are, the lower is HRQL. It has to be emphasized that HRQL is highly influenced by many non-menopausal factors, such as basic socio-cultural conditions, education, mood, concomitant physical diseases, and the personal attitude against menopause [22].

MHT may reverse a decline of HRQL if the deterioration is due to postmenopausal hormonal changes. Low HRQL will be significantly improved by MHT in women suffering from severe VMS, sleeping problems, musculo-skeletal pain or depressive mood induced by menopausal oestrogen-deficiency [22, 93, 191–193]. In a RCT in 367 women suffering from climacteric symptoms, use of sequential transdermal MHT (E2 50 μg/day weeks 1 and 2; E2 50 μg/day + NETA 250 μg/day weeks 3 and 4) raised the global mean HRQL score ("Women's Health Questionnaire", 22 questions adapted from Hunter [194]) from 2.97 (basal) to 3.15 at three and 3.21 at 6 months ($p < 0.001$) [95].

However, MHT does not increase HRQL in peri- and postmenopausal women without climacteric symptoms [22, 195]. In asymptomatic postmenopausal women, all measures ameliorating unfavourable non-hormonal factors may improve HRQL among postmenopausal women. These measures include partnership and sexual counselling, psychosocial measures as well as the optimal medical treatment of concomitant diseases such as diabetes mellitus, cardiovascular diseases or psychiatric disorders not linked to menopause.

References

1. Archer DF, Sturdee DW, Baber R et al (2011) Menopausal hot flushes and night sweats: where are we now? Climacteric 14:515–528
2. Li C, Borgfeldt C, Samsioe G et al (2005) Background factors influencing somatic and psychological symptoms in middle-age women with different hormonal status. A population-based study of Swedish women. Maturitas 52:306–318
3. Santoro N, Epperson CN, Mathews SB (2015) Menopausal symptoms and their management. Endocrinol Metab Clin N Am 44(3):497–515
4. Avis NE, Kaufert PA, Lock M, McKinlay SM, Vass K (1993) The evolution of menopausal symptoms. Ballières Clin Endocrinol Metab 7:17–32
5. Hunter MS, Gentry-Maharaj A, Ryan A et al (2012) Prevalence, frequency and problem rating of hot flushes persist in older postmenopausal women: impact of age, body mass index, hysterectomy, hormone therapy use, lifestyle and mood in a cross-sectional cohort study of 10,418 British women aged 54–65. BJOG 119:40–50
6. Avis NE, Crawford SL, Greendale G et al (2015) Duration of menopausal vasomotor symptoms over the menopause transition. JAMA Intern Med 175:531–539
7. Palacios S, Henderson VW, Siseles N et al (2010) Age of menopause and impact of climacteric symptoms by geographical region. Climacteric 13:419–428
8. Chedraui P, Blumel JE, Baron G et al (2008) Impaired quality of life among middle aged women: a multicentre Latin American study. Maturitas 61:323–329
9. Obermeyer CM (2000) Menopause across cultures. A review of the evidence. Menopause 7:184–192
10. Freeman EW, Sherif K (2007) Prevalence of hot flushes and night sweats around the world: a systematic review. Climacteric 10:197–214
11. Tan D, Haines CJ, Limpaphayom KK et al (2005) Relief of vasomotor symptoms and vaginal atrophy with three doses of conjugated estrogens and medroxy-progesterone acetate in postmenopausal Asian women from 11 countries: the Pan-Asia menopause (PAM) study. Maturitas 52:35–51
12. Lam PM, Leung TN, Haines C, Chung TK (2003) Climacteric symptoms and knowledge about hormone replacement therapy among Hong Kong Chinese women aged 40–60 years. Maturitas 45:99–107
13. Bairy L, Adiga S, Bhat P, Bhat R (2009) Prevalence of menopausal symptoms and quality of life after menopause in women from South India. Aust N Z J Obstet Gynaecol 49:106–109

14. Kapur P, Sinha B, Pereira BM (2009) Measuring climacteric symptoms and age at natural menopause in an Indian population using the Greene climacteric scale. Menopause 16:378–384
15. Lock M (1986) Ambiguity of ageing: Japanese menopause. Cult Med Psychiatry 10:23–47
16. Lock M, Kaufert P, Gelbert O (1988) Cultural construction of the menopause syndrome: the Japanese case. Maturitas 10:317–332
17. Melby MK, Lock M, Kaufert P (2005) Culture and symptom reporting at menopause. Hum Reprod Update 11:495–512
18. Genazzani AR, Schneider HP, Panay N, Nijland EA (2006) The European menopause survey 2005: women's perceptions on the menopause and postmenopausal hormone therapy. Gynecol Endocrinol 22:369–375
19. Avis NE, McKinlay SM (1991) A longitudinal analysis of women's attitudes toward the menopause: results from the Massachusetts women's health study. Maturitas 13:65–79
20. Bloch A (2002) Self-awareness during the menopause. Maturitas 41:61–68
21. Huang AJ, Grady D, Jacoby VL et al (2008) Persistent hot flushes in older postmenopausal women. Arch Intern Med 168(8):840–846
22. Schneider HPG, Birkhäuser M (2017) Quality of life in climacteric women. Climacteric 20(3):187–194. https://doi.org/10.1080/13697137.2017.1279599
23. Greene JG (1998) Constructing a standard climacteric scale. Maturitas 29:25–31
24. Hunter M (1992) The women's health questionnaire: a measure of mid-aged women's perceptions of their emotional and physical health. Psychol Health 7(1):45–54
25. Girod I, de la Loge C, Keininger D, Hunter MS (2006) Development of a revised version of the women's health questionnaire. Climacteric 9:4–12
26. Le Floch JP, Colau JCI, Zartarian M (1994) Validation d'une méthode d'évaluation de la qualité de vie en ménopause. Refs en Gynécol Obstétr 2:179–188
27. Hilditch JR, Lewis J, Peter A et al (1996) A menopause-specific quality of life questionnaire: development and psychometric properties. Maturitas 24:161–175
28. Schneider HPG, Doeren M (1996) Traits for long-term acceptance of hormone replacement therapy – results of a representative German survey. Eur Menopause J 3:94–98
29. Potthoff P, Heinemann LA, Schneider HP et al (2000) Menopause-Rating Skala (MRS): methodische Standardisierung in der deutschen Bevölkerung. Zentralbl Gynaekol 122:280–286
30. Perz JM (1997) Development of the menopause symptom list: a factor analytic study of menopause associated symptoms. Women Health 25:53–69
31. Jacobs P, Hyland ME, Ley A (2000) Self rated menopausal status and quality of life in women aged 40–63 years. Br J Health Psychol 5:395–411
32. Utian WH, Janata JW, Kingsberg SA, Schluchter M, Hamilton JC (2002) The Utian Quality of Life (UQOL) Scale: development and validation of an instrument to quantify quality of life through and beyond menopause. Menopause 9:402–410
33. Joffe H, Massler A, Sharkey KM (2010) Evaluation and management of sleep disturbance during the menopause transition. Semin Reprod Med 28:404–421
34. Oldenhave A, Jaszmann LJ, Haspels AA, Everaerd WT (1993) Impact of climacteric on well-being. A survey based on 5213 women 39 to 60 years old. Am J Obstet Gynecol 168:772–780
35. Gold EB, Sternfeld B, Kelsey JL et al (2000) Relation of demographic and lifestyle factors in symptoms in a multi-racial/ethnic population of women 40–55 years of age. Am J Epidemiol 152:463–473
36. Vikström J, Spetz Holm AC, Sydsjö G (2013) Hot flushes still occur in a population of 85-year old Swedish women. Climacteric 16:453–459
37. Ayers B, Hunter MS (2012) Health-related quality of life of women with menopausal hot flushes and night sweats. Climacteric 15:1–5
38. Birkhaeuser M (2013) Depression, anxiety and somatic symptoms in peri- and postmenopausal women. Menopause live-29 April, 2013 www.imsociety.org/updates_members.php?
39. Freeman EW, Sammel MD, Lin H et al (2011) Duration of menopausal hot flushes and associated risk factors. Obstet Gynecol 117:1095–1104
40. Pines A (2011) Vasomotor symptoms and cardiovascular disease risk. Climacteric 14:535–536

41. Silveira JS, Clapauch R, de Souza MC, Bouskela E (2016) Hot flashes: emerging cardiovascular risk factors in recent and late postmenopause and their association with higher blood pressure. Menopause 23(8):846–855
42. Mintziori G, Lambrinoudaki I, Dimitrios G, Goulis DG et al (2015) EMAS position statement: non-hormonal management of menopausal vasomotor symptoms. Maturitas 81:410–413
43. WHO (2015) Medical eligibility criteria for contraceptive use. A WHO family planning cornerstone, 5th edn. World Health Organization, Geneva
44. de Villiers TJ, Hall JE, Pinkerton JV et al (2016) Revised global consensus statement on menopausal hormone therapy. Climacteric 19(4):313–315. https://doi.org/10.1080/13697137.2016.1196047
45. MacLennan AH, Broadbent JL, Lester S, Moore V (2004) Oral oestrogen and combined oestrogen/progestogen therapy versus placebo for hot flushes. Cochrane Database Syst Rev 18(4):CD002978. https://doi.org/10.1002/14651858.CD002978.pub2
46. Santen RJ, Allred DC, Ardoin SP et al (2010) Postmenopausal hormone therapy: an Endocrine Society scientific statement. J Clin Endocrinol Metab 95:S1–S66
47. Nelson HD (2004) Commonly used types of postmenopausal estrogen for treatment of hot flashes: scientific review. JAMA 291:1610–1620
48. Martin KA, Barbieri RL (2016) Treatment of menopausal symptoms with hormone therapy. UpToDate, http://www.uptodate.com/contents/treatment-of-menopausal-symptoms
49. Kenemans P, Speroff L, For the International Tibolone Consensus Group (2005) Tibolone: clinical recommendations and practical guidelines. A report of the international tibolone consensus group. Maturitas 51:21–28
50. Cummings SR, Ettinger B, Delmas PD et al (2008) The effects of tibolone in older postmenopausal women. N Engl J Med 359:697–708
51. Stuenkel CA, Davis SR, Gompel A, Lumsden MA, Murad MH, Pinkerton JAV, Santen RJ (2015) Treatment of symptoms of the menopause: an endocrine society clinical practice guideline. J Clin Endocrinol Metab 100(11):3975–4011. https://doi.org/10.1210/jc.2015-2236
52. Formoso G, Perrone E, Maltoni S et al (2016) Short-term and long-term effects of tibolone in postmenopausal women. Cochrane Database Syst Rev 10:CD008536. https://doi.org/10.1002/14651858.CD008536.pub3
53. Kenemans P, Bundred NJ, Foidart J-M et al (2009) Safety and efficacy of tibolone in breast-cancer patients with vasomotor symptoms: a double-blind randomised non-inferiority trial. Lancet Oncol 10:135–146
54. Jane FM, Davis SR (2014) A practitioner's toolkit for managing the menopause. Climacteric 17:1–16
55. Birkhäuser MH, Panay N, Archer DF et al (2008) Updated practical recommendations for hormone replacement therapy in the peri- and postmenopause. Climacteric 11:108–123
56. Shapiro S, de Villiers TJ, Pines A et al (2014) Risks and benefits of hormone therapy: has medical dogma now been overturned? Climacteric 17:215–222
57. Stute P, Becker HG, Bitzer J et al (2014) Ultra-low dose – new approaches in menopausal hormone therapy. Climacteric 17:1–5
58. Baber RJ, Panay N, Fenton A (2016) The IMS writing group. 2016 IMS recommendations on women's midlife health and menopause hormone therapy. Climacteric 19:109–150. https://doi.org/10.3109/13697137.2015.1129166
59. Guttuso T Jr (2012) Effective and clinically meaningful non-hormonal hot flash therapies. Maturitas 72(1):6–12
60. Borrelli F, Ernst E (2010) Alternative and complementary therapies for the menopause. Maturitas 66:333–343
61. Albertazzi P (2007) Non-estrogenic approaches for the treatment of climacteric symptoms. Climacteric 10(Suppl 2):115–120
62. Lethaby A, Marjoribanks J, Kronenberg F et al (2013) Phytoestrogens for menopausal vasomotor symptoms. Cochrane Database Syst Rev 10(12):CD001395. https://doi.org/10.1002/14651858.CD001395.pub4

63. Schmidt M, Ardjomand-Wölkerkart K, Birkhaeuser M et al (2016) Consensus: soy isoflavones as a first-line approach to the treatment of menopausal vasomotor complaints. Gynecol Endocrinol 4:1–4
64. Frei-Kleiner S, Schaffner W, Rahlfs VW, Bodmer C, Birkhäuser M (2005) Cimicifuga racemosa dried ethanolic extract in menopausal disorders: a double-blind placebo-controlled clinical trial. Maturitas 51:397–404
65. Mohammad-Alizadeh-Charandabi S, Shahnazi M, Nahaee J, Bayatipayan S (2013) Efficacy of black cohosh (Cimicifuga racemosa L.) in treating early symptoms of menopause: a randomized clinical trial. Chin Med 8:20–26
66. Schellenberg R, Saller R, Hess L et al (2012) Dose-dependent effects of the Cimicifuga racemosa extract Ze 450 in the treatment of climacteric complaints: a randomized, placebo-controlled study. Evid Complement Alternat Med 2012:260301. https://doi.org/10.1155/2012/260301
67. Ismail R, Taylor-Swanson L, Thomas A et al (2015) Effects of herbal preparations on symptom clusters during the menopausal transition. Climacteric 18:11–28
68. Einbond LS, Soffritti M, Degli Esposti D et al (2012) Chemopreventive potential of black cohosh on breast cancer in Sprague-Dawley rats. Anticancer Res 32(1):21–30
69. Henneicke-von Zepelin HH, Becher H, Schröder-Bernhardi D, Stammwitz U (2005) Kongress der Deutschen Menopause Gesellschaft 2005, 17./18. Juni 2005, Münster. Abstracts von freien Vorträgen und Poster. Extended Abst J Menopause 12(2):18
70. Zhu X, Liew Y, Liu ZL (2016) Chinese herbal medicine for menopausal symptoms. Cochrane Database Syst Rev 3:CD009023. https://doi.org/10.1002/14651858.CD009023.pub2
71. Nedeljkovic M, Tian L, Ji P et al (2013) Effects of acupuncture and Chinese herbal medicine (Zhi mu 14) on hot flushes and quality of life in postmenopausal women: results of a four-arm randomized controlled pilot trial. Menopause 21:15–24
72. Dodin S, Blanchet C, Marc I et al (2013) Acupuncture for menopausal hot flushes. Cochrane Database Syst Rev 2013(7):CD007410. https://doi.org/10.1002/14651858.CD007410.pub2
73. Castelo Branco A, Luca d, da Fonseca AM et al (2011) Acupuncture-ameliorated menopausal symptoms: single-blind, placebo-controlled, randomized trial. Climacteric 14:140–145
74. Blumel JE, Cano A, Mezones-Holguin E et al (2012) A multinational study of sleep disorders during female mid-life. Maturitas 72:359–366
75. Ensrud KE, Stone KL, Blackwell TL et al (2009) Frequency and severity of hot flashes and sleep disturbance in postmenopausal women with hot flashes. Menopause 16:286–292
76. Tranah GJ, Parimi N, Blackwell T et al (2010) Postmenopausal hormones and sleep quality in the elderly: a population based study. BMC Womens Health 10:15–22
77. Brown JP, Gallicchio L, Flaws JA, Tracy JC (2009) Relations among menopausal symptoms, sleep disturbance and depressive symptoms in midlife. Maturitas 62:184–189
78. Attarian H, Hachul H, Guttuso T, Phillips B (2014) Treatment of chronic insomnia disorder in menopause: evaluation of literature. Menopause 22:674–684. https://doi.org/10.1097/gme.0000000000000348
79. Pines A (2012) Menopause Live. Better sleep but higher mortality risk, www.imsociety.com/
80. Glass J, Lanctot KL, Herrmann N et al (2005) Sedative hypnotics in older people with insomnia: meta-analysis of risks and benefits. BMJ 331:1169
81. Kripke DF, Langer RD, Kline LE (2012) Hypnotics' association with mortality or cancer: a matched cohort study. BMJ Open 2(1):e000850
82. Pinkerton JAV, Abraham L, Bushmakin AG et al (2016) Relationship between changes in vasomotor symptoms and changes in menopause-specific quality of life and sleep parameters. Menopause 23(10):1060–1066
83. Karsdal MA, Bay-Jensen AC, Henriksen K, Christiansen C (2012) The pathogenesis of osteoarthritis involves bone, cartilage and synovial inflammation: may estrogen be a magic bullet? Menopause Int 18:139–146
84. Christgau S, Tanko LB, Cloos PA et al (2004) Suppression of elevated cartilage turnover in postmenopausal women and in ovariectomized rats by estrogen and a selective estrogen-receptor modulator (SERM). Menopause 11:508–518

85. Fillingim RB, King CD, Ribeiro-Dasilva MC et al (2009) Sex, gender, and pain: a review of recent clinical and experimental findings. J Pain 10:447–485
86. Tsang A, Korff MV, Lee S, Alonso J et al (2008) Common chronic pain conditions in developed and developing countries: gender and age differences and comorbidity with depression-anxiety disorders. J Pain 9:883–891
87. Welton AJ, Vickers MR, Kim J et al (2008) Health related quality of life after combined hormone replacement therapy: randomised controlled trial. BMJ 337:550–553
88. Moilanen J, Aalto AM, Hemminki E et al (2010) Prevalence of menopause symptoms and their association with lifestyle among Finnish middle-aged women. Maturitas 67:368–374
89. Chedraui P, Aguirre W, Hidalgo L, Fayad L (2007) Assessing menopausal symptoms among healthy middle aged women with the menopause rating scale. Maturitas 57:271–278
90. Munce SE, Stewart DE (2007) Gender differences in depression and chronic pain conditions in a national epidemiologic survey. Psychosomatics 48:394–399
91. Barnabei VM, Cochrane BB, Aragaki AK et al (2005) Menopausal symptoms and treatment-related effects of estrogen and progestin in the women's health initiative. Obstet Gynecol 105:1063–1073
92. Chlebowski RT, Cirillo DJ, Eaton CB et al (2013) Estrogen alone and joint symptoms in the women's health initiative randomized trial. Menopause 20(6):600–608. https://doi.org/10.1097/GME.0b013e31828392c4
93. Ockene JK, Barad DH, Cochrane BB (2005) Symptom experience after discontinuing use of estrogen plus progestin. JAMA 294:183–193
94. Cirillo DJ, Wallace RB, Wu L, Yood RA (2006) Effect of hormone therapy on risk of hip and knee joint replacement in the women's health initiative. Arthritis Rheum 54:3194–3204
95. Birkhäuser M (1990) Long-term substitution with combined transdermal hormone therapy: efficacy in the control of postmenopausal somatic and psychological symptoms. In: Abstract Volume Sixth International Congress on the Menopause, Bangkok, 29.10–2
96. Kyllönen ES, Heikkinen JE, Väänänen HK et al (1998) Influence of estrogen-progestin replacement therapy and exercise on lumbar spine mobility and low back symptoms in a healthy early postmenopausal female population: a 2-year randomized controlled trial. Eur Spine J 7:381–386
97. Brincat MP, Calleja-Agius J, Muscat Baron Y (2007) The skin, carotid and intervertebral disc: making the connection! Climacteric 10:83–87
98. Castelo-Branco C, Francesc Figueras F, Martinez de Osaba M, Vanrell JA (1998) Facial wrinkling in postmenopausal women. Effects of smoking status and hormone replacement therapy. Maturitas 29:75–86
99. Masuda Y, Hirao T, Mizunuma H (2013) Improvement of skin surface texture by topical estradiol treatment in climacteric women. J Dermatol Treat 24:312–317
100. Akpek EK, Klimava A, Thorne JE, Martin D, Lekhanont K, Ostrovsky A (2009) Evaluation of patients with dry eye for presence of underlying Sjögren syndrome. Cornea 28(5):493–497
101. Golebiowski B, Badarudin N, Eden J et al (2017) The effects of transdermal testosterone and oestrogen therapy on dry eye in postmenopausal women: a randomised, placebo-controlled, pilot study. Br J Ophthalmol 101(7):926–932. https://doi.org/10.1136/bjophthalmol-2016-309498
102. Schaumberg DA, Buring JE, Sullivan DA et al (2001) Hormone replacement therapy and dry eye syndrom e. JAMA 286:2114–2119
103. Sator MO, Joura EA, Golaszewski T et al (1998) Treatment of menopausal keratoconjunctivitis sicca with topical oestradiol. Br J Obstet Gynaecol 105:100–102
104. Zetterberg M (2016) Age-related eye disease and gender. Maturitas 83:19–26
105. Birkhäuser M (2010) Depression und Östrogene. Besteht eine kausale Beziehung? Gynäkol Endokrinol 8:82–88. https://doi.org/10.1007/s10304-009-0317-6
106. Clayton AH, Ninan PT (2010) Depression or menopause? Presentation and management of major depressive disorder in perimenopausal and postmenopausal women. Prim Care Companion J Clin Psychiatry 12(1):PCC.08r00747. https://doi.org/10.4088/PCC.08r00747blu

107. Juang KD, Wang SJ, Lu SR, Lee SJ, Fuh JL (2005) Hot flashes are associated with psychological symptoms of anxiety and depression in peri- and post- but not premenopausal women. Maturitas 52:119–126
108. Terauchi M, Hiramitsu S, Akiyoshi M et al (2013) Associations among depression, anxiety and somatic symptoms in peri- and postmenopausal women. J Obstet Gynaecol Res 39(5):1007–1013
109. Freeman EW, Sammel MD, Hui Lin H (2009) Temporal associations of hot flashes and depression in the transition to menopause. Menopause 16:728–734. https://doi.org/10.1097/gme.0b013e3181967e16
110. Weber MT, Maki PM, McDermott MP (2014) Cognition and mood in perimenopause: a systematic review and meta-analysis. J Steroid Biochem Mol Biol 142:90–98
111. Deecher D, Andree TH, Sloan D, Schechter LE (2008) From menarche to menopause: exploring the underlying biology of depression in women experiencing hormonal changes. Psychoneuroendocrinology 33:3–17
112. Freeman EW, Sammel MD, Lin H, Nelson DB (2006) Associations of hormones and menopausal status with depressed mood in women with no history of depression. Arch Gen Psychiatry 63:375–382
113. Rocca WR, Grossardt BR, Geda YE (2008) Long-term risk of depressive and anxiety symptoms after early bilateral oophorectomy. Menopause 15:1050–1059
114. Daly RC, Danaceau MA, Rubinow DR, Schmidt PJ (2003) Concordant restoration of ovarian function and mood in perimenopausal depression. Am J Psychiatry 160:1842–1846
115. Ryan J, Burger H, Szoeke C (2009) A prospective study of the association between endogenous hormones and depressive symptoms in postmenopausal women. Menopause 16(3):509–517. https://doi.org/10.1097/gme.0b013e31818d635f
116. Freeman EW, Sammel MD, Liu L et al (2004) Hormones and menopausal status as predictors of depression in women in transition to menopause. Arch Gen Psychiatry 61:62–70
117. Zweifel JE, O'Brien WH (1997) A meta-analysis of the effect of hormone replacement therapy upon depressed mood (published erratum appears in Psychoneuroendo-crinology 1997;22:655). Psychoneuroendocrinology 22:189–212
118. Schmidt PJ, Rubinow DR (2009) Sex hormones and mood in the perimenopause. Ann N Y Acad Sci 1179:70–85
119. Sherwin BB (1988) Affective changes with estrogen and androgen replacement therapy in surgically menopausal women. J Affect Disord 14:177–187
120. Soares CN, Prouty J, Born L, Steiner M (2005) Treatment of menopause-related mood disturbances. CNS Spectr 10:489–497
121. de Lignières B, Vincens M (1982) Differential effects of exogenous oestradiol and progesterone on mood in post-menopausal women: individual dose/effect relationship. Maturitas 4:67–72
122. Wisniewski AB, Migeon CJ, HFL M-B et al (2000) Complete androgen and insensitivity syndrom: long-term medical, surgical, and psychosexual outcome. J Clin Endocrinol Metab 85:2664–2669
123. Hlatky MA, Boothroyd D, Vittinghoff E et al (2002) Quality-of-life and depressive symptoms in postmenopausal women after receiving hormone therapy: results from the heart and estrogen/progestin replacement study (HERS) trial. JAMA 287:591–597
124. Cohen LS, Soares CN, Poitras JR, Prouty J, Alexander AB, Shifren JL (2003) Short-term use of estradiol for depression in perimenopausal and postmenopausal women: a preliminary report. Am J Psychiatry 160:1519–1522
125. Pearlstein T, Rosen K, Stone AB (1997) Mood disorders and menopause. Endocrinol Metab Clin N Am 26:279–294
126. Soares CN, Poitras JR, Prouty J (2003) Effect of reproductive hormones and selective estrogen receptor modulators on mood during menopause. Drugs Aging 20:85–100
127. Stahl SM (2001) Why drugs and hormones may interact in psychiatric disorders. J Clin Psychiatry 62:225–226

128. Studd J (1997) Depression and the menopause. Oestrogens improve symptoms in some middle aged women. BMJ 314:977–978
129. Soares CN, Almeida OP, Joffe H, Cohen LS (2001) Efficacy of estradiol for the treatment of depressive disorders in perimenopausal women: a double-blind, randomized, placebocontrolled trial. Arch Gen Psychiatry 58:529–534
130. Schmidt PJ, Nieman L, Danace au MA et al (2000) Estrogen replacement in perimenopause-related depression: a preliminary report. Am J Obstet Gynecol 183:414–420
131. Gleason CE, Dowling NM, Wharton W et al (2015) Effects of hormone therapy on cognition and mood in recently postmenopausal women: findings from the randomized, controlled KEEPS-cognitive and affective study. PLoS Med 12:e1001833206
132. Whooley MA, Deborah Grady D, Caule JA (2000) Postmenopausal estrogen therapy and depressive symptoms in older women. J Gen Intern Med 15:535–541
133. Maki PM, Gast MJ, Vieweg A, Burriss SW, Yaffe K (2007) Hormone therapy in menopausal women with cognitive complaints: a randomized, double-blind trial. Neurology 69:1322–1330
134. Sherwin BB (1991) The impact of different doses of estrogen and progestin on mood and sexual behavior in postmenopausal women. J Clin Endocrinol Metab 72:336–343
135. Hunter MS (1990) Emotional well-being, sexual behaviour and hormone replacement therapy. Maturitas 12:299–314
136. Hays J, Ockene JK, Brunner RL et al (2003) Effects of estrogen plus progestin on health-related quality of life. N Engl J Med 348:1839–1854
137. Morrison MF, Kallan MJ, Ten Have T et al (2004) Lack of efficacy of estradiol for depression in postmenopausal women: a randomized, controlled trial. Biol Psychiatry 55:406–412
138. Morgan ML, Cook IA, Rapkin AJ, Leuchter AF (2005) Estrogen augmentation of antidepressants in perimenopausal depression: a pilot study. J Clin Psychiatry 66:774–780
139. Schneider LS, Small GW, Hamilton SH, Bystritsky A, Nemeroff CB, Meyers BS (1997) Estrogen replacement and response to fluoxetine in a multicenter geriatric depression trial. Fluoxetine collaborative study group. Am J Geriatr Psychiatry 5:97–106
140. Amsterdam J, Garcia-Espana F, Fawcett J et al (1999) Fluoxetine efficacy in menopausal women with and without estrogen replacement. J Affect Disord 55:11–17
141. Henderson VW (2011) Gonadal hormones and cognitive aging: a midlife perspective. Women Health 7:81–93
142. Yaffe K, Lui L-Y, Grady D et al (2000) Cognitive decline in women in relation to non-protein-bound estradiol concentrations. Lancer 356:708–712
143. Rocca WA, Grossardt BR, Shuster LT (2011) Oophorectomy, menopause, estrogen treatment, and cognitive aging: clinical evidence for a window of opportunity. Brain Res 1379:188–198
144. Maki PM (2013) The critical window hypothesis of hormone therapy and cognition: a scientific update on clinical studies. Menopause 20(6):695–709. https://doi.org/10.1097/GME.0b013e3182960cf8
145. Edward D, Panay N (2016) Treating vulvovaginal atrophy/genitourinary syndrome of menopause: how important is vaginal lubricant and moisturizer composition? Climacteric 19:151–161
146. Pastore LM, Carter RA, Hulka BS, Wells E (2004) Self-reported urogenital symptoms in postmenopausal women: women's health initiative. Maturitas 49:292–303
147. Sturdee D, Panay N (2010) Recommendations for the management of postmenopausal vaginal atrophy. Climacteric 13:509–522
148. Nappi RE, Kokot-Kierepa M (2012) Vaginal health: insights, views & attitudes (VIVA) results from an international survey. Climacteric 15:36–44
149. Simon JA, Kokot-Kierepa M, Goldstein J, Nappi RE (2013) Vaginal health in the United States: results from the vaginal health: insights, views & attitudes survey. Menopause 20(10):1043–1048. https://doi.org/10.1097/GME.0b013e318287342d
150. Castelo-Branco C, Biglia N, Nappi RE et al (2015) Characteristics of post-menopausal women with genitourinary syndrome of menopause: implications for vulvovaginal atrophy diagnosis and treatment selection. Maturitas 81:462–469

151. Kingsberg SA, Wysocki S, Magnus L, Krychman ML (2013) Vulvar and vaginal atrophy in postmenopausal women: findings from the REVIVE (Real Women's Views of Treatment Options for Menopausal Vaginal Changes) survey. J Sex Med 10(7):1790–1799. https://doi.org/10.1111/jsm.12190
152. Stute P, May TW, Masur C, Schmidts-Winkler IM (2015) Efficacy and safety of non-hormonal remedies for vaginal dryness: open, prospective, randomized trial. Climacteric 18:1–8
153. The American College of Obstetricians and Gynecologists (2016) Committee opinion no 659. The use of vaginal estrogen in women with a history of estrogen-dependent breast cancer. Obstet Gynecol 127:e93–e96
154. Mueck AO, AG Hormone des Berufsverbands der Frauenärzte (BVF) (2015) Anwendungsempfehlungen zur Hormonsubstitution in Klimakterium und Postmenopause Aktualisierte gemeinsame Empfehlungen, August 2015. Gynakol Endokrinol 13:270–273
155. Labrie F, Archer DF, Koltun WMD et al (2015) Efficacy of intravaginal dehydroepiandrosterone (DHEA) on moderate to severe dyspareunia and vaginal dryness, symptoms of vulvovaginal atrophy, and of the genitourinary syndrome of menopause. Maturitas 82:315–316
156. Palacios S, Cancelo MJ (2016) Clinical update on the use of ospemifene in the treatment of severe symptomatic vulvar and vaginal atrophy. Int J Women Health 8:617–626
157. Wierman ME, Arlt W, Basson R et al (2014) Androgen therapy in women: a reappraisal: an Endocrine Society clinical practice guideline. J Clin Endocrinol Metab 99:3489–3510
158. Wahlin-Jacobsen S, Pedersen AT, Kristensen E et al (2015) Is there a correlation between androgens and sexual desire in women? J Sex Med 12:358–373
159. Laumann EO, Paik A, Rosen RC (1999) Sexual dysfunction in the United States: prevalence and predictors. JAMA 281:537–544
160. Dunn KM, Croft PR, Hackett GI (1999) Sexual problems: the study of the prevalence and need for health care in the general population. J Epidemiol Community Health 53:144–148
161. Santoro N, Torrens J, Crawford S et al (2005) Correlates of circulating androgens in mid-life women: the study of women's health across the nation. J Clin Endocrinol Metab 90:4836–4845
162. Leiblum SR, Koochaki PE, Rodenberg CA, Barton IP, Rosen RC (2006) Hypoactive sexual desire disorder in postmenopausal women: US results from the women's international study of health and sexuality (WISHeS). Menopause 13(1):10–11
163. Dennerstein L, Koochaki P, Barton I, Graziottin A (2006) Hypoactive sexual desire disorder in menopausal women: a survey of western European women. J Sex Med 3(2):212–222
164. West SL, D'Aloisio AA, Agans RP et al (2008) Prevalence of low sexual desire and hypoactive sexual desire disorder in a nationally representative sample of US women. Arch Intern Med 168(13):1441–1449
165. Avis NE, Brockwell S, Randolph JF et al (2009) Longitudinal changes in sexual functioning as women transition through menopause: results from the study of Women's health across the nation. Menopause 16:442–452
166. Dennerstein L, Dudley E, Burger H (2001) Are changes in sexual functioning during midlife due to aging or menopause? Fertil Steril 76:456–460
167. Kling J, Manson JE, Naughrton MJ et al (2017) Association of sleep disturbances and sexual function in postmenopausal women. Menopause 24(6):604–612. https://doi.org/10.1097/GME.0000000000000824
168. Burger HG, Hale GE, Robertson DM, Dennerstein L (2007) A review of hormonal changes during the menopausal transition: focus on findings from the Melbourne women's midlife health project. Hum Reprod Update 13:559–565
169. Modelska K, Litwack S, Ewing SK, Yaffe K (2004) Endogenous estrogen levels affect sexual function in elderly post-menopausal women. Maturitas 49:124–133
170. Burger HG, Hale GE, Dennerstein L, David M, Robertson DM (2008) Cycle and hormone changes during perimenopause: the key role of ovarian function. Menopause 15:605–614
171. Burger HG, Dudley EC, Robertson DM, Dennerstein L (2002) Hormonal changes in the menopause transition. Recent Prog Horm Res 57:257–275

172. Burger HG, Dudley EC, Cui J et al (2000) A prospective longitudinal study of serum testosterone, dehydroepiandrosterone sulfate, and sex hormone-binding globulin levels through the menopause transition. J Clin Endocrinol Metab 85:2832–2838
173. Haring R, Hannemann A, John U et al (2012) Age-specific reference ranges for serum testosterone and androstene-dione concentrations in women measured by liquid chromatography-tandem mass spectrometry. J Clin Endocrinol Metab 97:408–415
174. Lasley BL, Crawford S, McConnell DS (2011) Adrenal androgens and the menopausal transition. Obstet Gynecol Clin N Am 38(3):467–475. https://doi.org/10.1016/j.ogc.2011.06.001
175. Kingsberg SA, Eoodard T (2015) Female sexual dysfunction focus on low desire. Obstet Gynecol 125:477–486
176. Jaspers L, Feys F, Bramer WM et al (2016) Efficacy and safety of flibanserin for the treatment of hypoactive sexual desire disorder in women. A systematic review and meta-analysis. JAMA Intern Med 176(4):453–462. https://doi.org/10.1001/jamainternmed.2015.8565
177. Nastri CO, Lara LA, Ferriani RA, Rosa-e-Silva ACJS, Figueiredo JBP, Martins WP (2013) Hormone therapy for sexual function in perimenopausal and postmenopausal women. Cochrane Database Syst Rev 6:CD009672. https://doi.org/10.1002/14651858.CD009672.pub2
178. Syrjala KL, Roth-Roemer SL, Abrams JR et al (1998) Prevalence and predictors of sexual dysfunction in long-term survivors of marrow transplantation. J Clin Oncol 16:3148–3157
179. The North American Menopause Society (2005) The role of testosterone therapy in postmenopausal women: position statement of the North American Menopause Society. Menopause 12(5):496–511. quiz 649
180. Kingsberg SA, Simon JA, Goldstein I (2008) The current outlook for testosterone in the management of hypoactive sexual desire disorder in postmenopausal women. J Sex Med 5(suppl 4):182–193
181. Schwenkhagen A, Studd J (2009) Review: role of testosterone in the treatment of hypoactive sexual desire disorder. Maturitas 63:152–159
182. Davis SR, Moreau M, Kroll R et al (2008) Testosterone for low libido in postmenopausal women not taking estrogen. N Engl J Med 359:2005–2017
183. Elraiyah T, Sonbol MB, Wang Z et al (2014) Clinical review: the benefits and harms of systemic dehydroepiandrosterone (DHEA) in postmenopausal women with normal adrenal function: a systematic review and meta-analysis. J Clin Endocrinol Metab 99:3536–3542
184. Nappi RE, Davis SR (2012) The use of hormone therapy for the maintenance of urogynecological and sexual health post WHI. Climacteric 15:267–274
185. Liu JH (2005) Therapeutic effects of progestins, androgens, and tibolone for menopausal symptoms. Am J Med 118(Suppl 12B):88–92
186. Judd HL, Lucas WE, Yen SS (1973) Effect of oophorectomy on circulating testosterone and androstenedione levels in patients with endometrial cancer. Am J Obstet Gynecol 118:793–798
187. Laughlin GA, Barrett-Connor E, Kritz-Silverstein D, von Mühlen D (2000) Hysterectomy, oophorectomy, and endogenous sex hormone levels in older women: the rancho bernardo study. J Clin Endocrinol Metab 85:645–651
188. Davis SR, Panjari M, Stanczyk FZ (2011) Dehydroepiandrosterone (DHEA) replacement for postmenopausal women. J Clin Endocrinol Metab 96:1642–1653
189. Peixotoa C, Carrilhoc CG, Barros JA et al (2017) The effects of dehydroepiandrosterone on sexual function: a systematic review. Climacteric 20(2):129–137. https://doi.org/10.1080/13697137.2017.1279141
190. Harlow SD, Gass M, Hall JE et al (2012) Executive summary of the stages of reproductive aging workshop +10: addressing the unfinished agenda of staging reproductive aging. Climacteric 15:105–114
191. Wiklund I, Karlberg J, Mattson L-A (1993) Quality of life of postmeno-pausal women on a regimen of transdermal estradiol therapy: a double-blind placebo-controlled study. Am J Obstet Gynecol 168:824–830
192. Limouzin-Lamothe MA, Mairon N, Joyce JRB, Le Gal M (1994) Quality of life after the menopause: influence of hormonal replacement therapy. Am J Obstet Gynecol 170:618–624

193. Nielsen TF, Ravn P, Pitkin J, Christiansen C (2006) Pulsed estrogen therapy improves postmenopausal quality of life: a 2-year placebo-controlled study. Maturitas 53:184–290
194. Hunter M, Battersby R, Whitehead M (1988) Relationships between psychological symptoms, somatic complaints and menopausal status. Maturitas 8:217–228
195. Skarsgard C, Berg GE, Ekblad S, Wiklund I, Hammar ML (2000) Effects of estrogen therapy on well-being in postmenopausal women with-out vasomotor complaints. Maturitas 36:123–130

Part II

Fertility

Progress in Recommendations on Menopause, MHT and POI

5

Nick Panay

5.1 The New Recommendations

NICE UK uses the GRADE (Grading of Recommendations, Assessment, Development and Evaluations) systematic approach for assessing the quality of evidence and strength of recommendations in their guidelines. It is the first time that this organisation has considered the subject of menopause. Due to the rigorous nature of the data analysis and the cost-effective approach to treatment options, the guidance is usually closely adhered to in the UK and respected by other organisations and countries. In a press statement issued on 8 June 2015, Rod Baber, the then IMS President, commented "IMS believes that the guidance is based on the best available evidence and offers best practice advice on the care of menopausal women. We know this will resonate around the world…".

To oversee the guideline development process, NICE worked with a Guideline Development Committee, chaired by Professor Mary Ann Lumsden, current President of the IMS and comprising of 15 expert advisers in menopause management and post-reproductive care. The group included gynaecologists, specialist general practitioners, specialist menopause nurses and physicians; lay women in the group ensured the patient perspective was taken into account. There were 117 registered stakeholder organisations including the British Menopause Society whose opinions were taken into account in formulating the scope and the final version of the guidelines. The key issues in the scope of the guidelines included the diagnosis

N. Panay BSc FRCOG MFSRH
Consultant Gynaecologist, Specialist in Reproductive Medicine, Imperial College Healthcare, London, UK

Consultant Gynaecologist, Specialist in Reproductive Medicine, Chelsea and Westminster Hospital, London, UK

Honorary Senior Lecturer, Imperial College, London, UK
e-mail: nickpanay@msn.com

M. Birkhaeuser, A.R. Genazzani (eds.), *Pre-Menopause, Menopause and Beyond*, ISGE Series, https://doi.org/10.1007/978-3-319-63540-8_5

and classification of menopause stages, the evidence-based management of symptoms with hormone therapy and alternatives, the effect of HRT on long-term menopause conditions and the diagnosis and management of POI.

The guideline was published in full in November 2015; work is now concentrating on developing a number of quality standards as benchmarks of clinical excellence that health service providers will be expected to adhere to. This will hopefully drive funding of menopause services from the UK Department of Health to train more menopause specialists and to develop facilities to deliver these services. This is vitally important given the starvation of resources for menopause management over the last decade. Work is also continuing to secure funding for the research recommendations published by the group to achieve scientific advances in the field of menopause medicine. The limitation of the NICE recommendation is that due to NICE methodology and limited data, it was not possible to issue advice on the pros and cons of hormone therapy regimens with different types of oestrogen and progestogens/progesterone.

The ESHRE guidelines are the first to be produced on the evidence-based management of POI with a view to improving the holistic care of women with this condition. A special interest group in reproductive endocrinology collaborated to produce this best practice guideline. The scope of the guideline is to offer the best practice advice for the management of women with POI, including the management of older women who initially presented under the age of 40 years. The guideline aims to assist healthcare professionals in the initial assessment of POI including making the diagnosis, determining the causation and performing basic assessments. Guidance is also provided on the consequences of the condition and hormone therapy. Bone health, cardiovascular problems, life expectancy, psychosexual, psychological, neurological and fertility implications have all been considered. Fertility issues include not only fertility preservation and treatment but also assessment of fitness for pregnancy and obstetric risks specific to patients with POI.

The limitation of the ESHRE guidelines on POI is that there is a lack of long-term randomised prospective trial data upon which to base the management guidelines. Much of the guidance is therefore based on expert opinion rather than clinical trials. It is hoped that good quality long-term observational trial data from POI databases [1] and registries [2] (https://poiregistry.net/) can be used to support and develop the guidelines in the future. In the meantime, it is important that HCPs are provided with some information to achieve the best practice given current clinical knowledge.

The 2016 IMS recommendations are the first to be published since the guidelines of 2013 [3]. The recommendations constitute a more thorough analysis of the data through incorporation of levels of scientific evidence and systematic review of new data. Recommendations are graded according to the strength of the evidence. Authors of the document have been commissioned to provide each section based on their expertise as global opinion leaders and are drawn from both within and outside the International Menopause Society. The guidelines facilitate the state-of-the-art management of menopause symptoms and the prevention of chronic diseases of midlife and beyond. The IMS maintains its awareness of the geographical variations related to different priorities of medical care, different prevalence of diseases and country-specific attitudes of the public, the medical community and the health authorities towards menopause management.

As with the previous IMS guidelines, a consensus statement has also been published to provide key practice points which will be relevant across many global organisations [4]. The 2016 revised consensus on menopause hormone therapy (MHT) as with the 2013 version brought together menopause and other societies from the four corners of the globe. The original consensus was achieved as a result of an initiative by the IMS to update the 2011 recommendations on postmenopausal hormone therapy and simultaneously extract the key points for incorporation into a unified statement. In order to achieve as wide a coverage and uptake as possible, the global statement has been simultaneously published in *Maturitas* (the journal of the European Menopause Society) and will also be made available on the websites of NAMS, APMF, The Endocrine Society and IOF.

Statements and guidelines are only as good as knowledge in the field and the available data; for instance, it was clear from the discussions leading to the latest recommendations and consensus versions that considerable uncertainty and controversy remain as far as the issue of breast cancer and its relationship to MHT is concerned. In an ideal world, a much larger study than WHI would be conducted, using appropriate doses of state-of-the-art hormones in early postmenopausal women and in premature ovarian insufficiency [5]. Funding for such a study is not likely to be forthcoming in the near future. In the absence of such data, a pragmatic way forward could be through the establishment of global registries to facilitate evidence-based practice and refinement of guidelines. There is also concern that much of the data used to formulate the consensus have arisen from studies performed in the USA and Europe. The impact of menopause and the usage of MHT differ in many ways in Asia, Africa and South America; this limits the relevance of global recommendations in these areas and warrants further research to facilitate region-specific modifications of the guidelines.

The revised global consensus and recommendations are potentially very useful tools; how can these best be used to positively influence the care of menopausal women? In my view, these are the six points which should be acted upon to maximise their impact.

1. Regulators/health policy

   For global recommendations to have a significant impact, it is vital that the global consensus, recommendations and society-specific adaptations should be used to positively influence governmental departments of health and medical authorities such as the FDA, EMA and MHRA. It is only through such action that the negative advice currently being issued by the regulators will be changed. In the UK, possibly as a result of the recommendations issued by the BMS to the government in 2011, the Department of Health commissioned NICE to draw up the menopause diagnosis and management guidelines as previously discussed.

2. The prescribers—education and training of health professionals
   The revised consensus, recommendations and society-specific adaptations can be used as an opportunity to draw up, or modify, locally relevant guidelines and training courses in menopause management. It is ultimately through education and training of the main prescribers, in most countries the primary care physicians, that the aspirations of global and national societies can change clinical practice for the better. The WHI study did incalculable damage to the confidence of primary care to prescribe HRT—it will take many years of retraining to restore expertise and confidence in this area.
3. Media—engaging positively
   It is vitally important that we engage positively with the media; the messages are often complex and need to be stated clearly and made locally relevant. A global consensus will go some way to initiate the conversation. It is imperative that we inform the journalists and the public that expert opinion regarding the WHI has moved on. Breast cancer is a key issue because women fear this the most; we have to present the small risks in absolute numbers and put them into perspective for the media to report, so that the public is not unduly alarmed. Most journalists will publish well-balanced informative articles if they are given the correct information to begin with!
4. Pharma industry—withdrawal of R&D in MHT and alternatives
   There has been a huge reduction in the funding of research and development of MHT which has paralleled the downturn in MHT usage globally. The problem has been compounded by the withdrawal of many safe, efficacious products such as hormone implants and transdermal testosterone, purely due to commercial profitability reasons. There were no licenced alternatives when the withdrawal of hormone implants was announced; this left many women in a very difficult position as none of the alternatives had worked for them. Despite protestations from the menopause societies, the decision could not be reversed because although immoral, it was not illegal. A global consensus on MHT will go some way to demonstrate to the pharma industry the scale of the menopause problem and the need for a full range of products to facilitate individualisation of therapy. It is hoped that this will convince the pharma industry to further invest in research and development of new products.
5. The menopausal woman—sources/access to information
   Misinformation following the WHI has resulted in many women with severe menopause symptoms being too scared to use MHT due to fears of breast cancer and cardiovascular disease. Many have been unable to access treatment because of prescribing restrictions in primary care. The global consensus and recommendations should be used to cascade information from secondary to primary care through to menopausal women. This will give them the confidence to approach their primary care physician or gynaecologist for appropriate treatment. There are too many symptomatic women being told that menopause is a natural state; it is normal for them to suffer symptoms and that there is nothing that can be done to improve their quality of life.

6. Type of HRT
   Important progress has been made in clarifying that different types of MHT have different actions and different risk profiles. In particular the dose and duration should be individualised. Recent data are encouraging that with some MHT options, there is no significant increase in risk of any type of cancer even with long-term use. The revised consensus and recommendations highlight that optimum MHT is more refined than just prescribing a standard oral systemic oestrogen/progestogen combination. In addition to this, they emphasise that local symptoms are often best treated with local therapy and that androgens may be required if sexual desire is low.

Conclusion

The NICE, ESHRE, updated IMS recommendations and global consensus should form the template upon which to rebuild confidence in prescribing MHT. We believe that these new guidelines and recommendations will lead to genuine progress in the diagnosis and management of women with premature ovarian insufficiency and natural menopause. However, guidelines and recommendations are only as good as the information from which they are derived, and it is therefore vital that active research continues to provide the raw materials from which further guidelines can be developed and refined. The ongoing task is to ensure that the interpretation of new data and reanalysis of old data are as accurate as possible and that this information is translated into actions which optimise the health of our patients. New research is starting to demonstrate that benefits can be maintained and risks minimised through refinement of MHT preparations; this will hopefully stimulate further funding in the ongoing development of new refined preparations [6]. The excellent collaborative efforts of the menopause societies will only pay dividends if we work in harmony with governmental departments of health, regulators, pharma industry, media, primary care and women's advocacy groups to achieve our goal of optimisation of menopausal women's health.

References

1. Faubion SS, Kuhle CL, Shuster LT, Rocca WA (2015) Long-term health consequences of premature or early menopause and considerations for management. Climacteric 8(4):483–491
2. Panay N, Fenton A (2012) Premature ovarian insufficiency: working towards an international database. Climacteric 15(4):295–296
3. Baber RJ, Panay N (2016) Fenton A; IMS Writing Group. 2016 IMS Recommendations on women's midlife health and menopause hormone therapy. Climacteric 19(2):109–150
4. de Villiers TJ, Hall JE, Pinkerton JV, Cerdas Pérez S, Rees M, Yang C, Pierroz DD (2016) Revised global consensus statement on menopausal hormone therapy. Climacteric 19(4):313–315
5. Panay N, Fenton A (2011) Has the time for the definitive, randomized, placebo-controlled HRT trial arrived? Climacteric 14(2):195–196
6. Panay N, Fenton A (2016) Menopause in the 21st century: the need for research and development. Climacteric 19(3):213–214

Female Infertility and Autoimmunity

6

Paolo Giovanni Artini and Patrizia Monteleone

6.1 Autoimmune Disorders in Fertile Patients

Autoimmune diseases occur when the immune system attacks and destroys the organs and tissues of its own host. Eighty percent of autoimmune patients are women, and autoimmune disorders often start in women of childbearing age. These diseases are a heterogenous group of pathologies. Some are systemic, like systemic lupus erythematosus, antiphospholipid syndrome, polymyositis, and dermatomyositis, while others are organ specific, like thyroid autoimmune disease and celiac disease. The problem with autoimmune disease is that, once it has developed, a wider range of autoimmune reactions may be triggered, so that an individual may develop more than one autoimmune disorder. The following review focuses on thyroid autoimmunity and its association with other autoimmune diseases suspected of interfering with female reproductive outcome (Fig. 6.1).

6.2 Thyroid Autoimmunity

Thyroid autoimmunity (TAI) is characterized by the presence of antithyroid antibodies, which include anti-thyroperoxidase (TPO-Ab) and antithyroglobulin antibodies (TG-Ab), with or without clinical or subclinical thyroid dysfunction [1]. Thyroid insufficiency and TAI have independently been associated with unfavorable fertility and pregnancy outcomes. TAI represents the most common autoimmune disorder in women, affecting 5–20% of the females in childbearing age [2].

P.G. Artini (✉)
Department of Clinical and Experimental Medicine, Division of Obstetrics and Gynecology Oncology, University of Pisa, Pisa, Italy
e-mail: pgartini@gmail.com

P. Monteleone
Division of Obstetrics and Gynecology, Ospedale San Francesco, Barga, Lucca, Italy

M. Birkhaeuser, A.R. Genazzani (eds.), *Pre-Menopause, Menopause and Beyond*, ISGE Series, https://doi.org/10.1007/978-3-319-63540-8_6

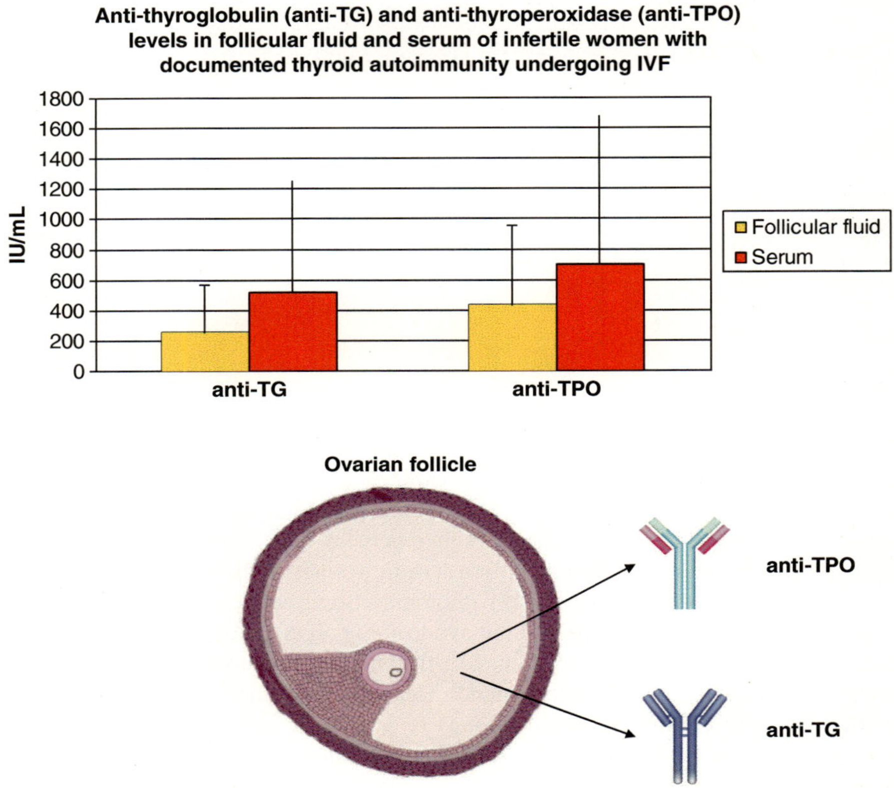

Fig. 6.1 Antithyroglobulin (anti-TG) and anti-thyroperoxidase (anti-TPO) levels in follicular fluid and serum of infertile women with documented thyroid autoimmunity undergoing IVF. From: Monteleone et al. [26]

Thyroid autoantibodies seem to interfere with female reproduction from conception to embryo implantation to early pregnancy.

The presence of thyroid antibodies in euthyroid patients is associated with unexplained subfertility [3]. No association, however, seems to exist between thyroid autoimmunity and the clinical pregnancy rates after in vitro fertilization (IVF) [3, 4]. It is possible that IVF, especially IVF/ICSI, allows to overcome the interference of thyroid antibodies with natural conception. A very large cross-sectional analysis reported a lack of association between TAI and ovarian reserve, evaluated as AMH [5]. However, a recent study found that thyroid autoimmunity has a negative effect on the outcome of controlled ovarian hyperstimulation in euthyroid women with a preserved ovarian follicle reserve undergoing assisted reproductive technology (ART) [6]. In this study, the presence of thyroid antibodies determined significantly lower ratio between serum estradiol concentration on the day of pickup and the total number of recombinant FSH (r-FSH) units administered, a significantly higher dose of administered r-FSH and lower number of retrieved metaphase II oocytes.

Past studies have affirmed that similar rates of pregnancy are present in euthyroid women with and without TAI and that the disorder is not deemed to alter implantation of the embryo [7, 8]. A very recent case-control study [9] has shown that thyroid autoimmunity, mainly due to positive TPO antibody status, was associated to poorer embryo quality in euthyroid women with low-normal TSH levels or high-normal TSH levels, suggesting that implantation may indeed be impaired in women with thyroid autoimmunity.

Thyroid autoimmune disorder without overt thyroid dysfunction is significantly associated with a three- to fivefold increase in overall miscarriage rate [3, 10, 11], and a recent meta-analysis confirmed the association of thyroid antibodies and recurrent miscarriage [3]. Following conflicting results in the literature [12–14], recently, Poppe et al. performed a prospective study to delineate the impact of TAI on the outcome of ART [15]. The results showed that the pregnancy success rates were comparable between women with and without TAI, but the miscarriage rate was significantly higher in women with TAI (53% vs. 23%; $p = 0{\cdot}016$). Together with previously published studies, it indicates a negative impact of TAI on the outcome of pregnancy following ART. Therefore if, on the one hand, it seems that ART can overcome the interference of thyroid antibodies with natural egg fertilization, it does not seem to annul the negative effect on embryo implantation.

How thyroid autoimmunity can affect reproductive outcome is still an unanswered question. Various mechanisms have been proposed. One hypothesis could be that despite euthyroidism at baseline, the presence of thyroid autoimmunity increases the risk for developing subclinical hypothyroidism in situations involving increased estrogen levels, such as ovarian hyperstimulation or pregnancy [16–19]. In other words, in conditions of increased demand, the thyroid of women with autoimmunity becomes insufficient and subclinical hypothyroidism ensues. A recent meta-analysis has revealed that levothyroxine supplementation versus placebo/no treatment determines a significant increase in delivery, increase in implantation of embryos, and decrease in miscarriage in women [20].

The second hypothesis is that thyroid antibodies can be considered an expression of a generalized autoimmune disorder, causing an immune imbalance that negatively affects fertility and pregnancy outcome [2]. Quantitative and qualitative changes in the profile of endometrial T cells and a shift in cytokine production, consisting of reduced IL-4 and IL-10 and increased interferon-γ, may hamper pregnancy outcome [21]. At the same time, polyclonal B cell activation is two to three times more frequent in thyroid autoimmunity [21] and is associated with increased titers of non-organ-specific autoantibodies [22]. Very recently, it was demonstrated that women with repeated implantation failure following IVF and thyroid autoimmunity present decreased percentage of $CD3^+CD8^+$ Tc cells, related to recurrent miscarriage, fetal growth restriction, and preeclampsia, and increased Th/Tc ratio with respect to women with repeated implantation failure but without TAI [23].

Thirdly, antithyroid antibodies may directly target zona pellucida, and placental antigens, thus affecting embryo implantation [2]. The zona pellucida and thyroid tissue seem to share similar antigens, as demonstrated by Kelkar et al. [24] in an experimental study where human anti-zona pellucida antibodies recognized antigens within murine thyroid tissue. The fact that IVF-ICSI, which requires no interaction between the sperm cell and the zona pellucida, produces a similar pregnancy outcome in TAI-positive and TAI-negative women [25] seems be in line with this hypothesis.

Finally a potential hypothesis was provided by our research group [26] based on the observation that antithyroid antibodies are present in the follicular fluid of euthyroid women undergoing IVF. We found that the follicular fluid concentrations of anti-TG and anti-TPO were measurable in all TAI-positive women and in concentrations approximately half with respect to those found in serum at oocyte retrieval. In our study, oocyte fertilization, grade A embryos, and pregnancy rates were lower in women with thyroid autoimmunity than in negative controls, while early miscarriage rates were higher. We hypothesized that the presence of antithyroid antibodies may cause antibody-mediated cytotoxicity in the growing ovarian follicle and damage the maturing oocyte, thereby reducing its quality and its developmental potential.

6.3 Thyroid Autoimmunity and Other Reproductive Disorders

In a study by Poppe et al. [27], a significantly higher prevalence of TPO-Ab was found in infertile women, compared to controls, precisely 18% vs. 8%, and, among these women, the highest prevalence of positive antibodies was observed in women with infertility due to endometriosis. Endometriosis and thyroid autoimmunity may share a common autoimmune dysfunction; endometriosis has frequently been associated with a variety of immunological changes, such as the presence of polyclonal B lymphocyte cell activation, abnormal B and T lymphocyte cell function, and chronic inflammatory tissue damage [28, 29].

Another association has been observed between TAI and polycystic ovary syndrome (PCOS) [30, 31]. These data have been confirmed by a recent case-control study in which the prevalence of TPO-Ab was significantly higher in PCOS patients than in controls [32]. Other non-organ-specific antibodies, such as antinuclear antibodies and smooth muscle antibodies, have been more frequently detected in PCOS patients [33] as well as anti-ovarian antibodies of all isotypes (immunoglobulin (Ig) G, IgA, IgM), almost as high as in patients with primary ovarian failure [34].

Finally, thyroid autoimmune disease seems to be the most common autoimmune disease associated with premature ovarian failure [35–38].

6.4 Thyroid Autoimmunity and Other Autoimmune Disorders

6.4.1 Antiphospholipid Antibody Positivity

There are reports of a significant association between thyroid autoimmunity and non-specific antibodies, such as antiphospholipid (aPL) antibodies, specifically lupus anticoagulant, anticardiolipin, and beta-2 glycoprotein I. These antibodies were shown to directly react with human placental trophoblast [39, 40]. The presence of antiphospholipid antibodies has been proven to cause pregnancy morbidity. Specifically, a history of three or more consecutive spontaneous abortions before 10 weeks of gestation, one or more unexplained fetal loss beyond 10 weeks of gestation, or one or more premature births of a morphologically normal neonate before 34 weeks of gestation due to eclampsia or preeclampsia, in the presence of antiphospholipid antibodies and no other known autoimmune disease, are diagnostic criteria for the antiphospholipid syndrome [41]. Treatment of this syndrome to avoid adverse obstetric outcome during pregnancy is well established [41]. Antiphospholipid antibody positivity on the other hand cannot be currently associated to infertility and is not predictive for success or failure of IVF [42]. Studies have explored the outcome of IVF in aPL-positive women and found no association between aPL positivity and the number of IVF cycles or fertility success rates [42]. Therefore, the assessment of antiphospholipid antibodies is not indicated among infertile couples undergoing IVF, and therapy is not justified based on existing data [42]. This area deserves further research, however, as there is very recent evidence that aPL positivity is associated with decreased levels of anti-Mullerian hormone, therefore of ovarian reserve, in infertile women [43].

6.4.2 Celiac Disease

The association of autoimmune thyroid disease with celiac disease has been well described in the literature [44–46].

Celiac disease is an autoimmune enteropathy caused by an abnormal immune response to dietary gluten and characterized by the production of antigliadin, anti-endomysial, and tissue transglutaminase antibodies. This disease may not cause gastrointestinal symptoms and go undiagnosed for a long while, leading to long-term complications on reproductive health. In a recent meta-analysis of the literature, it is reported that patients with unexplained infertility, recurrent miscarriage, or intrauterine growth restriction have a nearly five-, six-, or eightfold, respectively, increased risk of being affected by celiac disease compared with the general population. [47]. In vitro studies have indicated that anti-transglutaminase antibodies may cause placental damage at the fetomaternal interface by direct binding to trophoblast cells and endometrial endothelial cells [47]. It is important to suspect celiac disease in women suffering from the abovementioned reproductive disorders especially in light of the fact that adherence to a gluten-free diet may annul the negative impact of the disease on general and reproductive health [48, 49].

6.4.3 Systemic Autoimmune Disorders

Finally, thyroid autoimmunity has been frequently seen concurrently with systemic autoimmune diseases such as systemic lupus erythematosus and Sjogren syndrome [50].

Conclusion

It is becoming increasingly clear that autoimmune diseases, namely, thyroid autoimmunity, which are on the rise in the female population, contribute to the factors that negatively affect fertility and obstetric outcome. Thyroid autoimmunity may be present in women suffering from other reproductive disorders, such as endometriosis, polycystic ovary syndrome, and premature ovarian insufficiency. Moreover, women who develop thyroid autoimmunity are more susceptible to developing other autoimmune disorders that have also associated to poor reproductive outcome, such as celiac disease and antiphospholipid syndrome. The field of autoimmunity and female infertility has many unsolved questions. Further research focused on understanding the true prevalence of autoimmune disorders in infertile women, and the causal mechanisms is much needed to develop diagnostic and management strategies.

References

1. Poppe K, Velkeniers B, Glinoer D (2007) Thyroid disease and female reproduction. Clin Endocrinol 66:309–321
2. Poppe K, Velkeniers B, Glinoer D (2008) The role of thyroid autoimmunity in fertility and pregnancy. Nat Clin Pract Endocrinol Metab 4:394–405
3. van den Boogaard E, Vissenberg R, Land JA, van Wely M, Ven der Post JA, Goddijn M, Bisschop PH (2016) Significance of (sub)clinical thyroid dysfunction and thyroid autoimmunity before conception and in early pregnancy: a systematic review. Hum Reprod Update 22(4):532–533
4. Busnelli A, Paffoni A, Fedele L, Somigliana E (2016) The impact of thyroid autoimmunity on IVF/ICSI outcome: a systematic review and meta-analysis. Hum Reprod Update 22(6):775–790
5. Polyzos NP, Sakkas E, Vaiarelli A, Poppe K, Camus M, Tournaye H (2015) Thyroid autoimmunity, hypothyroidism and ovarian reserve: a cross-sectional study of 5000 women based on age-specific AMH values. Hum Reprod 30(7):1690–1696
6. Magri F, Schena L, Capelli V, Gaiti M, Zerbini F, Brambilla E, Rotondi M, De Amici M, Spinillo A, Nappi RE, Chiovato L (2015) Anti-Mullerian hormone as a predictor of ovarian reserve in ART protocols: the hidden role of thyroid autoimmunity. Reprod Biol Endocrinol 13(1):106
7. Grassi G et al (2001) Thyroid autoimmunity and infertility. Gynecol Endocrinol 15:389–396
8. Poppe K et al (2003) Assisted reproduction and thyroid autoimmunity: an unfortunate combination? J Clin Endocrinol Metab 88:4149–4152
9. Weghofer A, Himaya E, Kushnir VA, Barad DH, Gleicher N (2015) The impact of thyroid function and thyroid autoimmunity on embryo quality in women with low functional ovarian reserve: a case-control study. Reprod Biol Endocrinol 13:43
10. Stagnaro-Green A, Glinoer D (2004) Thyroid autoimmunity and the risk of miscarriage. Best Pract Res Clin Endocrinol Metab 18:167–181
11. Prummel MF, Wiersinga WM (2004) Thyroid autoimmunity and miscarriage. Eur J Endocrinol 150:751–755
12. Singh A, Dantas ZN, Stone SC, Asch RH (1995) Presence of thyroid antibodies in early reproductive failure: biochemical versus clinical pregnancies. Fertil Steril 63:277–281
13. Muller AF, Verhoeff A, Mantel MJ, Berghout A (1999) Thyroid autoimmunity and abortion: a prospective study in women undergoing in vitro fertilization. Fertil Steril 71:30–34

14. Bussen S, Steck T, Dietl J (2000) Increased prevalence of thyroid antibodies in euthyroid women with a history of recurrent in-vitro fertilization failure. Hum Reprod 15:545–548
15. Poppe K, Glinoer D, Tournaye H, Devroey P, van Steirteghem A, Kaufman L, Velkeniers B (2003) Assisted reproduction and thyroid autoimmunity: an unfortunate combination? J Clin Endocrinol Metab 88:4149–4152
16. Glinoer D, Riahi M, Grün JP, Kinthaert J (1994) Risk of subclinical hypothyroidism in pregnant women with asymptomatic autoimmune thyroid disorders. J Clin Endocrinol Metab 79:197–204
17. Poppe K, Glinoer D, Tournaye H, Schiettecatte J, Devroey P, van Steirteghem A, Haentjens P, Velkeniers B (2004) Impact of ovarian hyperstimulation on thyroid function in women with and without thyroid autoimmunity. J Clin Endocrinol Metab 89:3808–3812
18. Bagis T, Gokcel A, Saygili ES (2001) Autoimmune thyroid disease in pregnancy and the postpartum period: relationship to spontaneous abortion. Thyroid 11:1049–1053
19. Lazzarin N, Moretti C, De Felice G, Vaquero E, Manfellotto D (2012) Further evidence on the Role of Thyroid autoimmunity in women with recurrent miscarriage. Int J Endocrinol 7:171–185
20. Velkeniers B, Van Meerhaeghe A, Poppe K, Unuane D, Tournaye H, Haentjens P (2013) Levothyroxine treatment and pregnancy outcome in women with subclinical hypothyroidism undergoing assisted reproduction technologies: systematic review and meta-analysis of RCTs. Hum Reprod Update 19(3):251–258
21. Kim NY, Cho HJ, Kim HY, Yang KM, Ahn HK, Thornton S, Park JC et al (2011) Thyroid autoimmunity and its association with cellular and humoral immunity in women with reproductive failures. Am J Reprod Immunol 65:78–87
22. Pratt D, Novotny M, Kaberlein G, Dudkiewicz A, Gleicher N (1993) Antithyroid antibodies and the association with non-organ-specific antibodies in recurrent pregnancy loss. Am J Obstet Gynecol 168:837–841
23. Huang C, Liang P, Diao L, Liu C, Chen X, Li G, Chen C, Zeng Y (2015) Thyroid autoimmunity is associated with decreased cytotoxicity T cells in women with repeated implantation failure. Int J Environ Res Public Health 12(9):10352–10361
24. Kelkar RL, Meherji PK, Kadam SS, Gupta SK, Nandedkar TD (2005) Circulating autoantibodies against the zona pellucida and thyroid microsomal antigen in women with premature ovarian failure. J Reprod Immunol 66:53–67
25. Tan S, Dieterle S, Pechlavanis S, Janssen OE, Fuhrer D (2014) Thyroid autoantibodies per se do not impair intracytoplasmic sperm injection outcome in euthyroid healthy women. Eur J Endocrinol 170(4):495–500
26. Monteleone P, Parrini D, Faviana P, Carletti E, Casarosa E, Uccelli A, Cela V et al (2011) Female infertility related to thyroid autoimmunity: the ovarian follicle hypothesis. Am J Reprod Immunol 66:108–114
27. Poppe K, Glinoer D, Van Steirteghem A, Tournaye H, Devroey P, Schiettecatte J, Velkeniers B (2002) Thyroid dysfunction and autoimmunity in infertile women. Thyroid 12:997–1001
28. Matarese G, De Placido G, Nikas Y, Alviggi C (2003) Pathogenesis of endometriosis: natural immunity dysfunction or autoimmune disease? Trends Mol Med 9:223–228
29. Pasoto SG, Abrao MS, Viana VST, Bueno C, Leon EP, Bonfa E (2005) Endometriosis and systemic lupus erythematosus: a comparative evaluation of clinical manifestations and serological autoimmune phenomena. Am J Reprod Immunol 53(2):85–93
30. Janssen OE, Mehlmauer N, Hahn S, Offner AH, Gärtner R (2004) High prevalence of autoimmune thyroiditis in patients with polycystic ovary syndrome. Eur J Endocrinol 150:363–369
31. Yu Q, Wang JB (2016) Subclinical hypothyroidism in PCOS: impact on presentation, insulin resistance, and cardiovascular risk. Biomed Res Int 2016:2067087
32. Kachuei M, Jafari F, Kachuei A, Keshteli AH (2012) Prevalence of autoimmune thyroiditis in patients with polycystic ovary syndrome. Arch Gynecol Obstet 285:853–856
33. Reimand K, Talja I, Metskula K, Kadastik U, Matt K, Uibo R (2001) Autoantibody studies of female patients with reproductive failure. J Reprod Immunol 51:167–176

34. Fenichel P, Gobert B, Carre Y, Barbarino-Monnier P, Hieronimus S (1999) Polycystic ovary syndrome in autoimmune disease. Lancet 353:2210
35. Abalovich M, Mitelberg L, Allami C, Gutierrez S, Alcaraz G, Otero P, Levalle O (2007) Subclinical hypothyroidism and thyroid autoimmunity in women with infertility. Gynecol Endocrinol 23(5):279–283
36. Ayesha, Jha V, Goswami D (2016) Premature ovarian failure: an association with autoimmune diseases. J Clin Diagn Res 10(10):QC10–QC12
37. Goswami R, Marwaha RK, Goswami D, Gupta N, Ray D, Tomar N, Singh S (2006) Prevalence of thyroid autoimmunity in sporadic idiopathic hypoparathyroidism in comparison to type 1 diabetes and premature ovarian failure. J Clin Endocrinol Metab 91(11):4256–4259
38. Poppe K, Glinoer D, Van Steirteghem A, Tournaye H, Devroey P, Schiettecatte J et al (2002) Thyroid dysfunction and autoimmunity in infertile women. Thyroid 12:997–1001
39. Lyden TW, Vogt E, Ng AK, Johnson PM, Rote NS (1992) Monoclonal antiphospholipid antibody reactivity against human placental trophoblast. J Reprod Immunol 22:1–14
40. Di Simone N, Meroni PL, de Papa N, Raschi E, Caliandro D, De Carolis CS, Khamashta MA et al (2000) Antiphospholipid antibodies affect trophoblast gonadotropin secretion and invasiveness by binding directly and through adhered beta2-glycoprotein I. Arthritis Rheum 43:140–150
41. Miyakis S, Lockshin MD, Atsumi T, Branch DW, Brey RL, Cervera R, Derksen RH, de Groot PG, Koike T, Meroni PL et al (2006) International consensus statement on an update of the classification criteria for definite antiphospholipid syndrome (APS). J Thromb Haemost 4:295–306
42. Levine AB, Lockshin MD (2014) Assisted reproductive technology in SLE and APS. Lupus 23(12):1239–1241
43. Vega M, Barad DH, Yu Y, Darmon SK, Weghofer A, Kushnir VA, Gleicher N (2016) Anti-mullerian hormone levels decline with the presence of antiphospholipid antibodies. Am J Reprod Immunol 76(4):333–337
44. Barker JM, Gottelib PA, Elizabeth GS (2008) The immunoendocrinopathy syndromes. In: Melmed S, Polonsky KS, Larsen PR, Kronenberg HM (eds) Williams textbook of endocrinology, 12th edn. Saunders Elsevier, Philadelphia, pp 1768–1781
45. Collin P, Kaukinen K, Valmiki M et al (2002) Endocrine disorders and celiac disease. Endocr Rev 23:464–483
46. Marwaha RK, Garg MK, Tandon N et al (2013) Glutamic acid decarboxylase (anti-GAD) & tissue transglutaminase (anti-TTG) antibodies in patients with thyroid autoimmunity. Indian J Med Res 137:82–86
47. Tersigni C, Castellani R, de Waure C, Fattorossi A, De Spirito M, Gasbarrini A, Scambia G, Di Simone N (2014) Celiac disease and reproductive disorders: meta-analysis of epidemiologic associations and potential pathogenic mechanisms. Hum Reprod Update 20(4):582–593
48. Sher KS, Mayberry JF (1996) Female fertility, obstetric and gynaecological history in coeliac disease: acase control study. Acta Paediatr Suppl 412:76–77
49. Khashan AS, Henriksen TB, Mortensen PB, McNamee R, McCarthy Pedersen MG, Kenny LC (2010) The impact of maternal celiac disease on birthweight and preterm birth: a Danish population-based cohort study. Hum Reprod 25:528–534
50. Szyper-Kravitz M, Marai I, Shoenfeld Y (2005) Coexistence of thyroid autoimmunity with other autoimmune diseases: friend or foe? Additional aspects on the mosaic of autoimmunity. Autoimmunity 38:247–255

Part III

Thyroid Disorders, Polycystic Ovary and Metabolic Syndrome

7 Oocyte Donation in Perimenopausal and Menopausal Women

Basil Tarlatzis and Julia Bosdou

7.1 Menopause and Fertility

For most women, the menopause is a natural and permanent pause of menstruation due to ovarian ageing and natural loss of ovarian function. It is considered as a biological and not just a chronological phenomenon, usually occurring in the late 40s or early 50s [1, 2]. Reproductive menopause is recognized as a pause of reproductive ability due to the decline of ovarian reserve with age. Menopause has been classified as primary in Turner's syndrome or secondary including natural or premature menopause. Premature menopause describes definitive loss of ovarian function before the age of 40. It can be either spontaneous or induced by surgical treatment, radiotherapy, chemotherapy or treatment with gonadotropin-releasing hormone analogues [3].

Premature menopause represents temporary or permanent loss of ovarian function in women before the age of 40. In these women, the possibility of natural conception falls to approximately 2%, whereas the possibility of conception after in vitro fertilization (IVF) is less than 4% [4].

The time period preceding menopause, called perimenopause, involves a transition period of variations in the menstrual cycle and endocrine levels. A decrease in the levels of ovarian steroid hormones is observed due to the loss of ovarian follicular function [1]. During perimenopause, women experience a quantitative as well as a qualitative decline of ovarian reserve with age [5, 6]. Evidently, this is reflected by an observed decrease in the number of follicles and an increase in oocyte aneuploidy rates. Since oocyte number and quality are significantly affected by advanced maternal age, the ovarian follicle reserve seems to be an important factor

B. Tarlatzis (✉) • J. Bosdou
Unit for Human Reproduction, First Department of OB/GYN, Medical School, Aristotle University of Thessaloniki, Thessaloniki, Greece
e-mail: basil.tarlatzis@gmail.com

M. Birkhaeuser, A.R. Genazzani (eds.), *Pre-Menopause, Menopause and Beyond*, ISGE Series, https://doi.org/10.1007/978-3-319-63540-8_7

determining the outcome of assisted reproductive technologies (ART), irrespective of maternal chronological age.

As expected, a decrease in the probability of clinical pregnancy is observed with advanced maternal age. Based on the latest European IVF Monitoring (EIM) data published in 2016, the effect of women's age on fertility outcome is clearly shown. Pregnancy rates per aspiration after IVF or intracytoplasmic sperm injection (ICSI) declined from 29.6% and 29.3% in women aged less than 35 years to 13.5% and 12.6% in those aged 40 years or more, respectively [7]. Moreover, the probability of live birth in women >40 years of age is small and decreases significantly with each additional year [8, 9].

While fertility declines with age, perimenopausal conception remains a challenge regarding the chances of pregnancy achievement, taking into consideration the health risks as well as the socio-ethical issues raised. Ovarian stimulation for IVF remains one of the most popular treatment options available for achieving a pregnancy in perimenopausal women. Approximately 20% of all IVF cycles are performed in patients aged 40 years or more. However, advanced age is associated with poor IVF outcome, a poor response to ovarian stimulation and increased rates of cycle cancellation. Moreover, there are fewer oocytes retrieved, fewer embryos available for transfer, lower embryo quality, lower implantation rate and higher miscarriage rate [10].

Although IVF is widely used in the management of infertility in women of advanced age, the extremely low pregnancy rates achieved in these patients necessitate to consider alternative options with higher success rates, such as oocyte donation.

7.2 Oocyte Donation

7.2.1 Pregnancy Outcomes

Since the first successful pregnancy achieved in 1984 with donated oocytes in a woman with premature ovarian failure [11], oocyte donation represents an efficacious and well-established treatment option in ART, especially in women of advanced maternal age [12]. Although initially used for treating women with a variety of disorders, including premature ovarian failure, Turner's syndrome, avoidance of genetic disease transmission or poor oocyte quality following conventional assisted reproduction, oocyte donation was soon expanded in the management of perimenopausal or menopausal infertility.

Higher pregnancy and delivery rates, as well as lower miscarriage rates, have been reported with the use of donated oocytes in women of advanced age [12–15]. Based on the latest EIM data published in 2016 regarding oocyte donation [7, 16], a substantial increase in pregnancy and delivery rates was shown with the use of donor oocytes as compared to own oocytes in women of ≥40 years old (Table 7.1). However, it should be noted that, although the probability of live birth after oocyte donation is high in older IVF recipients, it seems to decline with increasing maternal age [17].

Table 7.1 IVF pregnancy and delivery rates with own and donor oocytes in Europe [7, 16]

	Pregnancy rates (%)		Delivery rates (%)	
Year	2011	2012	2011	2012
Own oocytes ≤34 years	37.0	29.6	28.6	22.7
Own oocytes ≥40 years	16.4	13.5	9.9	8.1
Donor oocytes	41.6	45.1	24.6	28.2

Regarding endometrial preparation for fresh embryo transfer in oocyte donation cycles, no difference has been reported in live birth rates when comparing a constant dose versus an increasing dose of oestrogens either with oral or transdermal supplementation [18]. Thus, oestrogen dose and administration route did not seem to affect pregnancy outcomes in oocyte donation cycles after fresh embryo transfer.

Considering pregnancy outcomes in oocyte donation cycles using cryopreserved donor oocytes, a recently published study showed similar efficiency in terms of oocyte-to-baby rates, by using vitrified versus fresh oocytes. Moreover, the probability of live birth using vitrified oocytes appeared to increase progressively with the number of oocytes consumed by the recipients [19].

In another recently published retrospective cohort study, evaluating donor thyroid function with recipient pregnancy outcome in fresh donor oocyte cycles, donor TSH levels ≥2.5 mIU/L were found to be associated with decreased recipient implantation and clinical pregnancy rate, suggesting that thyroid function may negatively impact the probability of pregnancy achievement among donor oocyte recipients [20].

7.2.2 Pregnancy Complications

Pregnancy complications are considerably increased in women of advanced maternal age. The factors affected by age include increased rate of oocyte chromosomal anomalies, hypertension, diabetes, placenta praevia, a higher incidence of caesarean section as well as increased maternal and foetal mortality and morbidity [10]. Moreover, obstetrical and perinatal risks seem to be increased in pregnancies with oocyte donation due to the unique condition of pregnancy achievement with an immunologically allogeneic embryo. Due to the inadequate immune response between the mother and the foreign foetus leading to reduced trophoblastic invasion of the spiral arteries, oocyte donation appears to be an independent risk factor for preeclampsia. Hence, increased risks for preeclampsia have been reported after oocyte donation compared to natural conception, especially in women of advanced maternal age [21, 22].

Several studies have reported on the obstetrical and perinatal outcomes after oocyte donation, the assessment of which remains of significance importance. In one of the first studies published, evaluating pregnancy outcomes after oocyte donation, a high incidence of obstetric and neonatal complications was reported, including first trimester bleeding, preeclampsia, intrauterine growth restriction (IUGR) and caesarean section [23]. Subsequent studies, comparing obstetrical and perinatal complication rates between women who conceived with donated oocytes and those who conceived through IVF with autologous oocytes, showed that pregnancies after oocyte donation were associated with a significantly higher risk of first trimester bleeding, abnormal placentation, preeclampsia, pregnancy-induced hypertension and caesarean section compared with IVF pregnancies using autologous oocytes [24, 25].

In a recently published systematic review of relevant studies regarding maternal and foetal complications from pregnancies conceived through oocyte donation, the risk of placental disorders, such as gestational hypertension and preeclampsia, appeared to be higher in oocyte donation pregnancies when compared to IVF pregnancies. In addition, twin pregnancies were associated with poorer outcomes, especially when combined with concomitant obstetric complications [21].

In agreement with previous studies, a retrospective population-based cohort study from Sweden, evaluating perinatal outcomes in singletons after oocyte donation vs. IVF/ICSI and spontaneous conception during a 10-year period (2003–2012), demonstrated that singleton oocyte donation pregnancies were associated with a significantly increased risk for preeclampsia [adjusted odds ratio (aOR), 3.1; 95% CI, 2.2–4.2], postpartum haemorrhage (>1000 mL) (aOR, 2.7; 95% CI, 2.0–3.5), preterm birth (<37 weeks) (aOR, 1.8; 95% CI, 1.3–2.5) and low birthweight (<2500 g) (aOR, 1.7; 95% CI, 1.2–2.4) as compared with IVF/ICSI and spontaneous conception pregnancies. Moreover, the rate of large-for-gestational age babies was significantly increased in singletons born after oocyte donation with frozen cycles when compared with fresh cycles (OR: 5.3, 95% CI: 1.3–21.5) [26].

The recently published systematic review and meta-analysis of obstetric and neonatal complications after oocyte donation vs. IVF/ICSI showed elevated risk for preeclampsia in singleton and in multiple pregnancies, preterm birth and low birthweight in singletons [27], (Table 7.2).

Similarly, studies evaluating women of advanced maternal age (aged ≥40 years, >43 years, ≥45 years or ≥50 years) demonstrated high rate of complications in all groups, especially among twin pregnancies achieved by IVF with oocyte donation [28–30]. Given the increased risks of adverse maternal and neonatal outcomes associated with multiple pregnancies after oocyte donation, it seems necessary to provide proper counselling of the intended parents prior to fertility treatment with donated oocytes and to encourage single embryo transfer, especially in women of advanced maternal age.

Primary ovarian failure is a common feature of Turner's syndrome. This syndrome is associated in most cases with ovarian dysgenesis, and only a few spontaneous pregnancies have been reported in the literature [31]. However, the progress in

Table 7.2 Meta-analysis of obstetric and neonatal complications after OD vs. IVF/ICSI [27]

		AOR	95% CI
Preeclampsia	Singleton	2.11	1.42–3.15
	Multiples	3.31	1.61–6.80
Preterm birth	Singleton	1.75	1.39–2.20
Low birthweight	Singleton	1.53	1.16–2.01

reproductive medicine has made it feasible for women with Turner's syndrome to achieve successful pregnancies using oocyte donation. Considerable success rates of pregnancy achievement have been reported in patients with Turner's syndrome after oocyte donation. However, it should be highlighted that these pregnancies are associated with substantial maternal and obstetrical complications, including cardiovascular complications, preeclampsia, gestational hypertension, foetal growth restriction and caesarean section [32–35]. For these reasons, it has been suggested that women with Turner's syndrome should be screened for abnormalities of the aorta, the aortic valve and the cardiovascular system before undergoing oocyte donation and be followed closely during their pregnancy.

Oocyte donation has proven to be an effective option of infertility treatment, particularly in perimenopausal and menopausal women. However, obstetrical and neonatal complications seem to be increased in pregnancies with oocyte donation, raising ethical and social considerations associated with pregnancy achievement in women of advanced maternal age. In order to minimize the risk of serious complications, appropriate management strategies with regard to oocyte donation should be evaluated after careful selection of patients. Moreover, a detailed medical evaluation and a thorough counselling of patients interested in receiving donated oocytes need to be offered.

Conclusions

- Maternal age is the single most important factor affecting oocyte number and quality.
- Biological age, e.g. ovarian reserve, seems to affect ART outcome independently of maternal chronological age.
- Poor ART results in women with advanced age are mainly due to chromosomally abnormal oocytes.
- Using donor oocytes, excellent ART results can be achieved in older women.
- Obstetrical and neonatal complications seem to be increased in pregnancies with oocyte donation.
- Women with Turner's syndrome, before applying oocyte donation, should be screened for abnormalities of the aorta, the aortic valve and the cardiovascular system and should be followed closely during pregnancy.
- The ethical and social issues associated with pregnancies in women of advanced age need to be addressed.

References

1. Harlow SD et al (2012) Executive summary of the Stages of Reproductive Aging Workshop +10: addressing the unfinished agenda of staging reproductive aging. Climacteric 15(2):105–114
2. Vujovic S et al (2010) EMAS position statement: managing women with premature ovarian failure. Maturitas 67(1):91–93
3. Armeni E et al (2016) Maintaining postreproductive health: a care pathway from the European Menopause and Andropause Society (EMAS). Maturitas 89:63–72

4. Speroff L, Glass RH, Kase NG (1999). Clinical Gynecologic Endocrinology and Infertility. 6th ed. Baltimore: Lippincott, Williams and Wilkins
5. te Velde ER, Dorland M, Broekmans FJ (1998) Age at menopause as a marker of reproductive ageing. Maturitas 30(2):119–125
6. Broekmans FJ et al (2004) Antral follicle counts are related to age at natural fertility loss and age at menopause. Menopause 11(6 Pt 1):607–614
7. European IVF-Monitoring Consortium (EIM), ESHRE et al (2016) Assisted reproductive technology in Europe, 2011: results generated from European registers by ESHRE. Hum Reprod 31(2):233–248
8. Ciray HN et al (2006) Outcome of 1114 ICSI and embryo transfer cycles of women 40 years of age and over. Reprod Biomed Online 13(4):516–522
9. Serour G et al (2010) Analysis of 2,386 consecutive cycles of in vitro fertilization or intracytoplasmic sperm injection using autologous oocytes in women aged 40 years and above. Fertil Steril 94(5):1707–1712
10. Marcus SF, Brinsden PR (1996) In-vitro fertilization and embryo transfer in women aged 40 years and over. Hum Reprod Update 2(6):459–468
11. Lutjen P et al (1984) The establishment and maintenance of pregnancy using in vitro fertilization and embryo donation in a patient with primary ovarian failure. Nature 307(5947):174–175
12. Edwards RG et al (1991) High fecundity of amenorrhoeic women in embryo-transfer programmes. Lancet 338(8762):292–294
13. Serhal PF, Craft IL (1989) Oocyte donation in 61 patients. Lancet 1(8648):1185–1187
14. Sauer MV, Paulson RJ (1995) Oocyte and embryo donation. Curr Opin Obstet Gynecol 7(3):193–198
15. Navot D et al (1991) Poor oocyte quality rather than implantation failure as a cause of age-related decline in female fertility. Lancet 337(8754):1375–1377
16. European IVF-Monitoring Consortium (EIM) for the ESHRE et al (2016) Assisted reproductive technology in Europe, 2012: results generated from European registers by ESHRE. Hum Reprod 31(8):1638–1652
17. Yeh JS et al (2014) Pregnancy outcomes decline in recipients over age 44: an analysis of 27,959 fresh donor oocyte in vitro fertilization cycles from the Society for Assisted Reproductive Technology. Fertil Steril 101(5):1331–1336
18. Madero S et al (2016) Endometrial preparation: effect of estrogen dose and administration route on reproductive outcomes in oocyte donation cycles with fresh embryo transfer. Hum Reprod 31(8):1755–1764
19. Cobo A et al (2015) Six years' experience in ovum donation using vitrified oocytes: report of cumulative outcomes, impact of storage time, and development of a predictive model for oocyte survival rate. Fertil Steril 104(6):1426–1434.e8
20. Karmon AE et al (2016) Donor TSH level is associated with clinical pregnancy among oocyte donation cycles. J Assist Reprod Genet 33(4):489–494
21. Savasi VM et al (2016) Maternal and fetal outcomes in oocyte donation pregnancies. Hum Reprod Update 22(5):620–633
22. Bos M et al (2017) Loss of placental thrombomodulin in oocyte donation pregnancies. Fertil Steril 107(1):119–129. e5
23. Pados G et al (1994) The evolution and outcome of pregnancies from oocyte donation. Hum Reprod 9(3):538–542
24. Stoop D et al (2012) Obstetric outcome in donor oocyte pregnancies: a matched-pair analysis. Reprod Biol Endocrinol 10:42
25. Tarlatzi TB et al (2017) Does oocyte donation compared with autologous oocyte IVF pregnancies have a higher risk of preeclampsia? Reprod Biomed Online 34(1):11–18
26. Nejdet S et al (2016) High risks of maternal and perinatal complications in singletons born after oocyte donation. Acta Obstet Gynecol Scand 95(8):879–886
27. Storgaard M et al (2017) Obstetric and neonatal complications in pregnancies conceived after oocyte donation: a systematic review and meta-analysis. BJOG 124(4):561–572

28. Le Ray C et al (2012) Association between oocyte donation and maternal and perinatal outcomes in women aged 43 years or older. Hum Reprod 27(3):896–901
29. Soares SR et al (2005) Age and uterine receptiveness: predicting the outcome of oocyte donation cycles. J Clin Endocrinol Metab 90(7):4399–4404
30. Guesdon E et al (2017) Oocyte donation recipients of very advanced age: perinatal complications for singletons and twins. Fertil Steril 107(1):89–96
31. Bernard V et al (2016) Spontaneous fertility and pregnancy outcomes amongst 480 women with Turner syndrome. Hum Reprod 31(4):782–788
32. Chevalier N et al (2011) Materno-fetal cardiovascular complications in Turner syndrome after oocyte donation: insufficient prepregnancy screening and pregnancy follow-up are associated with poor outcome. J Clin Endocrinol Metab 96(2):E260–E267
33. Alvaro Mercadal B et al (2011) Pregnancy outcome after oocyte donation in patients with Turner's syndrome and partial X monosomy. Hum Reprod 26(2068):2061–2068
34. Tarani L et al (1998) Pregnancy in patients with Turner's syndrome: six new cases and review of literature. Gynecol Endocrinol 12(2):83–87
35. Pasqualini-Adamo J (1988) Turner's syndrome and pregnancy. Rev Fr Gynecol Obstet 83(11):717–721

Thyroid Disorders in Climacteric Women

8

Anna Brona, Andrzej Milewicz, Justyna Kuliczkowska-Płaksej, and Marek Bolanowski

8.1 Introduction

The appearance of menopause is combined with the incidence of many diseases typical of middle age, i.e., thyroid disorders, osteoporosis, and cardiovascular diseases. Thyroid disorders, especially subclinical hypothyroidism and subclinical hyperthyroidism, are frequent medical conditions among postmenopausal women. The prevalence of metabolic syndrome and osteoporosis significantly increases in postmenopausal women [1]. Many symptoms appear due to decreased estrogen level; however, chronic diseases influence quality of life as well. One of them is thyroid diseases, which are associated with risk factors for osteoporosis and cardiovascular diseases. Some symptoms of chronic diseases may mimic or modify the clinical expression of climacteric symptoms. Menopause and thyroid disease may present with similar symptoms, i.e., sweating, heart palpitations, insomnia, irritability, or mood changes, which suggest menopause, hyperthyroidism, or both. In addition, weight gain, constipation, skin atrophy, and hair atrophy are climacteric symptoms as well as symptoms of hypothyroidism [2]. With aging, the level of thyroid-stimulating hormone (TSH) remains within normal range and occasionally has a tendency to increase [3]. Reduction of thyroid iodine uptake, free thyroid hormone synthesis, and catabolism of free thyroxine (FT4) are observed. In addition, reverse triiodothyronine (rT3) level increases [3].

A. Brona
Department of the Biological and Motoric Basis of Sport, University School of Physical Education, Wrocław, Poland

A. Milewicz (✉) • J. Kuliczkowska-Płaksej • M. Bolanowski
Department of Endocrinology, Diabetes and Isotope Therapy, Wroclaw Medical University, Wrocław, Poland
e-mail: andrzej.milewicz@umed.wroc.pl

M. Birkhaeuser, A.R. Genazzani (eds.), *Pre-Menopause, Menopause and Beyond*, ISGE Series, https://doi.org/10.1007/978-3-319-63540-8_8

8.2 Thyroid and Bone Metabolism

The decrease in bone mass with age in postmenopausal women is well documented [4]. Thyroid hormones are important regulators of bone formation and remodeling. Triiodothyronine (T3) stimulates osteoblast activity both directly and indirectly through various growth factors and cytokines. It also has a direct impact on osteoclast differentiation [5, 6]. Changes in thyroid hormone levels within normal range are associated with bone mineral density (BMD) and fracture in healthy euthyroid postmenopausal women. It has been shown that FT4 and free triiodothyronine (FT3) in upper laboratory range is related to decreased BMD and FT4 in upper laboratory range is associated with increased bone loss at the hip [7].

Abe et al. demonstrated direct effects of TSH on skeletal remodeling, osteoblastic bone formation, and osteoclastic bone resorption, via the TSH receptor present on osteoblast and osteoclast precursors [8]. Other authors suggested that TSH bone-protective action is mediated by inhibiting osteoclastogenesis [9]. Vestergaard et al. indicated an increased fracture risk within the first 5 years after diagnosis of hyperthyroidism and the first 10 years after diagnosis of hypothyroidism [10].

8.2.1 Thyroid Function and Osteoprotegerin and Osteocalcin

The relationship between increased follicle-stimulating hormone (FSH) and luteinizing hormone (LH) with the markers of bone turnover was found in postmenopausal women, i.e., a higher release of osteocalcin in the systemic circulation [11].

Osteoprotegerin (OPG) and osteocalcin (OC) are produced by the osteoblast. OPG is a decoy receptor of the receptor activator of nuclear factor kappa-B ligand (RANKL) and influences osteoclast differentiation and activation. OC is a secretory glycoprotein, produced mainly by bone osteoblast. Age and various other factors have an impact on circulating OPG and OC levels. Thyroid function exerts effect on bone remodeling and bone cell metabolism, as well as the serum levels of these molecules [12].

Polovina et al. indicated a positive association between the serum osteocalcin level and TSH in euthyroid and subclinical hypothyroid postmenopausal women, but they did not find differences in osteocalcin levels in these groups [13].

Shinkov et al. demonstrated an almost linear positive association between OC and the thyroid hormones in the postmenopausal women [12]. They also reported lower OPG levels in the euthyroid subjects compared to those with elevated or suppressed TSH [12]. The higher OPG level in hyperthyroidism may be explained by the increased bone turnover due to elevated thyroid hormones and reduced TSH [14]. The increased OPG level in hypothyroidism is poorly understood.

8.2.2 Hyperthyroidism and Fractures

Thyroid hormones stimulate bone resorption, and overt hyperthyroidism is associated with increased bone turnover and an increased risk of osteoporosis and fractures [15].

Many studies reported a decreased BMD in women after menopause with subclinical hyperthyroidism [15, 16].

Abrahamsen et al. demonstrated the relationship between a single first measurement of decreased TSH and an increased long-term risk of hip fractures in older women [17]. In another study, they indicated that the higher risk of major osteoporotic fractures in hypothyroid postmenopausal women was associated with excessive levothyroxine dosing (LT-4) [18].

Data from the available prospective cohort studies suggest an increased risk of hip fractures and non-spine fractures in subclinical hyperthyroidism. Higher fracture risk was reported in adults with grade 2 subclinical hyperthyroidism [6, 19]. Thus, the European Thyroid Association recommends performing BMD (and possibly biochemical markers of bone turnover) in women after menopause with TSH below 0.1 mIU/l (grade 2 subclinical hyperthyroidism) [6, 19].

Prospective studies showed an improvement in BMD after ATDs or RAI therapy in postmenopausal women with subclinical hyperthyroidism and a continuous decrease of BMD in untreated patients [15, 16]. Femoral and lumbar spine BMDs increased by 1.9% and 1.6% respectively, 1 year after RAI treatment. However, there are no data showing that treatment of subclinical hyperthyroidism reduces the risk of fracture [15, 16].

8.2.3 Hypothyroidism and Fractures

Hypothyroid patients tend to exhibit higher bone density. Despite somewhat higher bone quantity, hypothyroidism is related to an increased fracture risk before and after diagnosis [13].

The results of studies examining the influence of subclinical hypothyroidism and L-T4 replacement therapy on bone have generated considerable interest but also controversy [5]. Some studies indicated that treatment with replacement doses of L-T4 caused a decrease in BMD [5]. Other showed the relationship between this treatment and accelerated decrease in BMD but not typical of osteoporosis [5].

Baqi et al. [20] reported a favorable bone status in postmenopausal women with normal TSH levels compared to those with low TSH levels [5]. The available data suggest that the preservation of bone after menopause depends on TSH [5]. Polovina et al. found evidence for association between FRAX score and TSH in postmenopausal women. They indicated that the main FRAX score and hip FRAX score were significantly higher in the group with subclinical hypothyroidism than in the controls [13].

In a large, population-based study, Abrahamsen et al. indicated that increased risk of hip and major osteoporotic fractures in postmenopausal women is strongly associated with the cumulative duration of low TSH, probably from excessive thyroid hormone replacement therapy. They did not identify any independent clinically significant effects of hypothyroidism itself on fracture risk in women [18].

Fadejev et al. [21] found that the combination of L-T4 and levotriiodothyronine (L-T3) in the treatment of primary hypothyroidism leads to a higher rate of bone resorption [13].

Pedrera-Zamorano et al. studied a group of 180 postmenopausal women treated with L-T4 and estimated bone mass in the phalanx using the quantitative ultrasound (QUS) measurements of the phalanx. They reported no differences between the treated patients and untreated controls [5]. La Vignera et al., in a study of 99 postmenopausal women between 50 and 56 years of age and treated with L-T4 for 1 year, indicated a slight but significant reduction in the BMD of the lumbar vertebrae measured by DXA, which was more pronounced in patients on suppressive therapy than in those on replacement therapy [22]. Other authors observed no reduction in BMD in postmenopausal women with subclinical hypothyroidism who were on L-T4 treatment [5].

8.3 Subclinical Hypothyroidism and Cardiovascular Risk

There is ongoing debate on cardiovascular risk and subclinical thyroid disease [23]. The mechanisms relating subclinical hypothyroidism to cerebrovascular conditions such as stroke are yet not completely understood. Studies demonstrated association between subclinical hypothyroidism and increased carotid arterial stiffness, elevated serum low-density lipoprotein cholesterol and apolipoprotein-B, elevated mean platelet volume, and altered low-density lipoprotein-C oxidizability [24]. However, the results of studies examining these associations are contraindicatory [25].

Like overt hypothyroidism, subclinical hypothyroidism has been related to increased risk for heart failure and atherosclerotic disease [23]. In the literature it is suggested that subclinical hypothyroidism is associated with higher risk of incident coronary heart disease (CHD) events and deaths, but evidence has not been consistent [23]. In some patients with subclinical hypothyroidism, FT4 levels are very close to those typical of overt hypothyroidism. These lower FT4 levels in more severe forms of subclinical hypothyroidism could be associated with an increase vascular resistance. This effect may be mediated via impaired inhibition of collagen-induced platelet aggregation [24].

Data on the relationship between subclinical hypothyroidism and myocardial infarction (MI) from one large cross-sectional study [26] and three follow-up studies are inconclusive [23]. Le Grys et al. examined the association between subclinical hypothyroidism and subsequent risk for MI in a large prospective cohort of postmenopausal US women aged 50–79 years [23]. Specifically their objective was to determine whether subclinical hypothyroidism at baseline is independently associated with risk for incident MI in the 7 years after enrollment in the Women's Health Initiative Observational Study (WHI-OS). They did not find evidence for an association between subclinical hypothyroidism and risk for MI. The lack of association between subclinical hypothyroidism and MI was not changed by the presence or absence of TPOAb and also did not vary by the severity of subclinical hypothyroidism (mild TSH 4.69–6.99 mU/l or moderate/severe TSH $\geq$ 7.00 mU/l) [23]. They did not have information on lipid levels but found that the proportion of antihyperlipidemic medication used to be similar, regardless of subclinical hypothyroidism status. They suggested that if the primary mechanism of MI progression in subclinical hypothyroidism is through increased LDL-C, the lack of association may be due to the predominantly older population in the study (approximately 70% of study population [including women] was 65 years of age or older at baseline) [23]. Lipid levels are strong predictors of cardiovascular disease including MI among middle-aged adults, but not among older adults, in which this association remains controversial [23, 27].

In another study, the same authors investigated an association between subclinical hypothyroidism and risk for incident ischemic stroke in the same group of postmenopausal women from the WHI-OS, but there was no evidence for such association [24]. Several studies have demonstrated an improvement in cardiovascular outcomes associated with subclinical hypothyroidism after treatment with LT-4, although evidence has not been consistent [24].

The influence of estrogen on LT-4 intake in postmenopausal women should be taken into account due to the antagonistic effect of estrogen use on efficacy of LT-4 therapy [28].

8.4 Hyperthyroidism and Cardiovascular Risk

In two large prospective studies, an increased risk of atrial fibrillation (AF) was found in elderly subjects with subclinical hyperthyroidism [15].

A recent systematic review, including six prospective studies, did not confirm an increased risk of stroke in subclinical hyperthyroidism [29]. Meta-analysis performed by the Thyroid Studies Collaboration Group did not show higher risk of stroke in subclinical hyperthyroidism patients in comparison to euthyroid controls [30].

The results of a population cohort study have shown that subclinical and overt hyperthyroidism is associated with increased all-cause mortality compared to euthyroid individuals [15]. In another prospective cohort studies, patients with subclinical hyperthyroidism had an increased risk of total mortality, CHD mortality, and incident AF. The risk of CHD mortality and AF were higher among adults with grade 2 subclinical hyperthyroidism [30, 31].

8.5 Risk of Thyroid Cancer

Thyroid cancer incidence is three times higher in women than in men and is the ninth most frequent among females worldwide [32]. It has been suggested that hormonal and reproductive factors may determine or modulate the risk of thyroid cancer [32]. Experimental data have shown that estrogens exert the promoting effect on the growth of thyroid cancer cells through a pathway mediated by estrogen receptors alpha and beta [32, 33].

Caini et al. performed a meta-analysis and indicated that increasing age at first pregnancy or birth and hysterectomy were associated with increased thyroid cancer risk. In their study women with younger age at menopause had a borderline significant reduced thyroid cancer risk [27].

Estrogen receptors (ERs) are present on both normal and neoplastic thyroid cells [27, 28]. ERs are likely to have an impact on the function of the thyroid gland mainly at puberty, in early pregnancy, and breastfeeding [27]. Endocrine disruptors may activate ERs [27]. It is suggested that a continuous activation of the ERs may cause the growth of thyroid and promote development and progression of well-differentiated thyroid cancers [27].

The role of estrogens in the physiology and pathology of both the thyroid gland and the uterus may explain the frequent association of uterine leiomyomas (a leading cause of hysterectomy) and thyroid nodules [34].

The activation of ERs of thyroid gland cells is not probably the only cause of development and progression of well-differentiated thyroid cancers. Except this, overweight and obesity may play a role [32].

8.6 Subclinical Hyperthyroidism

The incidence of endogenous subclinical hyperthyroidism varies considerably, between 0.6 and 16% [15]. The differences result from diagnostic criteria, the age and sex of population studied, and the TSH assay used for evaluation and iodine intake [15]. It is estimated that subclinical thyroid diseases affect 23.2% of postmenopausal women; among them 26.2% are hyperthyroid [3].

One of the most important documents on thyroid diseases published recently was the European Thyroid Association Guideline on subclinical hyperthyroidism. Although it has not been written specially for postmenopausal women, the recommendations may be very useful for everyday practice.

The diagnosis of subclinical hyperthyroidism is based on biochemical findings, i.e., a decreased serum TSH level and normal thyroid hormone levels [15]. Subclinical hyperthyroidism comprises two categories: grade 1 subclinical hyperthyroidism with low but detectable serum TSH levels (e.g., TSH 0.1–0.39 mIU/l) and grade 2 subclinical hyperthyroidism with suppressed serum TSH levels (<0.1 mIU/l) [15].

The most common forms of subclinical hyperthyroidism comprise Graves' disease in younger patients (≤65 years) in iodine-replete areas and toxic adenoma and toxic multinodular goiter in older patients (>65 years) and in iodine-deficient areas [35].

The management of subclinical hyperthyroidism depends on age and comorbidities. Recent meta-analyses indicate that subclinical hyperthyroidism is associated with increased risk of CHD mortality, incident AF, heart failure, fractures, and excess mortality in patients with serum TSH levels <0.1 mIU/l (grade 2 subclinical hyperthyroidism) [15].

Furthermore, there is evidence that treatment is indicated in patients older than 65 years with grade 2 subclinical hyperthyroidism to potentially avoid these serious cardiovascular events, fractures, and risk of progression to overt hyperthyroidism [15].

According to the task force's statement, treatment could be considered in patients older than 65 years with TSH levels 0.1–0.39 mIU/l (grade 1 subclinical hyperthyroidism) because of their increased risk of AF and might also be reasonable in younger (≤65 years) symptomatic patients with grade 2 subclinical hyperthyroidism because of the risk of progression, especially in the presence of symptoms and/or underlying risk factors or comorbidity [15].

The task force's final conclusion is that there are no data to support treating subclinical hyperthyroidism in younger asymptomatic patients with grade 1 subclinical hyperthyroidism. These patients should be followed without treatment due to the low risk of progression to overt hyperthyroidism and the weaker evidence for adverse health outcomes [15].

Subclinical hyperthyroidism may progress to overt hyperthyroidism. In grade 1 subclinical hyperthyroidism, it is uncommon, about 0.5–0.7% of patients over 7 years. In grade 2 subclinical hyperthyroidism, it is more frequent, about 5–8% of patients each year [36, 37]. Subclinical hyperthyroidism may remain stable or resolve in euthyroidism. Progression to overt hyperthyroidism or normalization of TSH is more common than persistent subclinical hyperthyroidism in patients with GD [15].

8.7 Subclinical Hypothyroidism

Subclinical hypothyroidism is more common with advancing age and may affect 10–15% of postmenopausal women [24] (according to other authors 5–20%) [23]. Overt hypothyroidism may affect 1–3% of postmenopausal women [23]. A higher prevalence was found in the LAVOS study in which 24.2% of postmenopausal women had TSH level >5.5 mIU/mL [1]. In the PolSenior study, 7.95% of women over 55 years had elevated serum TSH [1]. Subclinical hypothyroidism is defined as a serum concentration of TSH above the upper limit of the reference range when the concentration of serum-free T4 (FT4) is within the reference range [5].

Important questions about subclinical hypothyroidism are if it increases cardiovascular risk and which subjects should be treated with LT-4 [38]. There are no special guidelines for postmenopausal women; therefore, it is necessary to find relevant information in guidelines for general population.

Subclinical hypothyroidism comprises two categories: mildly increased TSH levels (4.0–10.0 mU/l) and more severely increased TSH levels (>10.0 mU/l), both with FT4 within reference range [38]. Subclinical hypothyroidism with mildly increased TSH comprises about 90% of subclinical hypothyroidism cases in general population [38].

Most patients with subclinical hypothyroidism do not have typical hypothyroid symptoms. The Colorado thyroid disease prevalence study demonstrated that subclinical hypothyroid patients complained of drier skin, poorer memory, slower thinking, weaker muscles, greater tiredness, more muscle cramps, more feeling cold, deeper and hoarser voice, puffier eyes, and more constipation compared to euthyroid controls [39].

European Thyroid Association recommends considering a trial of LT-4 replacement therapy in younger subclinical hypothyroidism patients (<65 years, TSH < 10 mU/l) with symptoms suggestive of hypothyroidism [38].

Replacement therapy is also recommended for younger subclinical hypothyroidism patients (<65 years) with TSH level > 10 mU/l even if there are no symptoms of hypothyroidism, [38].

Replacement therapy is recommended for patients with persistent subclinical hypothyroidism and diffuse or nodular goiter in order to normalize serum TSH levels [38].

LT-4 should be administered daily, approximately 1.5 μg/kg/day (e.g. 75 or 100 μg/day for a woman). Treatment in patients with cardiac disease and in the elderly should be started with 25 or 50 μg of LT-4 daily. The dose of LT-4 should be increased by 25 μg/day every 14–21 days until a full replacement dose is reached [38].

Several foods specifically impair LT-4 absorption: milk, coffee, soya products, and papaya [38, 40]. Medications that interfere with LT-4 absorption (iron salts, calcium salts, cholestyramine, raloxifene and antacids, sucralfate, H2 receptor blockers, and proton pump inhibitors) should be avoided or taken 4 h or more after LT-4 ingestion [41].

References

1. Siemińska L, Wojciechowska C, Walczak K, Borowski A, Marek B et al (2015) Associations between metabolic syndrome, serum thyrotropin, and thyroid antibodies status in postmenopausal women, and the role of interleukin-6. Endokrynol Pol 66:394–403
2. Roberts CG, Ladenson PW (2004) Hypothyroidism. Lancet 363:793–803
3. Schindler AE (2003) Thyroid function and postmenopause. Gynecol Endocrinol 17:79–85
4. Bączyk G, Opala T, Kleka P, Chuchracki M (2012) Multifactorial analysis of risk factors for reduced bone mineral density among postmenopausal women. Arch Med Sci 8:332–341
5. Pedrera-Zamorano JD, Roncero-Martin R, Calderon-Garcia JF, Santos-Vivas M, Vera V et al (2015) Treatment of subclinical hypothyroidism does not affect bone mass as determined by dual-energy X-ray absorptiometry, peripheral quantitative computed tomography and quantitative bone ultrasound in Spanish women. Arch Med Sci 11:1008–1014
6. Blum MR, Bauer DC, Collet TH, Fink HA, Cappola AR, da Costa BR et al (2015) Subclinical thyroid dysfunction and fracture risk: a meta-analysis. JAMA 313:2055–2065
7. Murphy E, Gluer CC, Reid DM et al (2010) Thyroid function within the upper normal range is associated with reduced bone mineral density and an increased risk of nonvertebral fractures in healthy euthyroid postmenopausal women. J Clin Endocrinol Metab 95:3173–3181
8. Abe E, Marians RC, Yu W et al (2003) TSH is a negative regulator of skeletal remodeling. Cell 115:151–162
9. Ma R, Morshed S, Latif R, Zaidi M, Davies TF (2011) The influence of thyroid-stimulating hormone and thyroid-stimulating hormone receptor antibodies on osteoclastogenesis. Thyroid 21:897–906
10. Vestergaard P, Rejnmark L, Mosekilde L (2005) Influence of hyper and hypothyroidism, and the effects of treatment with antithyroid drugs and levothyroxine on fracture risk. Calcif Tissue Int 77:139–144
11. García-Martín A, Reyes-García R, García-Castro JM, Rozas-Moreno P, Escobar-Jiménez F, Muñoz-Torres M (2012) Role of serum FSH measurement on bone resorption in postmenopausal women. Endocrine 41:302–308
12. Shinkov AD, Borissova AM, Kovatcheva RD, Atanassova IB, Vlahov JD, Dakovska LN (2014) Age and menopausal status affect osteoprotegerin and osteocalcin levels in women differently, irrespective of thyroid function. Clin Med Insights Endocrinol Diabetes 7:19–24

13. Polovina S, Popovic V, Duntas L, Milic N, Micic D (2013) Frax score calculations in postmenopausal women with subclinical hypothyroidism. Hormones (Athens) 12:439–448
14. Mysliwiec J, Adamczyk M, Nikolajuk A, Gorska M (2011) Interleukin-6 and its considerable role in the pathogenesis of thyrotoxicosis-related disturbances of bone turnover in postmenopausal women. Endokrynol Pol 62:299–302
15. Biondi B, Bartalena L, Cooper DS, Hegedüs L, Laurberg P, Kahaly GJ (2015) The 2015 European thyroid association guidelines on diagnosis and treatment of endogenous subclinical hyperthyroidism. Eur Thyroid J 4:149–163
16. Faber J, Jensen IW, Petersen L, Nygaard B, Hegedus L, Siersbaek-Nielsen K (1998) Normalization of serum thyrotropin by mean of radioiodine treatment in subclinical hyperthyroidism. Effect of bone loss in postmenopausal women. Clin Endocrinol 48:285–290
17. Abrahamsen B, Jørgensen HL, Laulund AS, Nybo M, Brix TH, Hegedüs L (2014) Low serum thyrotropin level and duration of suppression as a predictor of major osteoporotic fractures. The OPENTHYRO Register Cohort. J Bone Miner Res 29:2040–2050
18. Abrahamsen B, Jørgensen HL, Laulund AS, Nybo M, Bauer DC et al (2015) The excess risk of major osteoporotic fractures in hypothyroidism is driven by cumulative hyperthyroid as opposed to hypothyroid time: an observational register-based time-resolved cohort analysis. J Bone Miner Res 30:898–905
19. Wirth CD, Blum MR, da Costa BR, Baumgartner C, Collet TH et al (2014) Subclinical thyroid dysfunction and the risk for fractures: a systematic review and meta-analysis. Ann Intern Med 161:189–199
20. Baqi L, Payer J, Killinger Z, Susienkova K, Jackuliak P et al (2010) The level of TSH appeared favourable in maintaining bone mineral density in postmenopausal women. Endocr Regul 44:9–15.
21. Fadejev VV, Morgunova TB, Melnichenko GA, Dedov II (2010) Combined therapy with L-Thyroxine and L-Triiodthyronine compared to L-Thyroxine alone in the treatment of primary hypothyroidism. Hormones (Athens), 9:245–252.
22. La Vignera S, Vicari E, Tumino S et al (2008) L-thyroxin treatment and post-menopausal osteoporosis: relevance of the risk profile present in clinical history. Minerva Ginecol 60:475–484
23. Le Grys VA, Funk MJ, Lorenz CE, Giri A, Jackson RD et al (2013) Subclinical hypothyroidism and risk for myocardial infarction among postmenopausal women. J Clin Endocrinol Metab 98:2308–2317
24. Giri A, Edwards TL, LeGrys VA, Lorenz CE, Funk MJ et al (2014) Subclinical hypothyroidism and risk for incident ischemic stroke among postmenopausal women. Thyroid 24:1210–1217
25. Pearce EN (2012) Update in lipid alterations in subclinical hypothyroidism. J Clin Endocrinol Metab 97:326–333
26. Tunbridge WM, Evered DC, Hall R et al (1977) Lipid profiles and cardiovascular disease in the Whickham area with particular reference to thyroid failure. Clin Endocrinol 7:495–508
27. Psaty BM, Anderson M, Kronmal RA et al (2004) The association between lipid levels and the risks of incident myocardial infarction, stroke, and total mortality: the Cardiovascular Health Study. J Am Geriatr Soc 52:1639–1647
28. Arafah BM (2001) Increased need for thyroxine in women with hypothyroidism during estrogen therapy. New Engl J Med 344:1743–1749
29. Chaker L, Baumgartner C, Ikram MA, Dehghan A, Medici M et al (2014) Subclinical thyroid dysfunction and the risk of stroke: a systematic review and meta-analysis. Eur J Epidemiol 29:791–800
30. Collet TH, Gussekloo J, Bauer DC et al (2012) Thyroid Studies Collaboration: subclinical hyperthyroidism and the risk of coronary heart disease and mortality. Arch Intern Med 172:799–809
31. Gencer B, Collet TH, Virgini V et al (2012) Thyroid Studies Collaboration: subclinical thyroid dysfunction and the risk of heart failure events: an individual participant data analysis from 6 prospective cohorts. Circulation 126:1040–1049

32. Caini S, Gibelli B, Palli D, Saieva C, Ruscica M, Gandini S (2015) Menstrual and reproductive history and use of exogenous sex hormones and risk of thyroid cancer among women: a meta-analysis of prospective studies. Cancer Causes Control 26:511–518
33. Manole D, Schildknecht B, Gosnell B, Adams E, Derwahl M (2001) Estrogen promotes growth of human thyroid tumor cells by different molecular mechanisms. J Clin Endocrinol Metab 86:1072–1077
34. Kim MH, Park YR, Lim DJ, Yoon KH, Kang MI et al (2010) The relationship between thyroid nodules and uterine fibroids. Endocr J 57:615–621
35. Bülow Pedersen I, Knudsen N, Jørgensen T, Perrild H, Ovesen L, Laurberg P (2002) Large differences in incidences of overt hyper- and hypothyroidism associated with a small difference in iodine intake: a prospective comparative register-based population survey. J Clin Endocrinol Metab 87:4462–4469
36. Schouten BJ, Brownlie BEW, Frampton CM, Turner JG (2001) Subclinical thyrotoxicosis in an outpatient population—predictors of outcome. Clin Endocrinol 74:257–261
37. Rosario PW (2008) The natural history of subclinical hyperthyroidism in patients below the age of 65 years. Clin Endocrinol 68:491–492
38. Pearce SHS, Brabant G, Duntas LH, Monzani F, Peeters RP et al (2013) 2013 ETA guideline: management of subclinical hypothyroidism. Eur Thyroid J 2:215–228
39. Canaris GJ, Manowitz NR, Mayor G, Ridgway EC (2000) The Colorado thyroid disease prevalence study. Arch Intern Med 160:526–534
40. Benvenga S, Bartolone L, Pappalardo MA et al (2008) Altered intestinal absorption of L-thyroxine caused by coffee. Thyroid 18:293–301
41. Liwanpo L, Hershman JM (2009) Conditions and drugs interfering with thyroxine absorption. Best Pract Res Clin Endocrinol Metab 23:781–792

9 Thyroid Function and Pregnancy Outcome After ART: What Is the Evidence?

Gesthimani Mintziori, Dimitrios G. Goulis, and Basil C. Tarlatzis

Thyroid function is a crucial player on both fertility and early embryo development. Nowadays, it has been proved that thyroid hormone receptors are present in almost all reproductive organs, implying an important role of thyroid hormones on reproductive function [1]. It is known that thyroid hormones are necessary for brain development, as they direct the neuronal and glial cell differentiation and proliferation and influence axonal and dendritic development, synapse formation, cell migration, and myelination [2]. The role of thyroid function on fertility and early pregnancy has been recognized by nearly all international scientific societies involved with reproduction and endocrinology, and specific guidelines have been developed [3–6].

Subclinical hypothyroidism during pregnancy has been associated with adverse reproductive outcomes [7, 8]. Similarly, the presence of thyroid autoimmunity (TAI) is associated with an increased risk of unexplained infertility, spontaneous miscarriage, repeated miscarriage, premature birth, and postpartum thyroiditis [7, 8]. A Cochrane meta-analysis showed a favorable role of levothyroxine (LT_4) in regard to spontaneous miscarriages and a beneficial role of selenium (Se) for thyroid function postpartum [9]. According to this meta-analysis, LT_4 can decrease the risk of spontaneous miscarriage [relative risk (RR) 0.19, 95% confidence interval (CI) 0.08–0.39)] and premature birth (RR 0.41, 95% CI 0.24–0.68) [9].

The association of thyroid function and assisted reproductive technology (ART) has attracted major interest. Ovarian stimulation (OS), a common part of ART, has been suggested to have an impact on thyroid function [10, 11]. OS results in increased serum estradiol (E_2) concentrations that lead to an increase of thyroxin-binding globulin (TBG) production (Fig. 9.1). Thus, the number of circulating

G. Mintziori • D.G. Goulis • B.C. Tarlatzis (✉)
Units of Human Reproduction and Reproductive Endocrinology, First Department of Obstetrics and Gynecology, Medical School, Aristotle University of Thessaloniki, Thessaloniki, Greece
e-mail: basil.tarlatzis@gmail.com

M. Birkhaeuser, A.R. Genazzani (eds.), *Pre-Menopause, Menopause and Beyond*, ISGE Series, https://doi.org/10.1007/978-3-319-63540-8_9

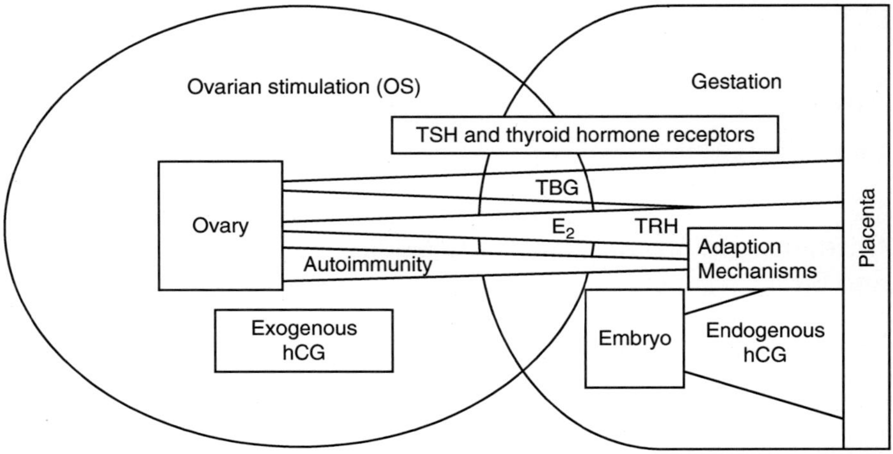

Fig. 9.1 Main events affecting thyroid function and autoimmunity during ovarian stimulation (OS) and early gestation. OS increases serum estradiol (E2) concentrations leading to increased thyroxin-binding globulin (TBG). TSH and thyroid hormone receptors are also present in ovaries and the endometrium, possibly playing a crucial role in the process

thyroxin-binding sites is also increased. As a result, free thyroxin (fT_4) concentrations are decreased and TSH production is induced [12].

Data from observational studies suggest that TSH concentrations are influenced by OS. Poppe et al. [13] have reported high TSH and low total thyroxine (T_4) concentrations after OS; however, other studies have failed to demonstrate such an effect [14, 15]. It has been suggested that TSH may be increased during or within 1 month after OS; however, a recent systematic review has been proved inconclusive [16]. In another study by Poppe et al. [17], 77 women free of thyroid disease were studied. Though in vitro fertilization (IVF) or intracytoplasmic sperm injection (ICSI) procedures were reported to have an impact on thyroid function, these changes had no influence on the outcome of pregnancy.

TAI is an entity that has been suggested to influence the reproductive outcome of fertile or infertile women, either in association or independently from thyroid function. It has been reported that women with the presence of TAI have an increased risk of spontaneous miscarriage after OS [18]. The exact mechanism of this association is not known. A meta-analysis of published studies on infertile women that have achieved pregnancy following ART has demonstrated that the presence of TAI is associated with an increased risk of spontaneous miscarriage (RR 1.99, 95% CI 1.42–2.79) in comparison with the absence of TAI. In a following meta-analysis of 13 studies that involved 966 patients with TAI and 7331 controls [7, 8], subclinical hypothyroidism, as compared to normal thyroid function, was associated with increased risk of preeclampsia and perinatal mortality [7, 8]. In the same study, TAI was associated with an increased risk of unexplained subfertility, miscarriage, recurrent miscarriage, preterm birth, and postpartum thyroid disease. However, when pregnancies achieved by IVF and spontaneous pregnancies were studied separately, early miscarriages in the former were not associated with the presence of TAI, though they were increased in the latter given the presence of TAI [7, 8]. Geva et al. [19] have shown a decreased pregnancy rate in subfertile women with TAI following IVF, in comparison to those without TAI (13.6% vs. 25.0%, $p < 0.05$). However, this observation was not always confirmed [20, 21]; on the contrary, the opposite has also been suggested [22]. In a recent meta-analysis, Busnelli et al. have concluded that in euthyroid women undergoing IVF/ICSI cycles, TAI is associated with a significant decreased live birth rate (OR 0.73; 95% CI 0.54–0.99, $p = 0.04$) [23–26].

A number of retrospective studies have been published on thyroid function and reproductive outcomes following ART. In a retrospective study by Fumarola et al. [27], women with TSH concentrations lower than 2.5 μIU/ml had increased rates of clinical pregnancy comparing to those with TSH higher than this threshold (22.3% vs. 8.9%, respectively, $p = 0.045$). In another study that involved 158 euthyroid women (TSH 0.5–4.5 μIU/ml) following IVF, lower TSH was not associated with favorable reproductive outcomes [28]. Karmon et al. [29], in a study of egg donors, evaluated the association between TSH concentrations in donors and reproductive outcome in the recipients. Only fresh donor oocyte IVF cycles were used. The authors concluded that donor's TSH was associated with clinical pregnancy rate, implying a role of thyroid function directly to the oocyte.

In a study of 540 women that had underwent ICSI, LT_4 replacement in those with TSH >2.5 μIU/ml together with age and ovulation induction with human chorionic gonadotropin (hCG) were predictive factors for pregnancy rate [30]. However, in another study, replacement with LT_4 for clinical or subclinical hypothyroidism was not associated with implantation or the live birth rate [31]. A meta-analysis of randomized controlled trials (RCTs) on the role of replacement with LT_4 for subclinical hypothyroidism in women undergoing ART has shown that LT_4 replacement is associated with significantly higher delivery rate, with a pooled RR of 2.76 (95% CI 1.20–6.44; $p = 0.018$; $I^2 = 70\%$) [32]. In the same meta-analysis, LT_4 replacement was associated with a significantly lower miscarriage rate with a pooled RR of 0.45 (95% CI 0.24–0.82; $p = 0.010$; $I^2 = 26$). LT_4 replacement was also associated with a significantly higher number of fertilized oocytes [two trials; standardized mean difference (SMD) 0.55, 95% CI 0.03–1.08; $p = 0.039$] and implantation rate (one trial; RR 1.81, 1.01–3.25; $p = 0.049$). No association was found between LT_4 replacement and clinical pregnancy rate, number of retrieved oocytes, number of mature oocytes, number of embryos transferred, or number of embryos cryopreserved.

Gizzo et al. [33] tried to see whether specific drugs used for hypothalamic inhibition in ART settings may have a specific impact on the thyroid function of euthyroid women and whether this difference is clinically significant, in regard to pregnancy rates. Indeed, they have found that TSH concentrations were increased after GnRH antagonist administration, though the same was not true for GnRH agonists. The presence of GnRH receptors (GnRH-Rs) in both thyrotroph cells of the adenohypophysis and the ovarian granulosa cells [34, 35] provide some insight of a possible mechanism for this association.

In conclusion, the evidence of the influence of thyroid function or the presence of TAI to ART outcome is limited; however, there is evidence to support the use of LT_4 intervention in case of suboptimal thyroid function and/or the presence of TAI. The need for thyroid function screening in women attempting undergoing ART is generally recognized and should include TSH measurement prior to any ART application and TAI assessment in selected cases (i.e., personal history of autoimmunity, family history of thyroid disease).

References

1. Colicchia M, Campagnolo L, Baldini E, Ulisse S, Valensise H, Moretti C (2014) Molecular basis of thyrotropin and thyroid hormone action during implantation and early development. Hum Reprod Update 20(6):884–904
2. Moog NK, Entringer S, Heim C, Wadhwa PD, Kathmann N, Buss C (2017) Influence of maternal thyroid hormones during gestation on fetal brain development. Neuroscience 342:68–100
3. Abalovich M, Amino N, Barbour LA, Cobin RH, De Groot LJ, Glinoer D et al (2007) Management of thyroid dysfunction during pregnancy and postpartum: an Endocrine Society Clinical Practice Guideline. J Clin Endocrinol Metab 92:S1–47
4. Alexander EK, Pearce EN, Brent GA, Brown RS, Chen H, Dosiou C et al (2017) 2017 Guidelines of the American Thyroid Association for the diagnosis and management of thyroid disease during pregnancy and the postpartum. Thyroid 27(3):315–389
5. Lazarus J, Brown RS, Daumerie C, Hubalewska-Dydejczyk A, Negro R, Vaidya B (2014) 2014 European thyroid association guidelines for the management of subclinical hypothyroidism in pregnancy and in children. Eur Thyroid J 3:76–94
6. Practice Committee of the American Society for Reproductive Medicine (2015) Electronic address, A.a.o.: Subclinical hypothyroidism in the infertile female population: a guideline. Fertil Steril 104:545–553
7. van den Boogaard E, Vissenberg R, Land JA, van Wely M, Ven der Post JA, Goddijn M et al (2016) Significance of (sub)clinical thyroid dysfunction and thyroid autoimmunity before conception and in early pregnancy: a systematic review. Hum Reprod Update 22:532–533
8. van den Boogaard E, Vissenberg R, Land JA, van Wely M, van der Post JA, Goddijn M et al (2011) Significance of (sub)clinical thyroid dysfunction and thyroid autoimmunity before conception and in early pregnancy: a systematic review. Hum Reprod Update 17:605–619
9. Reid SM, Middleton P, Cossich MC, Crowther CA, Bain E (2013) Interventions for clinical and subclinical hypothyroidism pre-pregnancy and during pregnancy. Cochrane Database Syst Rev 5:CD007752
10. Mintziori G, Anagnostis P, Toulis KA, Goulis DG (2012) Thyroid diseases and female reproduction. Minerva Med 103:47–62
11. Stuckey BG, Yeap D, Turner SR (2010) Thyroxine replacement during super-ovulation for in vitro fertilization: a potential gap in management? Fertil Steril 93:2414–2413
12. Krassas GE, Poppe K, Glinoer D (2010) Thyroid function and human reproductive health. Endocr Rev 31:702–755
13. Poppe K, Glinoer D, Tournaye H, Devroey P, Velkeniers B (2008) Impact of the ovarian hyperstimulation syndrome on thyroid function. Thyroid 18:801–802
14. Mintziori G, Goulis DG, Kolibianakis EM, Slavakis A, Bosdou J, Grimbizis G et al (2017) Thyroid function and autoimmunity during ovarian stimulation for intracytoplasmic sperm injection. Reprod Fertil Dev 29(3):603–608
15. Reh A, Chaudhry S, Mendelsohn F, Im S, Rolnitzky L, Amarosa A et al (2011) Effect of autoimmune thyroid disease in older euthyroid infertile woman during the first 35 days of an IVF cycle. Fertil Steril 95:1178–1181
16. Mintziori G, Goulis DG, Toulis KA, Venetis CA, Kolibianakis EM, Tarlatzis BC (2011) Thyroid function during ovarian stimulation: a systematic review. Fertil Steril 96:780–785

17. Poppe K, Glinoer D, Tournaye H, Schiettecatte J, Haentjens P, Velkeniers B (2005) Thyroid function after assisted reproductive technology in women free of thyroid disease. Fertil Steril 83:1753–1757
18. Toulis KA, Goulis DG, Venetis CA, Kolibianakis EM, Negro R, Tarlatzis BC et al (2010) Risk of spontaneous miscarriage in euthyroid women with thyroid autoimmunity undergoing IVF: a meta-analysis. Eur J Endocrinol 162:643–652
19. Geva E, Vardinon N, Lessing JB, Lerner-Geva L, Azem F, Yovel I et al (1996) Organ-specific autoantibodies are possible markers for reproductive failure: a prospective study in an in-vitro fertilization-embryo transfer programme. Hum Reprod 11:1627–1631
20. Kutteh WH, Schoolcraft WB, Scott RT Jr (1999) Antithyroid antibodies do not affect pregnancy outcome in women undergoing assisted reproduction. Hum Reprod 14:2886–2890
21. Poppe K, Glinoer D, Tournaye H, Devroey P, van Steirteghem A, Kaufman L et al (2003) Assisted reproduction and thyroid autoimmunity: an unfortunate combination? J Clin Endocrinol Metab 88:4149–4152
22. Muller AF, Verhoeff A, Mantel MJ, Berghout A (1999) Thyroid autoimmunity and abortion: a prospective study in women undergoing in vitro fertilization. Fertil Steril 71:30–34
23. Busnelli A, Paffoni A, Fedele L, Somigliana E (2016) The impact of thyroid autoimmunity on IVF/ICSI outcome: a systematic review and meta-analysis. Hum Reprod Update 22:775–790
24. Busnelli A, Paffoni A, Fedele L, Somigliana E (2016) Reply: the impact of thyroid autoimmunity on IVF/ICSI outcome: re-evaluation of the findings. Hum Reprod Update 22:792
25. Busnelli A, Paffoni A, Fedele L, Somigliana E (2016) The impact of thyroid autoimmunity on IVF/ICSI outcome: a systematic review and meta-analysis. Hum Reprod Update 22:793–794
26. Mintziori G, Tarlatzis BC, Goulis DG (2016) The impact of thyroid autoimmunity on IVF/ICSI outcome: re-evaluation of the findings. Hum Reprod Update 22:791
27. Fumarola A, Grani G, Romanzi D, Del SM, Bianchini M, Aragona A et al (2013) Thyroid function in infertile patients undergoing assisted reproduction. Am J Reprod Immunol 70:336–341
28. Mintziori G, Goulis DG, Gialamas E, Dosopoulos K, Zouzoulas D, Gitas G et al (2014) Association of TSH concentrations and thyroid autoimmunity with IVF outcome in women with TSH concentrations within normal adult range. Gynecol Obstet Investig 77:84–88
29. Karmon AE, Cardozo ER, Souter I, Gold J, Petrozza JC, Styer AK (2016) Donor TSH level is associated with clinical pregnancy among oocyte donation cycles. J Assist Reprod Genet 33:489–494
30. Jatzko B, Vytiska-Bistorfer E, Pawlik A, Promberger R, Mayerhofer K, Ott J (2014) The impact of thyroid function on intrauterine insemination outcome—a retrospective analysis. Reprod Biol Endocrinol 12:28
31. Busnelli A, Somigliana E, Benaglia L, Leonardi M, Ragni G, Fedele L (2013) In vitro fertilization outcomes in treated hypothyroidism. Thyroid 23:1319–1325
32. Velkeniers B, Van MA, Poppe K, Unuane D, Tournaye H, Haentjens P (2013) Levothyroxine treatment and pregnancy outcome in women with subclinical hypothyroidism undergoing assisted reproduction technologies: systematic review and meta-analysis of RCTs. Hum Reprod Update 19:251–258
33. Gizzo S, Noventa M, Quaranta M, Vitagliano A, Esposito F, Andrisani A et al (2016) The potential role of GnRH agonists and antagonists in inducing thyroid physiopathological changes during IVF. Reprod Sci 23:515–523
34. Hong IS, Klausen C, Cheung AP, Leung PC (2012) Gonadotropin-releasing hormone-I or -II interacts with IGF-I/Akt but not connexin 43 in human granulosa cell apoptosis. J Clin Endocrinol Metab 97:525–534
35. La Rosa S, Celato N, Uccella S, Capella C (2000) Detection of gonadotropin-releasing hormone receptor in normal human pituitary cells and pituitary adenomas using immunohistochemistry. Virchows Arch 437:264–269

PCOS: Implications of Cardiometabolic Dysfunction

10

Bart C.J.M. Fauser

10.1 Introduction

Polycystic ovary syndrome (PCOS) represents the most common endocrine disorder in women of reproductive age with a reported incidence of 6–15%, depending on the criteria used for defining this heterogeneous condition [1–4]. According to the Rotterdam criteria, at least two of the three following features must be present: ovulatory dysfunction, clinical or biochemical hyperandrogenism and polycystic ovarian morphology [2, 3]. Other possible underlying pathologies must be excluded. Familial clustering of this heterogeneous condition has clearly been shown although the aetiology and the genetic determinants of PCOS remain uncertain [5–7]. Needs for medical intervention in women with PCOS vary significantly depending on the stage of life (Fig. 10.1).

An association between PCOS and cardiometabolic dysfunction (such as hyperinsulinemia, dyslipidaemia, hypertension and obesity) is common. Numerous studies have convincingly demonstrated in recent years that—not surprisingly—even singleton pregnancies in women with PCOS are more often complicated by gestational diabetes and pregnancy-induced hypertension (Fig. 10.2). As woman age, an increased incidence of type 2 diabetes mellitus emerges [8, 9]. Considering the presence of metabolic risk factors already present in many women with PCOS at a young age, it is generally believed that chances for developing cardiovascular disease in later life are significantly increased (Fig. 10.3). Evidence generated so far, however, remains inconclusive. A large heterogeneity exists in women with PCOS, and therefore, cardiovascular risk profiles may vary with PCOS phenotype, age and ethnicity.

Features such as hyperandrogenemia and obesity in women with PCOS were clearly associated with metabolic syndrome (MetS) and insulin resistance (IR)

B.C.J.M. Fauser
Department of Reproductive Medicine and Gynaecology, University Medical Center, Utrecht, The Netherlands
e-mail: B.C.Fauser@umcutrecht.nl

M. Birkhaeuser, A.R. Genazzani (eds.), *Pre-Menopause, Menopause and Beyond*, ISGE Series, https://doi.org/10.1007/978-3-319-63540-8_10

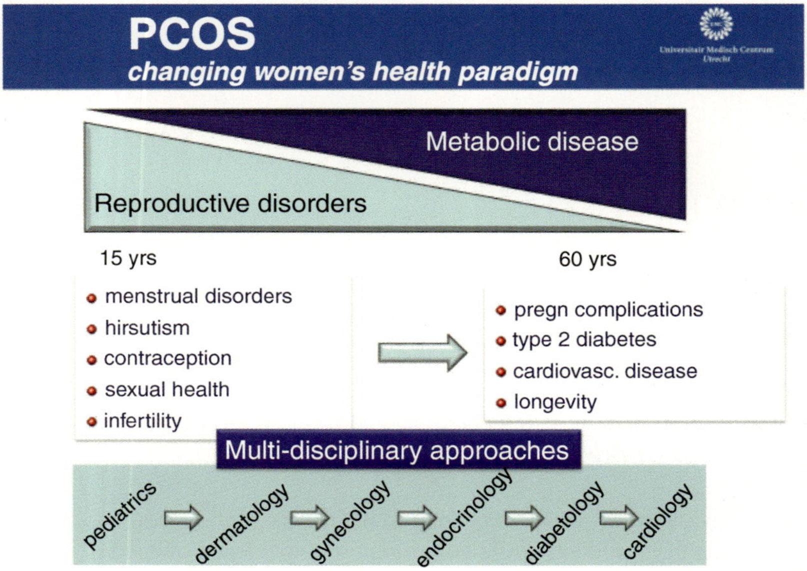

Fig. 10.1 Changing women's health perspective in women with PCOS depending on their stage of life

Fig. 10.2 Concept of metabolic dysfunction in women with PCOS, subsequent pregnancy complications and compromised children outcomes

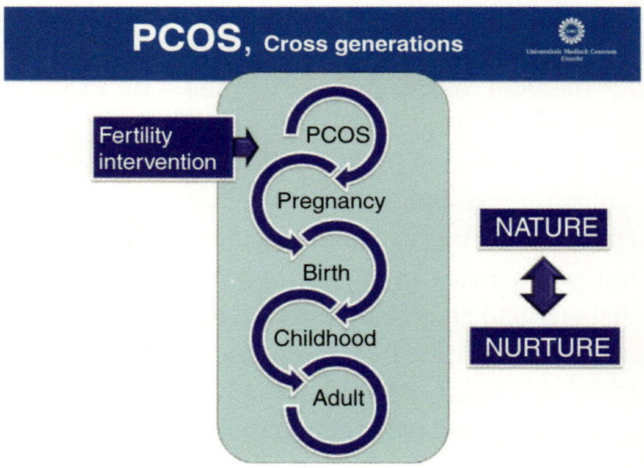

([10–12]). Metabolic features of women with PCOS compared to healthy controls were assessed in a meta-analysis in which 35 studies were included. Women with PCOS had a less favourable metabolic profile in comparison to healthy controls, even when matched for body weight. The latter suggests that BMI in itself does not solely explain the observed metabolic abnormalities in women with PCOS [13].

A large proportion of women with PCOS will undergo infertility treatment to establish a pregnancy. Several pregnancy complications are more common in women with PCOS [14, 15], such as gestational diabetes mellitus (GDM), preeclampsia and

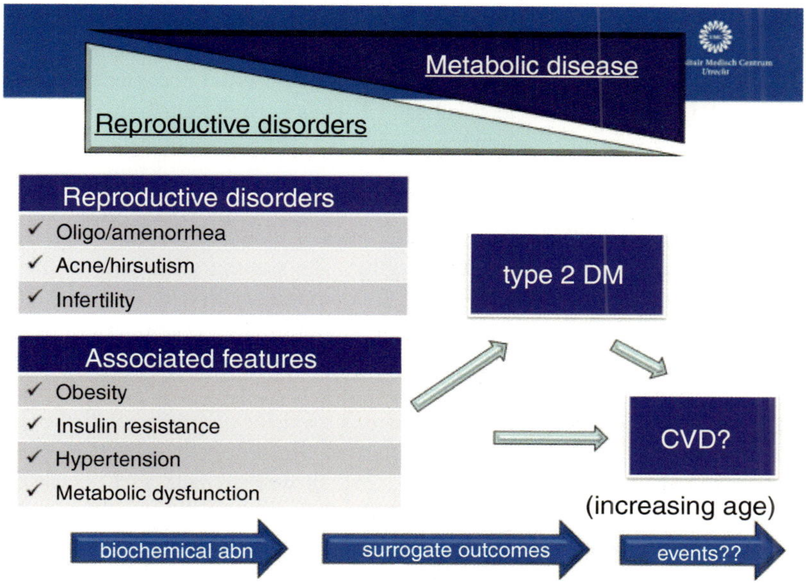

Fig. 10.3 Women with PCOS reproductive dysfunction is most prominent during early life, whereas features associated with metabolic dysfunction dominate later in life

preterm birth [16, 17]. Some preliminary studies even suggest that PCOS offspring has an increased risk for unfavourable cardiometabolic features such as increased fasting serum glucose, insulin, triglyceride, total cholesterol and LDL.

10.2 Surrogate Markers for Subclinical Cardiovascular Disease

The metabolic dysfunction described in the different stage of life implicates an increased risk for cardiovascular disease. Endothelial dysfunction is the starting point of progression towards cardiovascular disease. The flow-mediated dilation (FMD) is a technique developed to measure vascular dysfunction. This assessment is used to measure artery dilator response to reactive hyperaemia induced by a brief period of artificial limb ischaemia. A decreased FMD is a prognostic marker for cardiovascular disease in general, but more specifically it independently predicts occult coronary artery disease [18]. FMD in women with PCOS is reported extensively in a large meta-analysis in which 21 published studies were included (908 women with PCOS versus 566 controls). A sub-analysis involved seven of the four mentioned studies in which cases and controls were matched on BMI. The pooled mean FMD was 3.4% (95% confidence interval (CI) =1.9–4.9) lower in PCOS compared to controls, with substantial heterogeneity between studies. In the sub-analysis, the PCOS-mediated reduction in FMD was 4.1% (95% CI = 2.7–5.5).

Heterogeneity remained substantial (I(2) =81%). Moreover, the size of the FMD difference was not significantly influenced by BMI or age [19].

Measuring carotid intima media thickness (CIMT) is an accepted non-invasive method for diagnosing atherosclerosis [20]. CIMT is a structural change in the vascular system visualized by ultrasonography which is a strong predictor of cardiovascular events in both males and females [21]. In a meta-analysis regarding CIMT in the PCOS population, a total of 19 studies were included: 1123 women with PCOS conform NIH criteria versus 923 controls. Mean ages of included women range from 21 to 39 years old and BMI from 21 to 41 kg/m^2. The summary estimate of the mean difference in CIMT among women with PCOS compared with controls was 0.072 mm (95% CI: 0.040–0.105 with p-value < 0.0001) for highest quality studies and 0.084 mm (95% CI 0.042–0.126 with p-value = 0.0001) for good quality studies [22].

A third parameter which is a non-invasive method for the evaluation of vascular health is the Agatston score [23]. This score is used for quantification of coronary artery calcium (CAC). Coronary atherosclerosis on its turn is related to coronary heart disease and all-cause mortality [24, 25]. In women with PCOS, we do see more often any versus non-coronary atherosclerosis in comparison with non-PCOS controls [26]. When looking at continuous data of Agatston scores, higher Agatston scores are reported in women with PCOS, compared to controls [27, 28]. Another small study of 48 patients reports that obese PCOS patients and obese controls with quite similar cardiovascular risk profiles do differ in prevalence of coronary atherosclerosis, in disadvantage of the obese PCOS patient group [27]. This finding suggests that PCOS influences atherosclerosis, disregarding BMI, adiposity distribution, inflammation and metabolic markers. This all leads to the hypothesis that older women with PCOS have an increased risk for developing cardiovascular disease.

10.3 Long-Term Cardiovascular Outcomes and Implications

The long-term health implications of metabolic dysfunction in women with PCOS remain uncertain until now. PCOS is diagnosed during the reproductive lifespan: mostly in woman's early 20s and 30s when there is a wish to conceive. However, cardiovascular disease becomes manifest three to four decades later. Due to this large time gap, large well-phenotyped cohorts of women with PCOS with sufficient long-term follow-up are lacking. We are restricted to using surrogate outcomes or small follow-up studies in women previously diagnosed with PCOS or cross-sectional studies in postmenopausal women with a presumed PCOS history. Selecting the best suitable surrogate outcomes for cardiovascular disease (CVD) is only possible when we fully understand the mechanism underlying CVD in women. This mechanism differs from the pathophysiology seen in males. Unfortunately the majority of conducted research was based on the male concept of cardiovascular disease. It is generally known that cardiovascular disease in women is present approximately 10 years.

Several retrospective cohort studies were published on long-term health outcomes (for overview, see Table 10.1). Three small retrospective studies found no evidence

Table 10.1 Summary of retrospective studies concerning cardiovascular outcomes in women with PCOS

Publication	Study design	Intermediate outcomes	CVD outcomes
Pierpoint et al. [29]	786 PCOS, compared to national rates Mean age = 26.4 years, mean FU at 30 years Histological evidence of PCO, clinical signs and/or ovarian dysfunction and androgen excess	Similar diabetes mellitus	Similar mortality, all cause and CV Increased diabetes-related mortality in PCOS
Wild et al. [30]	61 PCOS vs. 63 controls Mean age 56.7 years (38–98), FU at 31 years AE, Rotterdam criteria	More diabetes, hyperlipidaemia, obesity, hypertension	CHD similar
Elting et al. [31]	345 PCOS vs. 8950 controls Mean age 38.7 at FU Oligo- or amenorrhoea and elevated LH	More hypertension and diabetes mellitus	Similar cardiac complaints
Hart and Doherty [32]	2.566 PCOS vs. 25.660 controls Median age = 35.8 years Rotterdam criteria used from 2004 (not for inclusions between 1997 and 2004)	More diabetes mellitus, obesity, hypertensive disorders, depression	More ischaemic heart disease, CVA, all-cause mortality

of an increased risk for coronary heart disease (CHD) and mortality in women with PCO. These studies were all prone to selection and/or information bias due to their design and heterogeneous inclusion criteria. The largest retrospective study on this subject was conducted by retrieving all women of which a PCOS diagnosis ($n = 2560$) was registered at hospitalization in Western Australia. A similar number of age-matched controls were selected from the same source. These data were combined with national registries on pregnancy, cancer and mortality. In contrast to the previous three mentioned smaller studies, Hart et al. show that ischaemic heart disease (IHD) (HR 2.89 (95%CI 1.68–4.97)) and all-cause mortality (HR 1.89 (95%CI: 1.12–3.17)) were higher in women with PCOS [32]. However, the use of a hospital registry as starting point for this study may give rise to inclusion bias.

Data on CVD and mortality in peri- and postmenopausal women with PCOS remains scarce and inconsistent. In 1992, Dahlgren et al. [33] estimated that the risk for a myocardial infarction was increased seven times in peri- and postmenopausal women with PCOS compared to healthy controls. After re-analysis of this data and extended follow-up, no significant difference was found in CVD between women with PCOS and healthy controls [34]. A small study of 28 PCOS patients and 752 controls in which an increased rate of NIDDM was seen in PCOS patients supports that women with PCOS have an increased risk for CAD. In a larger study ($n = 713$) of postmenopausal women, the number of present features of the putative PCOS phenotype, in women without diabetes mellitus, is also associated with

CAD. However, this association is not significant in the total PCOS population consisting of women with and without diabetes [35]. Postmenopausal women ($n = 497$) with a history of irregular menses and hyperandrogenism, with disregard of ovarian morphology, show an increased risk for self-reported MI and stroke, compared to controls ($n = 20,249$).

There are multiple possible hypotheses concerning possible mechanisms behind the absence of increased CVD in postmenopausal women with PCOS despite the metabolic derangements present early in life. The increased androgen levels in women with PCOS could have an influence on CVD in a later life. In a large cohort in Sweden consisting of 6440 perimenopausal women (age between 50–59 years), lower serum androgen levels were found in women with PCOS who have CAD compared to women without CAD. This might suggest that androgens have a protective role in progression to CAD in women with PCOS [36]. In the general Dutch female population (34–55 years old), the prevalence of diabetes mellitus increases with age. This was also the case in women with PCOS. However, cardiac complaints were not more often reported by women with PCOS but were more often reported in the general Dutch population as age increases. Another remarkable observation was that BMI differences between PCOS patients and the general population lose its significance as age increases [31]. This phenomenon could also play a role in similar CVD risk among woman with PCOS and healthy controls. It should be noted in this context that the normalization of regular menstrual cycles with increasing age along with a later age of menopause in women with PCOS may also affect cardiovascular risk. Finally, other—as yet unknown—protective factors may exist.

Conclusion

Woman with PCOS have increased risk for cardiovascular disease based on an unfavourable cardiovascular profile and surrogate markers for cardiovascular disease such as FDM, IMT and CAC. Whether these women truly have an increased risk for cardiovascular disease and mortality is still unknown. Large cohorts, all subjected to multiple biases, show contrasting results on the increased prevalence of CVD in peri- and postmenopausal women. The role of androgens in later life in women with PCOS remains unclear and must be clarified. More importantly is the need for large prospective cohort studies with well-phenotyped women with PCOS and standardized follow-up.

References

1. March WA, Moore VM, Willson KJ, Phillips DI, Norman RJ, Davies MJ (2010) The prevalence of polycystic ovary syndrome in a community sample assessed under contrasting diagnostic criteria. Hum Reprod 25(2):544–551
2. Rotterdam ESHRE/ASRM-Sponsored PCOS Consensus Workshop Group (2004a) Revised 2003 consensus on diagnostic criteria and long-term health risks related to polycystic ovary syndrome. Fertil Steril 81(1):19–25
3. Rotterdam ESHRE/ASRM-Sponsored PCOS consensus workshop group (2004b) Revised 2003 consensus on diagnostic criteria and long-term health risks related to polycystic ovary syndrome (PCOS). Hum Reprod 19(1):41–47

4. Williams DM, Palaniswamy S, Sebert S, Buxton JL, Blakemore AI, Hypponen E, Jarvelin MR (2016) 25-Hydroxyvitamin D concentration and leukocyte telomere length in young adults: findings from the northern finland birth cohort 1966. Am J Epidemiol 183:191–198
5. Legro RS, Kunselman AR, Demers L, Wang SC, Bentley-Lewis R, Dunaif A (2002) Elevated dehydroepiandrosterone sulfate levels as the reproductive phenotype in the brothers of women with polycystic ovary syndrome. J Clin Endocrinol Metab (87):2134–2138
6. Legro RS, Spielman R, Urbanek M, Driscoll D, Strauss JF 3rd, Dunaif A (1998) Phenotype and genotype in polycystic ovary syndrome. Recent Prog Horm Res 53:217–256
7. Urbanek M, Legro RS, Driscoll DA, Azziz R, Ehrmann DA, Norman RJ, Strauss JF 3rd, Spielman RS, Dunaif A (1999) Thirty-seven candidate genes for polycystic ovary syndrome: strongest evidence for linkage is with follistatin. Proc Natl Acad Sci U S A 96:8573–8578
8. Fauser BC, Tarlatzis BC, Rebar RW, Legro RS, Balen AH, Lobo R, Carmina E, Chang J, Yildiz BO, Laven JS, Boivin J, Petraglia F, Wijeyeratne CN, Norman RJ, Dunaif A, Franks S, Wild RA, Dumesic D, Barnhart K (2012) Consensus on women's health aspects of polycystic ovary syndrome (PCOS): the Amsterdam ESHRE/ASRM-Sponsored 3rd PCOS Consensus Workshop Group. Fertil Steril 97:28–38.e25
9. Wild RA, Carmina E, Diamanti-Kandarakis E, Dokras A, Escobar-Morreale HF, Futterweit W, Lobo R, Norman RJ, Talbott E, Dumesic DA (2010) Assessment of cardiovascular risk and prevention of cardiovascular disease in women with the polycystic ovary syndrome: a consensus statement by the Androgen Excess and Polycystic Ovary Syndrome (AE-PCOS) Society. J Clin Endocrinol Metab 95(5):2038–2049
10. Broekmans FJ, Knauff EA, Valkenburg O, Laven JS, Eijkemans MJ, Fauser BC (2006) PCOS according to the Rotterdam consensus criteria: change in prevalence among WHO-II anovulation and association with metabolic factors. BJOG 113(10):1210–1217
11. Goverde AJ, van Koert AJ, Eijkemans MJ, Knauff EA, Westerveld HE, Fauser BC, Broekmans FJ (2009) Indicators for metabolic disturbances in anovulatory women with polycystic ovary syndrome diagnosed according to the Rotterdam consensus criteria. Hum Reprod 24(3):710–717
12. Legro RS, Castracane VD, Kauffman RP (2004) Detecting insulin resistance in polycystic ovary syndrome: purposes and pitfalls. Obstet Gynecol Surv 59(2):141–154
13. Moran LJ, Misso ML, Wild RA, Norman RJ (2010) Impaired glucose tolerance, type 2 diabetes and metabolic syndrome in polycystic ovary syndrome: a systematic review and meta-analysis. Hum Reprod Update 16(4):347–363
14. Boomsma CM, Eijkemans MJ, Hughes EG, Visser GH, Fauser BC, Macklon NS (2006) A meta-analysis of pregnancy outcomes in women with polycystic ovary syndrome. Hum Reprod Update 12:673–683
15. Hart R, Norman R (2006) Polycystic ovarian syndrome—prognosis and outcomes. Best Pract Res Clin Obstet Gynaecol 20(5):751–778
16. de Wilde MA, Veltman-Verhulst SM, Goverde AJ, Lambalk CB, Laven JS, Franx A, Koster MP, Eijkemans MJ, Fauser BC (2014) Preconception predictors of gestational diabetes: a multicentre prospective cohort study on the predominant complication of pregnancy in polycystic ovary syndrome. Hum Reprod, 29:1327–1336
17. Palomba S, de Wilde MA, Falbo A, Koster MP, La Sala GB, Fauser BC (2015) Pregnancy complications in women with polycystic ovary syndrome. Hum Reprod Update 21:575–592
18. Mutlu B, Tigen K, Gurel E, Ozben B, Karaahmet T, Basaran Y (2011) The predictive value of flow-mediated dilation and carotid artery intima-media thickness for occult coronary artery disease. Echocardiography (Mount Kisco, NY) 28(10):1141–1147
19. Sprung VS, Atkinson G, Cuthbertson DJ, Pugh CJ, Aziz N, Green DJ, Cable NT, Jones H (2013) Endothelial function measured using flow-mediated dilation in polycystic ovary syndrome: a meta-analysis of the observational studies. Clin Endocrinol 78(3):438–446
20. Kaya MG, Yildirim S, Calapkorur B, Akpek M, Unluhizarci K, Kelestimur F (2015) Metformin improves endothelial function and carotid intima media thickness in patients with PCOS. Gynecol Endocrinol 31(5):401–405

21. Lorenz MW, Markus HS, Bots ML, Rosvall M, Sitzer M (2007) Prediction of clinical cardiovascular events with carotid intima-media thickness: a systematic review and meta-analysis. Circulation 115(4):459–467
22. Meyer ML, Malek AM, Wild RA, Korytkowski MT, Talbott EO (2012) Carotid artery intima-media thickness in polycystic ovary syndrome: a systematic review and meta-analysis. Hum Reprod Update 18(2):112–126
23. Agatston AS, Janowitz WR, Hildner FJ, Zusmer NR, Viamonte M Jr, Detrano R (1990) Quantification of coronary artery calcium using ultrafast computed tomography. J Am Coll Cardiol 15(4):827–832
24. Detrano R, Guerci AD, Carr JJ, Bild DE, Burke G, Folsom AR, Liu K, Shea S, Szklo M, Bluemke DA, O'Leary DH, Tracy R, Watson K, Wong ND, Kronmal RA (2008) Coronary calcium as a predictor of coronary events in four racial or ethnic groups. N Engl J Med 358(13):1336–1345
25. Raggi P, Gongora MC, Gopal A, Callister TQ, Budoff M, Shaw LJ (2008) Coronary artery calcium to predict all-cause mortality in elderly men and women. J Am Coll Cardiol 52(1):17–23
26. Talbott EO, Zborowski JV, Rager JR, Boudreaux MY, Edmundowicz DA, Guzick DS (2004) Evidence for an association between metabolic cardiovascular syndrome and coronary and aortic calcification among women with polycystic ovary syndrome. J Clin Endocrinol Metab 89(11):5454–5461
27. Shroff R, Kerchner A, Maifeld M, Van Beek EJ, Jagasia D, Dokras A (2007) Young obese women with polycystic ovary syndrome have evidence of early coronary atherosclerosis. J Clin Endocrinol Metab 92(12):4609–4614
28. Talbott EO, Zborowski J, Rager J, Stragand JR (2008) Is there an independent effect of polycystic ovary syndrome (PCOS) and menopause on the prevalence of subclinical atherosclerosis in middle aged women? Vasc Health Risk Manag 4(2):453–462
29. Pierpoint T, McKeigue PM, Isaacs AJ, Wild SH, Jacobs HS (1998) Mortality of women with polycystic ovary syndrome at long-term follow-up. J Clin Epidemiol 51(7):581–586
30. Wild S, Pierpoint T, Jacobs H, McKeigue P (2000) Long-term consequences of polycystic ovary syndrome: results of a 31 year follow-up study. Hum Fertil (Camb) 3(2):101–105
31. Elting MW, Korsen TJ, Bezemer PD, Schoemaker J (2001) Prevalence of diabetes mellitus, hypertension and cardiac complaints in a follow-up study of a Dutch PCOS population. Hum Reprod 16(3):556–560
32. Hart R, Doherty DA (2015) The potential implications of a PCOS diagnosis on a woman's long-term health using data linkage. J Clin Endocrinol Metab 100(3):911–919
33. Dahlgren E, Janson PO, Johansson S, Lapidus L, Oden A (1992) Polycystic ovary syndrome and risk for myocardial infarction. Evaluated from a risk factor model based on a prospective population study of women. Acta Obstet Gynecol Scand 71(8):599–604
34. Schmidt J, Landin-Wilhelmsen K, Brannstrom M, Dahlgren E (2011) Cardiovascular disease and risk factors in PCOS women of postmenopausal age: a 21-year controlled follow-up study. J Clin Endocrinol Metab 96(12):3794–3803
35. Krentz AJ, von Muhlen D, Barrett-Connor E (2007) Searching for polycystic ovary syndrome in postmenopausal women: evidence of a dose-effect association with prevalent cardiovascular disease. Menopause (New York, NY) 14(2):284–292
36. Khatibi A, Agardh CD, Shakir YA, Nerbrand C, Nyberg P, Lidfeldt J, Samsioe G (2007) Could androgens protect middle-aged women from cardiovascular events? A population-based study of Swedish women: The Women's Health in the Lund Area (WHILA) Study. Climacteric 10(5):386–392

Why Metformin Is so Important for Prevention and Therapy in Climacteric Women

11

Justyna Kuliczkowska-Plaksej, Andrzej Milewicz, Anna Brona, and Marek Bolanowski

Metformin (MET) is the most widely used oral antidiabetic agent, currently recommended as first-line therapy not only for all newly diagnosed type 2 diabetes mellitus (DM2) patients but also for prediabetic syndromes associated with insulin resistance (IR). MET has been used in the treatment of DM2 for over 50 years and has been found to be safe and efficacious both as monotherapy and in combination with other oral antidiabetic agents and insulin. Its major clinical advantage is not causing hypoglycemia or weight gain. Besides its use in DM2, there is interest in the use of MET for the treatment of polycystic ovary syndrome, diabetic nephropathy, and gestational diabetes [1]. This drug also counteracts the cardiovascular complications associated with DM2 [2]. Another possible benefit for MET use is the prevention of DM2 in obese prediabetic patients, antiproliferative effect associated with decreased cancer risk and improved cancer prognosis, and anabolic impact on bones [3, 4].

MET exerts its antihyperglycemic effect mainly by decreasing hepatic glucose production through suppression of gluconeogenesis and by reduction of intestinal glucose absorption. New data suggests that MET could also be implicated in down-regulation of gluconeogenic genes by a transcription-independent process [1]. Moreover, MET improves glucose uptake and utilization by peripheral tissues such as skeletal muscles and adipose tissue. Although the exact mechanism of MET action is still not fully elucidated, it acts mainly via activation of AMP-activated protein kinase (AMPK), a critical energy sensor of cellular energy homeostasis that integrates multiple signaling networks. MET decreases cellular respiration via

J. Kuliczkowska-Plaksej • A. Milewicz (✉) • M. Bolanowski
Department of Endocrinology, Diabetology and Isotope Therapy, Wroclaw Medical University, Wrocław, Poland
e-mail: andrzej.milewicz@umed.wroc.pl

A. Brona
Department of the Biological and Motoric Basis of Sport, University School of Physical Education, Wrocław, Poland

M. Birkhaeuser, A.R. Genazzani (eds.), *Pre-Menopause, Menopause and Beyond*, ISGE Series, https://doi.org/10.1007/978-3-319-63540-8_11

inhibition of the respiratory chain complex 1 [5]. All of these effects lead to improved insulin sensitivity and decrease in basal and postprandial glucose levels. Although MET exerts its effects mostly via AMPK, this mechanism may not explain all of the therapeutic effects of the drug.

After menopause, women exhibit a higher prevalence of metabolic syndrome (MS) and higher risk of cardiovascular disorders (CVD). Moreover, several cancer subtypes are more frequent in obese postmenopausal women due to obesity itself and hyperestrogenism caused by excessive peripheral aromatization in the adipose tissue. The prevalence of DM2 over the past three decades has increased fourfold, and there is also global obesity epidemic. Taking into account the negative impact of DM2 and obesity on chronic health concerns of aging women such as CVD, osteoporosis, and cancer, the newest data about pleiotropic effects of MET make this promising drug potentially useful not only in the treatment of DM2 but also in case of many other disorders.

11.1 Metformin in Prediabetic States and Obesity

Obesity is a major cause of morbidity and mortality, closely associated with DM2 and CVD [6]. As obesity is usually associated with IR, it seems reasonable that improvement in insulin sensitivity could play a crucial role in the weight loss. As MET is known not only for its antihyperglycemic and IR lowering effects but also for associated weight loss, it could be an ideal drug for obese patients not only with DM2 but also with MS. For that reason, these effects of MET have been studied in obese subjects without DM2. Despite the main effects of MET such as reduction of gluconeogenesis and intestinal glucose absorption, MET is engaged in many other metabolic pathways. MET is involved in restoring of leptin sensitivity and reducing of leptin resistance, decreasing of ghrelin level, and increasing of glucagon-like peptide-1 (GLP-1) which contributes to anorectic effect [7]. MET is also involved in irisin secretion from skeletal muscles which is associated with beneficial effects of physical activity on metabolism [8]. Besides these mechanisms, there are evidences that MET can act centrally by increasing proopiomelanocortin and decreasing neuropeptide Y expression and thus contributes to diminished appetite and food intake [6]. In the study on 199 obese subjects, MET use was associated with a mean weight loss of 5.8 kg, whereas control group has a mean weight gain of 0.8 kg. 16.2% of patients lost greater than 10% of their body weight [9]. In the BIGPRO1 study on obese subjects without DM2 treated with 850 mg of MET for 1 year, there was a mean loss of weight of 1.2 kg [10]. In the study of Malin et al., a 12-week therapy with 2000 mg of MET induced a weight loss of 3 kg in prediabetic patients [7]. In the meta-analysis of studies on overweight/obese subjects without DM2, MET monotherapy was associated with a mean of 1.92 kg weight loss and a 38% reduction of the incidence of developing DM2 [11]. In the Diabetes Prevention Study (DPP), the use of MET in prediabetic patients promoted significant weight loss greater than 5% of the initial body weight in 29% subjects compared to 13% in the placebo group, although intensive lifestyle changes were the most efficacious.

Subjects treated with MET reduced their body weight of 2.1 kg and reduced their incidence of developing DM2 by 31% [12]. In the DPP Outcome Study, the extension of DPP Study in order to evaluate the long-term benefits of MET therapy after 10 years, MET was found to be safe and well tolerated and was associated with significant and durable weight loss and 18% reduction of the incidence of DM2 in comparison with control group. Although patients from control group maintained a stable body weight, their waist circumferences increased during follow-up [13]. Many other studies have demonstrated significant reduction in the incidence of DM2 with metformin use [5, 6]. These results indicate that MET is not only useful in DM2 treatment but also is effective in the prevention of obesity and DM2 in population of obese prediabetic patients.

11.2 Metformin and Cardiovascular Diseases

CVD are associated with 52% deaths among DM2 patients, and approximately 30% of DM2 patients will develop diabetic cardiomyopathy and heart failure [14]. Many studies have shown that MET use is associated with decreased risk of micro- and macrovascular complications of diabetes and significantly reduced rate of diabetes-related mortality, all-cause mortality, and myocardial infarction [5]. In the UK Prospective Diabetes Study (UKPDS), patients treated with MET had reduced risk of any diabetes-related end points by 32%, diabetes-related death by 42%, and all-cause mortality by 36% in comparison with patients on sulfonylurea or insulin therapy [15]. Diabetes-related end points included sudden death, death from hyperglycemia or hypoglycemia, fatal or nonfatal myocardial infarction, angina, heart failure, stroke, renal failure, and ophthalmological complications. In the 10-year follow-up of UKPDS, MET-treated obese patients continued to show a reduction in myocardial infarction (33%) and death from any cause (33%) [16]. Numerous studies have confirmed the UKPDS conclusions. In the study of Kooy et al., MET treatment for 4.3 years was followed by improvement in the secondary, macrovascular end point—composite of myocardial infarction, heart failure, acute coronary syndrome, stroke, peripheral artery disease, and sudden death [17]. In the study of Hong et al. on 304 patients with DM2 and coronary artery disease randomized to receive glipizide or MET, after 5 years of therapy, patients from MET group had fewer major cardiovascular events [18]. But despite these results, in the meta-analysis of 35 clinical trials, MET was not associated with significant reduction or increase of cardiovascular events overall [19]. MET seems to be more beneficial in longer trials on younger patients. According to several studies, MET monotherapy was associated with improved survival, whereas combined therapy with sulfonylurea was associated with reduced survival [19]. Studies concerning the impact of MET on CVD risk factors—lipid concentration and blood pressure—have brought conflicting results. Several data revealed no differences in lipids and blood pressure after MET, whereas the others have demonstrated significant reductions in total cholesterol, LDL, triglycerides levels, and diastolic blood pressure [6, 20].

There are numerous studies that clearly demonstrated that the use of MET in case of congestive heart failure and diabetic cardiomyopathy had beneficial effects. The main hypothesis that MET is absolutely contraindicated in case of heart failure and myocardial infarction due to increased risk of lactic acidosis and cardiac mortality has been questioned. The Food and Drug Administration (FDA) withdrew the absolute heart failure contraindication from MET [21]. Moreover, clinical practice guidelines recommend MET as a first-line therapy in DM2 patients with heart failure. There are numerous beneficial effects of MET on cardiovascular risk factors. MET improves mitochondrial respiration and ATP synthesis in myocardial cells which in turn improves left ventricular function and remodeling [5, 6]. Furthermore, MET improves cardiac contractility by suppressing glucose 6-phosphate accumulation and decreasing hyperinsulinemia and tumor necrosis factor α (TNFα) in the myocardium and circulation [5, 6]. In addition, newer data indicates that MET has direct anti-hypertrophic effect on cardiomyocytes and vascular anti-inflammatory effect [22]. Moreover, MET exhibits antithrombotic action by the impact on PAI-1, ICAM-1, and VCAM-1 production and by the inhibition of platelet aggregation [23]. MET given at the time of reperfusion has reduced myocardial infarct size in both diabetic and nondiabetic hearts [20]. In cardiomyocytes, MET reduced apoptosis by increasing antiapoptotic proteins.

11.3 Metformin and Pancreatic β-Cells

Among many newly described actions, MET also exerts beneficial effects on β-cell function such as insulin release, transcriptional regulation, and islet cell viability. MET is able to restore insulin secretion which is usually altered by chronic exposure to free fatty acids and hyperglycemia in human islets and cell lines. Human islet cell lines incubated with high glucose exhibit decreased glucose-stimulated insulin secretion that is associated with decreased ATP production—all of these effects can be reversed by MET via inhibition of the activity of mitochondrial complex 1. Under glucolipotoxicity condition, MET preserves β-cell viability by several mechanisms; all of them remained unclear and warranting further investigation [24].

11.4 Metformin and Bone Metabolism

Many clinical observations indicate that there is a significant decrease in bone quality in patients with type 2 diabetes mellitus (DM2) known as diabetic osteopathy. Despite normal bone mass density (BMD), diabetic patients have twofold increase in hip, vertebral, and extremity fractures [25]. There are many mechanisms explaining the etiopathogenesis of diabetic osteopathy such as low-grade chronic inflammation, hyperglycemia, abnormal cytokine and growth factor secretory pattern, and excessive accumulation of AGEs in extracellular matrix [26]. The newest data suggest that not only DM2 is associated with decreased bone quality but also MS and its components. Until recently, it was believed that obesity was rather protective against fracture. This hypothesis was mainly based on the observation that BMI was positively correlated with BMD and that obese subjects had lower incidence of hip fractures [27]. A study from the Fracture Liaison Service in the United Kingdom reported for the first time a high prevalence of obesity (27%) in postmenopausal women presenting with a fragility fracture [28]. Results of the Global Longitudinal Study of Osteoporosis in Women (GLOW) conducted in postmenopausal women as well as the results of the Million Women Study and NHANES have revealed a comparable prevalence and incidence of fractures in normal weight and obese women [29, 30]. Results of the studies on the role of the main components of MS, hyperinsulinemia, and IR on bone metabolism have brought contradictory results. Hyperinsulinemia might be protective; however, the bone can become insulin resistant; thus, the possible anabolic insulin effects are abolished [26, 28]. According to new data, insulin reduces the production of osteoprotegerin, leading to increased bone resorption [31]. Osteoporosis is a common problem in the population of postmenopausal women, caused mainly by the loss of protective effect of estradiol and as a result of aging. Low-trauma fractures affect one in three postmenopausal women and are associated with significant morbidity, mortality, and economic cost [28]. According to the fact that postmenopausal women are especially prone to develop MS and DM2, studies on the effect of commonly used antidiabetic agents on bone metabolism are especially important. Recently, in vitro and in vivo studies have proven the potential beneficial anabolic effects of MET [26]. In in vitro studies, it has been found that MET modulates the physiology of osteoblasts and osteoclasts. Corizo et al. showed a dose-dependent increase in osteoblast proliferation, differentiation, and mineralization after MET use [32]. MET increased the osteoblastic transcription of osteocalcin genes, stimulated osteoprotegerin, and simultaneously reduced receptor activation of nuclear factor κ-B ligand (RANKL) mRNA and protein synthesis by osteoblastic cells and thus prevented the increase in apoptosis, caspase-3, and alteration in intracellular oxidative stress induced by AGEs [26]. In the culture of stromal cells from the bone marrow, MET stimulated alkaline phosphatase and mineralization and shifted the balance toward osteogenesis [33, 34]. In animal studies in vivo, most of these effects were also confirmed [26]. MET treatment stimulated the repair of bone lesions in vivo in diabetic and nondiabetic rats, whereas in insulin-resistant mice, it was associated with higher BMD, total bone volume, and mineral apposition in comparison with animals treated with rosiglitazone [34]. MET treatment improved BMD and bone microarchitecture in ovariectomized rats [35], although it was not confirmed by another study [36]. There are only few clinical studies in humans. Randomized, placebo-controlled studies are still unavailable. Vestergaard et al. and Melton et al. have found the beneficial effect of MET on the risk of fracture at any site in diabetic patients [25, 37]. This effect was not confirmed by another case-control study, but it was probably related to an insufficient sample size [38]. A Diabetes Outcome Progression Trial (ADOPT) has shown that MET-treated group had a lower risk of fracture in comparison with rosiglitazone-treated patients, for every skeletal site assessed [39]. In a randomized double-blind study comparing the effects of MET alone or in combination with rosiglitazone, MET monotherapy was associated with a significantly higher BMD in the hip and lumbar spine [40]. Results of the study comparing the potential anti-osteoporotic effects of MET versus sitagliptine in postmenopausal women were inconclusive—MET had no effect on alkaline phosphatase and urinary D-pyridinoline levels in contrast to sitagliptine-treated group, but finally BMD was unchanged in both groups [41].

Taken together, preclinical and clinical studies have brought promising results concerning the influence of MET on bone metabolism. Although several studies have been unable to confirm the beneficial effects of MET, many other studies have provided evidence for anabolic action of MET. MET should not be considered an anti-osteoporotic drug, but as it is one of the most widely prescribed antidiabetic drug with micro- and macrovascular benefits, this anabolic effect on the bones could be an additional benefit in the context of frequent MS, DM2, and diabetic osteopathy in the population of postmenopausal women.

11.5 Metformin in Oncology

Numerous studies have confirmed the association between DM2 and increased risk of malignancy [3, 4]. The most probable mechanism of this association is the effect of IR and secondary hyperinsulinemia which may exert mitogenic effect via the insulin-like growth factor-1 (IGF-1) receptor [42]. Women without DM2 with increased fasting insulin level (in the upper quartile) have increased risk of distance recurrence and death in comparison with patients with insulin levels in the lowest quartile [3, 4]. Furthermore, increased levels of estrogen caused by extensive aromatization from excess adipose tissue in postmenopausal obese women lead to the growth of estrogen-responsive tumors [3, 4]. All of these observations support the necessity for studies on anticarcinogenic properties of antidiabetic drugs. Several studies have revealed reduced incidence (even a 30% lower) of cancer in MET-treated group in comparison with patients treated by other groups of antidiabetic drugs [43]. In vitro and in vivo studies suggested that MET was associated with reduced risk of several obesity-related types of cancer, but the obtained results are not always unequivocal. In a cohort study, MET use was associated with 44% lower cancer mortality compared with an age-matched general population [44]. Many data have proven that MET exerts antiproliferative effect against various types of cancer via insulin and non-insulin mechanisms. One of them is the activation of AMPK, which in turn blocks signaling via the phosphatidylinositol 3-kinase and mitogen-activated protein kinase (MAPK) pathways involved in downstream signaling of the insulin and IGF-1 receptors. Another mechanism is the inhibition of mammalian target of rapamycin (mTOR) signaling by activated AMPK which finally leads to inhibition of proliferation of cancer cells. Furthermore, the MET-induced AMPK activation is mediated by the tumor suppressor liver kinase B1 (LKB1) which has antitumor properties [45]. Moreover, MET is able to inhibit cell cycle progression by decreasing cyclin D1 expression and inhibiting telomerase activity [46, 47]. The indirect effects of MET are mediated by its glucose-lowering capabilities and subsequent reduction of insulin concentration.

11.6 Metformin and Ovarian Cancer

Obesity and hyperandrogenism are known risk factors of ovarian cancer [48]. Several studies conducted in humans have proven potentially beneficial effect of MET on the prevention and survival outcomes of ovarian cancer, but the majority of this evidence comes from observational studies. Zhang et al. in the review of 28 studies reported that MET decreased mortality associated with ovarian cancer [49]. In the study concerning epithelial ovarian cancer in diabetic patients, the 5-year disease-specific survival rate in the MET group was significantly increased in comparison with the control group. Even after adjustment for background factors such as BMI, tumor grade, histology, and chemotherapy, MET remained an independent predictor of survival [50]. In vitro studies have proven that combined therapy with MET could have additional beneficial effects by improving chemotherapeutic efficacy and circumventing chemoresistance in epithelial ovarian cancer. Micromolar MET therapy in combination with chemotherapy resulted in significant cytotoxicity in comparison with chemotherapy alone at concentrations that usually are not effective [51]. Further controlled clinical trials in humans are required to verify this potential beneficial synergistic effect of MET on ovarian cancer prevention and survival.

11.7 Metformin and Cervical Cancer

There are only few clinical studies concerning MET effect on cervical cancer. One study on cell culture system demonstrated that MET was able to inhibit the growth of certain cervical cancer cells via blockage of mTOR signaling exerted by activation of AMPK after MET application [52].

11.8 Metformin and Endometrial Cancer

The association between obesity and endometrial cancer is well recognized and concerns both pre- and postmenopausal women—40–50% of endometrial cancers may be due to obesity which is associated with a twofold to fivefold increased risk [53]. Women affected by DM2 have also an increased risk of endometrial cancer both before and after menopause, independently of obesity. There is also increased risk of endometrial cancer in women without DM2 but with hyperinsulinemia and IR. Insulin reduces the liver production of SHBG, and hyperinsulinemia is associated with higher levels of free testosterone. Furthermore, insulin has direct proliferative effect on the endometrium, working similar to IGF-1, and specific insulin receptors were found in normal endometrial and endometrial cancer cell lines [48, 54]. Over 80% of cases of endometrial cancer occur after menopause. After menopause, the endometrium is frequently exposed to endogenous hormonal stimulation according to women's metabolic pattern. Prospective studies showed that endometrial cancer risk in postmenopausal women is positively associated with levels of estrogens and androgens and inversely associated with SHBG level [54]. In in vitro studies, MET inhibits the growth of various endometrial cancer cells lines, attenuates the invasion and metastasis of endometrial cancer cell lines, and enhances chemosensitivity to cisplatin and paclitaxel [47]. In the studies of Cantrell et al. and Shao et al., MET inhibited cell growth in a dose-dependent manner, resulting in G1 phase cell cycle arrest and induction of apoptosis [47, 55]. Preclinical studies showed that AMPK activation by MET inhibits the activity of aromatase promoter in the adipose tissue [3, 4]. Xie et al. have observed that MET and progesterone had a synergistic effect in the treatment of endometrial cancer [56]. MET was responsible for increased progesterone receptor expression and inhibition of mTOR signaling which enhances the efficacy of medroxyprogesterone acetate in the treatment of endometrial cancer [57]. In one population-based study, women with endometrial and ovarian cancer treated with MET at the time of diagnosis exhibited lower risk of mortality in comparison with the non-MET-treated group [58]. In the retrospective study of Nevadunsky et al., MET therapy was associated with improved overall survival rates in case of non-endometrioid endometrial cancer compared to non-MET users; however, cancer progression and recurrence rates were not reported [59]. In Ko et al.'s study, MET treatment was associated with improved recurrence-free survival and overall survival but not time to recurrence [60]. These results were not confirmed by all studies. In a case-control analysis study using the UK-based General Practice Research Database including 2554 cases exhibiting endometrial cancer, the risk of endometrial cancer did not differ between patients who had ever used MET and those who had never used MET [61]. MET probably could be an adjuvant drug in the treatment of endometrial cancer and could be added to lifestyle modifications in other high-risk women—with prediabetes, MS, and obesity with or without proven endometrial hyperplasia.

11.9 Metformin and Breast Cancer

DM2 is known to be associated with increased risk of breast cancer and is also linked to adverse breast cancer outcome [62]. Patients with increased level of fasting insulin and C-peptide and higher values of HOMA are at increased risk of death from breast cancer [63]. Despite these observations, recently two large population-based cohort analyses have questioned the association between DM2 and increased risk of breast cancer. In the British Columbia Linked Health Database and in the Danish National Diabetes Register and Cancer Registry, incidence of breast cancer was not associated with DM2 [64, 65]. Despite these controversies, some observational studies described lower incidence of breast cancer with MET use. In the study of Chlebowski et al., 68,019 postmenopausal women including 3401 with DM2 were observed for a mean of 11.8 years, among them 3273 with invasive breast cancer. In women with DM2, MET use was associated with a lower incidence of breast cancers positive for both estrogen receptor and progesterone receptor and negative for human epidermal growth factor 2 (HER2) overexpression [66]. Breast cancers in MET users were more likely to be ductal and less likely to be poorly differentiated, but none of these differences were statistically significant. Ruiter et al. have reported statistically significantly lower incidence of breast cancer in women who used MET compared with those who used sulfonylurea [67]. Some preclinical studies suggested predominant MET has influence on triple-negative cancer, cancer that does not express the genes for estrogen and progesterone receptor and HER2 [68]. Typically, this type of breast cancer develops in perimenopausal women with high BMI and seems to be highly sensitive to MET therapy. Liu et al. have proven that MET was able to inhibit cell growth of triple-negative breast cancer at the similar dose that is used in the treatment of DM2 by suppressing Ki-67, arresting the cell cycle in G1 phase, and inducing apoptosis via caspase-8 and caspase-9 [68]. Although the use of MET was not associated with improved survival in patients with triple-negative breast cancer, there was a trend for decreased distant recurrence [3]. However, in Berstein et al.'s study in 90 women with breast cancer and DM2, the incidence of progesterone receptor-positive cancer was higher in MET users [69]. Jiralerspong et al. have demonstrated the efficacy of MET in diabetic women exhibiting breast cancer in a retrospective study [70]. The complete response was 24% in MET-treated women compared to 8% in non-MET-treated patients. The optimal dosage of MET to be effective as antitumor drug is not established, but in xenograft models, it was 1500–2250 mg per day [3].

In recent years, a vast number of studies have highlighted the therapeutic potential of MET in the context of many diseases. Metformin works through multiple diverse mechanisms, and many of them are still under investigation. Many recent data confirm the pleiotropic actions of metformin and its beneficial effects on CVD, pancreatic β-cells, bones, and cancer. There are many other novel aspects of metformin, including immunoregulatory and antiaging effects. Many clinical trials concerning these novel actions of MET are still conducted.

References

1. An H, He L (2016) Current understanding of metformin effect on the control of hyperglycemia in diabetes. J Endocrinol 228:R97–106
2. Yang X, Xu Z, Zhang C, Cai Z, Zhang J (2017) Metformin, beyond an insulin sensitizer, targeting heart and pancreatic β cells. Biochim Biophys Acta 1863(8):1984–1990
3. Irie H, Banno K, Yanokura M, Iida M, Adachi M, Nakamura K, Umene K, Nogami Y, Masuda K, Kobayashi Y, Tominaga E, Aoki D (2016) Metformin: a candidate for the treatment of gynecological tumors based on drug repositioning (review). Oncol Lett 11:1287–1293
4. Imai A, Ichigo S, Matsunami K, Takagi H, Yasuda K (2015) Clinical benefits of metformin in gynecologic oncology (review). Oncol Lett 10:577–582
5. Foretz M, Guigas B, Bertrand L, Pollak M, Viollet B (2014) Metformin: from mechanisms of action to therapies. Cell Metab 20:953–966
6. Igel LI, Sinha A, Saunders KH, Apovian CM, Vojta D, Aronne LJ (2016) Metformin: an old therapy that deserves a new indication for the treatment of obesity. Curr Atheroscler Rep 18:16–24
7. Malin SK, Kashyap SR (2014) Effects of metformin on weight loss: potential mechanisms. Curr Opin Endocrinol Diabetes Obes 21:323–329

8. Li D-J, Huang F, Lu W-J, Jiang G-J, Deng Y-P, Shen F-M (2015) Metformin promotes irisin release from murine skeletal muscle independently of AMP-activated protein kinase activation. Acta Physiol (Oxf) 13:711–721
9. Seifarth C, Schehler B, Schneider HJ (2013) Effectiveness of metformin on weight loss in non-diabetic individuals with obesity. Exp Clin Endocrinol Diabetes 121:27–31
10. Fontbonne A, Charles MA, Juhan-Vague I (1996) The effect of metformin on the metabolic abnormalities associated with upper-body fat distribution. BIGPRO Study Group. Diabetes Care 19:920–926
11. Peirson L, Douketis J, Ciliska D, Fitzpatrick-Lewis D, Ali MU, Raina P (2014) Treatment for overweight and obesity in adult populations: a systematic review and meta-analysis. CMAJ Open 2:E306–E317
12. Knowler WC, Barrett-Connor E, Fowler SE (2002) Reduction in the incidence of type 2 diabetes with lifestyle intervention or metformin. N Engl J Med 346:393–403
13. Diabetes Prevention Program Research Group (2012) Long-term safety, tolerability, and weight loss associated with metformin in the Diabetes Prevention Program Outcomes Study. Diabetes Care 35:731–737
14. Morrish NJ (2001) Mortality and causes of death in the WHO multinational study of vascular diseases in diabetes. Diabetologia 44(Suppl 2):S14–S21
15. Turner RC (1998) Risk factors for coronary artery disease in non-insulin dependent diabetes mellitus: United Kingdom Prospective Diabetes Study (UKPDS: 23). BMJ 316:823–828
16. Holman RR, Paul SK, Bethel MA, Matthews DR, Neil HA (2008) 10-years follow-up of intensive glucose control in type 2 diabetes. N Engl J Med 359:1577–1589
17. Kooy A, de Jager J, Lehert P (2009) Long-term effects of metformin on metabolism and microvascular and macrovascular disease in patients with type 2 diabetes mellitus. Arch Intern Med 169:616–625
18. Hong J, Zhang Y, Lai S (2013) Effects of metformin versus glipizide on cardiovascular outcomes in patients with type 2 diabetes and coronary artery disease. Diabetes Care 36:1304–1311
19. Lamanna C, Monami M, Marchionni N, Mannucci E (2011) Effect of metformin on cardiovascular events and mortality: a meta-analysis of randomized clinical trials. Diabetes Obes Metab 13:221–228
20. Pryor R, Cabreiro F (2015) Repurposing metformin: an old drug with new tricks in its binding pockets. Biochem J 471:307–322
21. Inzucchi SE, Matsoudi DK, McGuire DK (2007) Metformin in heart failure. Diabetes Care 12:e129
22. Horman S, Beauloye C, Vanoverschelde JL, Bertrand L (2012) AMP-activated protein kinase in the control of cardiac metabolism and remodelling. Curr Heart Fail Rep 9:164–173
23. De Jager J, Kooy A, Lehert P, Bets D, Wulffele MG, Teerlink T, Scheffer PG, Schalkwijk CG, Donker AJ, Stehouwer CD (2005) Effects of short-term treatment with metformin on markers of endothelial function and inflammatory activity in type 2 diabetes mellitus: a randomized, placebo-controlled trial. J Intern Med 257:100–109
24. Matchetti P (2004) Pancreatic islets from type 2 diabetic patients have functional defects and increased apoptosis that are ameliorated by metformin. J Clin Endocrinol Metab 11:5535–5541
25. Melton LJ, Leibson CL, Achenbach SJ, Therneau TM, Khosla S (2008) Fracture risk in type 2 diabetes: update of a population-based study. J Bone Miner Res 23:1334–1342
26. McCarthy AD, Cortizo AM, Sedlinsky C (2016) Metformin revisited: does this regulator of AMPK-activated protein kinase secondarily affect bone metabolism and prevent diabetic osteopathy? World J Diabetes 7:122–133
27. Zhao LJ, Jiang H, Papasian CJ, Maulik D, Drees B, Hamilton J et al (2008) Correlation of obesity and osteoporosis: effect of fat mass on the determination of osteoporosis. J Bone Miner Res 23(1):17–29
28. Premaor MO, Pilbrow L, Tonkin C, Parker RA, Compston J (2010) Obesity and fractures in postmenopausal women. J Bone Miner Res 25(2):292–297
29. Compston JE, Watts NB, Chapurlat R, Cooper C, Boonen S, Greenspan S et al (2011) Obesity is not protective against fracture in postmenopausal women: GLOW. Am J Med 124(11):1043–1050

30. Armstrong ME, Spencer EA, Cairns BJ, Banks E, Pirie K, Green J et al (2011) Body mass index and physical activity in relation to the incidence of hip fracture in postmenopausal women. J Bone Miner Res 26(6):1330–1338
31. Clemens TL, Karsenty G (2011) The osteoblast: an insulin target cell controlling glucose homeostasis. J Bone Miner Res 26(4):677–680
32. Corizo AM, Sedlinsky C, McCarthy AD, Blanco A, Schurman L (2006) Osteogenic actions of the anti-diabetic drug metformin on osteoblasts in culture. Eur J Pharmacol 536:38–46
33. Gao Y, Xue J, Li X, Jia Y, Hu J (2008) Metformin regulates osteoblast and adipocyte differentiation of rat mesenchymal stem cells. J Pharm Pharmacol 60:1695–1700
34. Molinuevo MS, Schurman L, McCarthy AD, Cortizo AM, Tolosa MJ, Gangoiti MV, Arnol V, Sedlinsky C (2010) Effect of metformin on bone marrow progenitor cell differentiation: in vivo and in vitro studies. J Bone Miner Res 25:211–221
35. Gao Y, Li Y, Xue J, Jia Y, Hu J (2010) Effect of the anti-diabetic drug metformin on bone mass in ovariectomized rats. Eur J Pharmacol 635:231–236
36. Jeyabalan J, Viollet B, Smitham P, Ellis SA, Zaman G, Bardin C, Goodship A, Roux JP, Pierre M, Chenu C (2013) The anti-diabetic drug metformin does not affect bone mass in vivo or fracture healing. Osteoporos Int 24:2659–2670
37. Vestergaard P, Rejnmark L, Mosekilde L (2005) Relative fracture risk in patients with diabetes mellitus, and the impact of insulin and oral antidiabetic medication on relative fracture risk. Diabetologia 48:1292–1299
38. Monami M, Cresci B, Colombini A, Pala L, Balzi D, Gori F, Chiasserini V, Marchionni N, Rotella CM, Mannucci E (2008) Bone fractures and hypoglycemic treatment in type 2 diabetic patients: a case-control study. Diabetes Care 31:199–203
39. Zinman B, Haffner SM, Herman WH, Holman RR, Lachin JM, Kravitz BG, Paul G, Jones NP, Aftring RP, Viberti G, Kahn SE (2010) Effect of rosiglitazone, metformin, and glyburide on bone biomarkers in patients with type 2 diabetes. J Clin Endocrinol Metab 95:134–142
40. Borges JL, Bilezikian JP, Jones-Leone AR, Acusta AP, Ambery PD, Nino AJ, Grosse M, Fitzpatrick LA, Cobitz AR (2011) A randomized, parallel group, double-blind, multicentre study comparing the efficacy and safety of Avandamet (rosiglitazone/metformin) and metformin on long-term glycaemic control and bone mineral density after 80 weeks of treatment in drug-naïve type 2 diabetes mellitus patients. Diabetes Obes Metab 13:1036–1046
41. Hegazy SK (2015) Evaluation of anti-osteoporotic effects of metformin and sitagliptin in postmenopausal diabetic women. J Bone Miner Metab 33:207–212
42. Weinstein D, Simon M, Yehezkel E, Laron Z, Werner H (2009) Insulin analogues display IGF1-like mitogenic and anti-apoptotic activities in cultured cancer cells. Diabetes Metab Res Rev 25:41–49
43. Bowker SL, Richardson K, Marra CA (2012) Risk of breast cancer after onset of type 2 diabetes: evidence of detection bias in postmenopausal women. Diabetes Care 34:2542–2544
44. Bo S, Ciccone G, Rosato R (2012) Cancer mortality reduction and metformin: a retrospective cohort study in type 2 diabetic patients. Diabetes Obes Metab 14:23–29
45. Gwinn DM, Shackelford DB, Egan DF, Mihaylova MM, Mery A, Vasquez DS, Turk BE, Shaw RJ (2008) AMPK phosphorylation of raptor mediates a metabolic checkpoint. Mol Cell 30:214–226
46. Ben Sahra I, Laurent K, Loubat A, Giorgetti-Peraldi S, Colosetti P, Auberger P, Tanti JF, Le Marchand-Brustel Y, Bost F (2008) The antidiabetic drug metformin exerts an antitumoral effect in vitro and in vivo through a decrease of cyclin D1 level. Oncogene 27:3576–3586
47. Cantrell LA, Zhou C, Mendivil A, Malloy KM, Gehring PA, Bae-Jump VL (2010) Metformin is a potent inhibitor of endometrial cancer cell proliferation—implications for a novel treatment strategy. Gynecol Oncol 116:92–98
48. Calle EE, Rodriguez C, Walker-Thurmond K, Thun MJ (2003) Overweight, obesity, and mortality from cancer in a prospectively studied cohort of U.S. adults. N Engl J Med 348:1625–1638
49. Zhang ZJ, Li S (2014) The prognostic value of metformin for cancer patients with concurrent diabetes: a systematic review and meta-analysis. Diabetes Obes Metab 16:707–710

50. Kumar S, Meuter A, Thapa P, Langstraat C, Giri S, Chien J, Rattan R, Cliby W, Shridhar V (2013) Metformin intake is associated with better survival in ovarian cancer: a case-control study. Cancer 119:555–562
51. Erices R, Bravo M, Gonzales P, Oliva B, Racordon D, Garrido M, Ibariez C, Kato S, Branse J, Pizarro J (2013) Metformin, at concentrations corresponding to the treatment of diabetes, potentiates the cytotoxic effects of carboplatin in cultures of ovarian cancer cells. Reprod Sci 20:1433–1446
52. Xiao X, He Q, Lu C, Werle KD, Zhao RX, Chen J, Davis BC, Cui R, Liang J, Xu ZX (2012) Metformin impairs the growth of liver kinase B1-intact cervical cancer cells. Gynecol Oncol 127:29–255
53. Fader AN, Arriba LN, Frasure HE, Von Gruenigen VE (2009) Endometrial cancer ad obesity: epidemiology, biomarkers, prevention and survivorship. Genycol Oncol 114:121–127
54. Campagnoli C, Abba C, Ambroggio S, Brucao T, Pasanisi P (2013) Life-style and metformin for the prevention of endometrial pathology in postmenopausal women. Gynecol Endocrinol 29:119–124
55. Shao R, Li X, Feng Y, Lin JF, Billing H (2014) Direct effects of metformin in the endometrium: a hypothetical mechanism for the treatment of women with PCOS and endometrial carcinoma. J Exp Clin Cancer Res 33:41
56. Xie Y, Wang YL, Yu L, Hu Q, Ji L, Zhang Y, Liao QP (2011) Metformin promotes progesterone receptor expression via inhibition of mammalian target of rapamycin (mTOR) in endometrial cancer cells. J Steroid Biochem Mol Biol 126:113–120
57. Tsuji K, Kisu I, Banno K, Yanokura M, Ueki A, Masuda K, Kobayashi Y, Yamagami W, Nomura H, Susumu N, Aoki D (2012) Metformin: a possible drug for treatment of endometrial cancer. Open J Obstet Gynecol 2:1–6
58. Currie CJ, Poole CD, Jenkins-Jones S, Gale EA, Johnson JA, Morgan CL (2012) Mortality after incident cancer in people with and without type 2 diabetes: impact of metformin on survival. Diabetes Care 35:299–304
59. Nevadunsky NS, Van Arsdale A, Strickler HD, Moadel A, Kaur G, Frimer M, Conroy E, Goldberg GL, Einstein MH (2014) Metformin use and endometrial cancer survival. Gynecol Oncol 132:236–240
60. Ko E, Walter P, Jackson A, Clark L, Franasiak J, Bolac C, Havrilesky LJ, Secord AA, Moore DT, Gehrig PA, Bae-Jump V (2014) Metformin is associated with improved survival in endometrial cancer. Gynecol Oncol 132:438–442
61. Becker C, Jick SS, Meier CK, Bodmer M (2013) Metformin and the risk of endometrial cancer: a case-control analysis. Gynecol Oncol 129:565–569
62. Miches KB, Solomon CG, Hu FB (2003) Type 2 diabetes and subsequent incidence of breast cancer in the Nurses' Health Study. Diabetes Care 26:1752–1758
63. Goodwin PJ, Ennis M, Pritchard KI (2002) Fasting insulin and outcome in early-stage breast cancer: results of a prospective cohort study. J Clin Oncol 20:42–51
64. Carstensen B, Witte DR, Friis S (2012) Cancer occurrence in Danish diabetic patients: duration and insulin effects. Diabetologia 55:948–958
65. Bowker SL, Yasui Y, Veugelers P, Johnson JA (2010) Glucose-lowering agents and cancer mortality rates in type 2 diabetes: assessing effects of time-varying exposure. Diabetologia 53:1631–1637
66. Chlebowski RT, McTiernan A, Wactawski-Wende J, Manson JE, Aragaki AK, Rohan T, Ipp E, Kaklamani VG, Vitolins M, Wallace R, Gunter M, Phillips LS, Strickler H, Margolis K, Euhus DM (2012) Diabetes, metformin, and breast cancer in postmenopausal women. J Clin Oncol 23:2844–2852
67. Ruiter R, Visser LE, van Herk-Sukel MP (2012) Lower risk of cancer in patients on metformin in comparison with those on sulfonylurea derivatives. Results from a large population-based follow-up study. Diabetes Care 35:119–124

68. Liu B, Fan Z, Edgerton SM, Deng XS, Alimova IN, Lind SE, Thor AD (2009) Metformin induces unique biological and molecular responses in triple negative breast cancer cell. Cell Cycle 8:2031–2040
69. Berstein LM, Boyarkina MP, Tsyrlina EV (2011) More favourable progesterone receptor phenotype of breast cancer in diabetes treated with metformin. Med Oncol 28:1260–1263
70. Jiralerspong S, Palla SL, Giordano SH, Meric-Bernstam F, Liedtke C, Barnett CM, Hsu L, Hung MC, Hortobagyi GN, Gonzales-Angulo AM (2009) Metformin and pathologic complete responses to neoadjuvant chemotherapy in diabetic patients with breast cancer. J Clin Oncol 27:3297–3302

Metabolic Changes and Metabolic Syndrome During the Menopausal Transition

12

Alessandro D. Genazzani, Alessia Prati, and Giulia Despini

12.1 Introduction

Menopausal transition represents a peculiar moment for all women since great and relevant changes take place, due to the ongoing phenomenon of ageing and in part due to the hormonal changes that take place starting from the early perimenopause. Indeed perimenopause and menopause are characterized by accelerated physical, psychological and neuroendocrine changes. The whole variety of adverse changes that occurs in response to the altered hormonal environment typical for the menopausal transition, such as the sharp reduction of oestrogen plasma levels, results in a dramatic increase in the risk of cardiovascular diseases (CVD) [1, 2]. Such risk increase is in great part coincident with the prevalence of specific metabolic and hemodynamic impairments triggered by the increase of insulin resistance [2, 3], of blood pressure [4], of visceral adiposity, of pro-inflammatory cytokines [5] and of oxidative stress [1, 6]. Interestingly, all these elements are specifically relevant factors of the metabolic syndrome (MS) and of obesity [7].

12.2 Obesity and Metabolic Syndrome (MS)

The WHO (World Health Organization) defines obesity as a chronic condition, characterized by an excessive weight gain due to an extreme fat mass deposition with great negative effects on health and quality of life (QoL). Obesity has multifactorial aetiology, with an increased incidence on overall population, in particular in the childhood and adolescents, and it will further increase its prevalence in the next decades.

A.D. Genazzani (✉) • A. Prati • G. Despini
Department of Obstetrics and Gynecology, Gynecological Endocrinology Center, University of Modena and Reggio Emilia, Via del Pozzo 71, 41100 Modena, Italy
e-mail: algen@unimo.it

M. Birkhaeuser, A.R. Genazzani (eds.), *Pre-Menopause, Menopause and Beyond*, ISGE Series, https://doi.org/10.1007/978-3-319-63540-8_12

More or less one third/one fourth of women are overweight or obese [8]. There are two different kinds of obesity: visceral or central obesity (android) and peripheral obesity (gynoid). The central obesity, typical of men and of postmenopausal women, is characterized by an increase of waist circumference, as measured with the waist/hip ratio (WHR) being normal below 0.80. In the gynoid obesity, typical of the fertile women, fat is mainly localised in the thighs and buttocks, and these different fat distributions reflect the different body structures between male and female, due to the ancestral different roles of the two genders: abdominal obesity permits manhunting, running and escaping, while the gynoid fat distribution in women protects the pregnancy (if present) from the mechanical and metabolic point of view [9]. Moreover, around menopausal transition, many women experience weight gain and increase in central adiposity. The central/visceral obesity is associated with important changes of lipids and glucose profiles, insulin-resistance and/or diabetes mellitus, with an increase of metabolic and cardiovascular risk. The central and the peripheral fat mass show also structural differences in the fat cell: the adipocyte of the gynoid obesity has a small size, a higher insulin sensibility and a more oestrogenic receptor density, thus promoting a higher fat mass deposition than in the android fat cells. On the contrary, the latter result more responsive to androgenic stimulation and produce and release a greater amount of pro-inflammatory adipocitokines in the portal circulation. The different oestrogenic or androgenic responsiveness of the fat cells, depending on the site of fat deposition, may explain the reason of the different obesity localisation in the two genders and during the women life [10].

A positive relationship exists between the waist girth increase and the worsening of cardiovascular profile, also in normal-weight people, especially in women [11]. In fact, more than BMI (body mass index), the main positive predictive factor of the negative obesity impact on health is the abdominal fat. According to the International Diabetes Federation (IDF) criteria, the waist circumference is the main diagnostic element of the metabolic syndrome (MS), which links the visceral adiposity with the worsening of metabolic profile (Table 12.1).

The MS represents a whole heterogeneous disorder, which correlates to high mortality and morbidity rates and high economics and social costs. The syndrome affects 20–25% of the general population with an increased prevalence with ageing, in particular among the 50–60-year-old people. The characteristics of MS are visceral obesity, abnormal lipid and glucose profiles and high blood pressure: the specific physiopathological feature is represented by the insulin resistance which can explain each of the metabolic impairments; the insulin resistance promotes the storage of fat tissue at visceral level which becomes less sensitive to insulin action, and as a consequence, a higher lipolytic activity takes place, and this increases the NEFA (non-esterified fatty acids) release into liver circulation. NEFA cause an abnormal glucose and triglycerides synthesis that in turn compromises the hepatic insulin clearance. Furthermore, the fat mass is not considered as a simple energetic store but an active endocrine tissue that releases a large number of adipocitokines, some of which have a pro-inflammatory and pro-atherogenic functions (such as TNF-α, IL-6, leptin, adiponectin, omentin) [5] with an active role on the modulation of the insulin sensitivity: in fact the reduced secretion of adiponectin has a crucial

Table 12.1 Criteria for metabolic syndrome (MS) diagnosis

	WHO (1999)	ATP-III (2001)	IDF (2005)
Fasting glucose	Diabetes mellitus, impaired glucose tolerance	>110 mg/dl	>100 mg/dl or previously type II diabetes
Blood pressure	≥140/90 mmHg or use of medication	>130/85 mmHg or use of medication	>130/85 mmHg or use of medication
Dyslipidemia (TG)	≥150 mg/dl	≥150 mg/dl	≥150 mg/dl
Dyslipidemia (HDL-CH)	<35 mg/dl for male <39 mg/dl for female	<40 mg/dl for male <50 mg/dl for female	<40 mg/dl for male <50 mg/dl for female
Central obesity	WHR > 0.9 in male >0.85 for female and/or BMI > 30	Waist circumference ≥102 cm for male ≥88 cm for female	Waist circumference >94 cm for male >80 cm for female of Caucasian race
Microalbuminuria	Urinary albumin excretion ratio ≥20 μg/min or albumin/creatinine ratio ≥30 mg/g		
Diagnostic criteria	MD type II or IGT and 2 criteria	3 or more criteria	Central obesity and 2 criteria

role in inducing insulin resistance and in determining the increase of triglycerides and of small, dense LDL particles. Increased leptin secretion may be responsible for sympathetic nervous system over activity and hypertension, while reduced omentin may have an important role in the development of atherogenic processes [12].

The insulin resistance, in turn, can be triggered also by other problems: an intrinsic/structural cell disorder, due to receptorial or post-receptorial function defects, or an acquired disorder, such as an excessive weight (overweight or obesity), that increases the amount of fat and induces a change of the receptor-binding ability of hormones. It can depend also on familial predisposition, especially when there are diabetic relatives and often on the combination of many elements above described.

Moreover insulin resistance promotes sodium retention at the kidney level, with a consequent negative impact on blood pressure homeostasis. Finally, when the pancreatic compensatory mechanisms to insulin resistance become inadequate, the fasting glucose increases, and, due to reduced glucose cell intake, the diabetes progressively appears: the metabolic syndrome is taking place, etc.

12.3 Relationship Between Obesity, MS and Menopausal Transition

As we know, the menopausal transition is characterized by an early (more or less 10 years before the menopause) and progressive increase of FSH levels, linked to a decrease of inhibin production by the ovaries; at the same time, the higher frequency of anovulatory cycles induces a progesterone fall during the luteal phase, thus resulting in a relative hyperestrogenism, followed by a stable hypoestrogenism when menopause finally takes place. At present, though a large number of publications have been produced, the change of body weight during menopausal transition represents an important topic of discussion.

In general weight changes depend on an increase of energetic input and/or a decrease of energy consumption, mostly due to physical activity and to the resting energy expenditure. It's well known that women after the 45–50 years old, in the presence of no changes of their lifestyle (feeding and physical activity), show a progressive body weight increase. What is the cause of this?

Whereas weight gain per se cannot be attributed to the menopause transition, the change in the hormonal milieu at menopause is associated with an increase in total body fat, and in particular there is an increase in abdominal fat [13]. Lovejoy et al. [14] showed that all along the perimenopausal interval, there is an increase of abdominal fat mass, concomitant with climacteric hypoestrogenism, with a slow increase of body weight despite the slight reduced amount of total calories intake.

From the clinical point of view, it's important to know the metabolic condition of our patients: during the reproductive life, they might have suffered for some metabolic disorders, including thyroid dysfunctions or diabetes mellitus and/or insulin resistance, as in the case of PCOS (polycystic ovary syndrome) or overweight/obesity. The exposure to environmental factors, till the beginning of childhood, can affect the normal weight and worsen it: in general, a number of systemic diseases might affect and induce the metabolic change(s) that will occur in menopausal transition.

The gonadal steroid hormones have specific metabolic effects during perimenopausal transition. As mentioned before, menopausal transition is characterized by low level of oestrogens and/or hyperestrogenism associated to low luteal progesterone levels. This event is greatly related to the higher amount of anovulatory menstrual cycles. Indeed, during the luteal phase of the menstrual cycle, the typical increase of P/E2 ratio induces the increase of body temperature of about 0.4 °C [15]: this temperature's rise causes an elevation of basal metabolism of about 200 Jk (50 kcal) a day [16]. On the contrary, the absence of progesterone increase, during the menopausal transition, determines the lack of such energy consumption in resting conditions typical of the luteal phase (about 50 kcal a day, for 12–14 days: approximately 600–700 kcal every month). This event is at the basis of the increased fat mass deposition during perimenopause [17] that can be interpreted as a reduction of the physiological burning of fat during the luteal phase.

This decline of the energetic consumption seems to be not exclusively dependant from the progesterone deficiency but also from other factors, such as the amount of lean mass, the sympathetic nervous system (SNS) activity, the endocrine status and the ageing-mediated physiological changes. In fact the decline of basal metabolism observed in postmenopausal women may depend also form ageing [18]. However, the basal metabolism decreases more during menopausal transition than what could be attributed to the ageing process [19]. Probably oestrogen depletion contributes to accelerate this decline. As the perimenopause becomes menopause, the progressive reduction of oestrogen levels induces a progressively worsening of the insulin resistance that is also increased by the concomitant cortisol rise (typical of ageing and menopause). This latter event physiologically induces gluconeogenesis, a typical compensatory mechanism that starts to occur to people above 55–60 years of age, and later promotes the increase of insulin resistance. In addition hypoestrogenism partly induces also the fall of GH levels that facilitates the storage of abdominal fat mass with a decrease of lipid metabolism [20, 21]. In addition the lack of oestrogens during the menopausal transition promotes the different fat storage: instead of mainly in the gluteal and femoral subcutaneous region, fat is mainly stored at the abdominal level [22], and thus oestrogen deficiency is expected to result in decreased peripheral fat mass [23].

Further confirmations in regard to the oestrogens' role on fat mass control come from experimental studies on animal models: the oestrogen treatment in ovariectomised mice reduces the fat mass and the adipocyte cell size, independently from the energy intake. In particular, oestradiol seems to accelerate the fat oxidation pathways in the muscles and the adipocyte lipolysis [24].

According to what was discussed up to now, the decrease of basal metabolism induces the gain in fat mass which, in turn, may contribute to improve the incidence of obesity-related diseases, such as worsening of cardiovascular profile and a higher risk to develop type II diabetes. The increase of visceral adiposity further worsens the insulin sensibility, in particular at the liver level so that higher amounts of insulin are needed to control glucose intake at tissue levels. All these changes determine the increase of the rate of incidence of the MS in overweight/obese women during the menopausal transition.

Recently, it has been suggested that another possible link between menopausal hypoestrogenism, appetite control and weight gain is the increase of orexin-A plasma levels [25]. This hypothalamic neuropeptide is involved in the regulation of feeding behaviour, of sleep-wake rhythm and of neuroendocrine homeostasis [26, 27]. In postmenopausal women, while oestrogens show low levels, plasma orexin-A levels are significantly higher, and this seems to participate in the increase of the cardiovascular risk factors, such as high glycaemia, abnormal lipid profile, increased blood pressure and high BMI [28].

12.4 The Management of Obesity and MS During Perimenopause

The management of overweight/obese premenopausal women has to start from a careful anamnesis investigating the age of the onset of obesity, and the weight changes occurred in the last months, if there are diabetic members of a family suffering from any other endocrinological diseases and/or obesity. The purpose of this check is to exclude any clinical cause that might need specific therapeutical approaches, like some uncommon secondary obesities, due to genetic, neurological or psychiatric conditions.

It's important to know if the patient suffered in the past for PCOS and/or premenstrual syndrome and premenstrual dysphoric disease (PMS and PMDD).

It is well recognised that insulin resistance is a frequent feature of the PCOS and that 50–60% of the patients are overweight/obese [29]. Recently we demonstrated [30] that patients with PCOS and insulin resistance have double chance to suffer from PMS/PMDD and mood disorders up to depression, during their reproductive life and more frequently during the menopausal transition. This condition seems to be due to a reduced production of neurosteroids, in particular of allopregnanolone, which is considered the most powerful endogenous anxiolytic and antidepressant substance derived from progesterone metabolism [31]. PCOS and hyperinsulinemic patients, during menopausal transition, have a higher risk to suffer from more intense climacteric symptoms, in particular those due to neurosteroids deficiency (i.e. allopregnanolone), like mood disorders, depression and anxiety, if they don't reduce insulin resistance and their weight [32].

In the presence of overweight/obesity, it is necessary to assess the presence of insulin resistance, even in nonobese women; in fact, perimenopausal women may have a normal weight, thanks to their lifestyle, though they have an insulin resistance predisposition, which can be disclosed only by an OGTT (oral glucose tolerance test). This test is usually done over 4 h, but it can be performed also with two blood samples, at time 0 (i.e. before drinking the glucose) and 60 or 90 min after glucose load of 75 g of sugar dissolved in a glass of water: a hyperinsulinism is diagnosed when insulin response is higher than 60 microU/ml [33, 34]. In women with a history of PCOS, an insulin resistance is frequently confirmed both during pre- and postmenopause [35].

The therapeutical approaches for women during menopausal transition have to consider the body weight at the moment of the perimenopausal transition: the normal-weight women and the overweight/obese women should be treated differently. In the first case, the approach is targeted to the weight gain's prevention, while in latter group, it is important to avoid a further weight increase and/or to treat the metabolic abnormalities. In both cases, the first recommendation is the modification of lifestyle, through the combination of a hypocaloric diet and a correct choice of nutrients with physical activity.

An endurance training (aerobic exercise for 45 min a day, three times a week) has been shown to promote body weight and fat mass losses and to reduce both waist girth and blood pressure in overweight/obese women [36]. Moreover, these interventions decrease plasma triglyceride, total cholesterol and low-density lipoprotein levels and increase high-density lipoprotein plasma concentrations [36]. The best improvement in metabolic risk profile has been observed in women with two or more determinants of the MS but still with no coronary heart disease [37]. In addition, the physical exercise amplifies the triggers on anorectic response limiting food's introduction [38]. Unfortunately, the association of diet and physical activity results effective in the short period and shows an increasing lower compliance and higher difficulty to maintain the weight loss in the long term. Quite often, in these cases, a psychological support is needed.

In normal-weight women with climacteric symptoms, the hormonal replacement therapy (HRT) has been successfully demonstrated to protect against perimenopausal changes of body composition [39, 40]. In these patients, no significant variations in weight, fat mass content and distribution has been observed probably also, thanks to the route of administration of HRT. In particular transdermal oestrogens seem to be more protective against fat mass increase and android fat distribution [41, 42]. Oral oestrogens have been associated with a small increase in fat mass and a decrease in lean mass [43]. Similar effects on body composition and on fat tissue have been observed when administering tibolone and raloxifene.

In obese women during menopausal transition, behavioural therapy is essential to achieve the weight control on long term, but there exists some medication like metformin, orlistat and inositol that might help and facilitate weight control and/or weight loss. Metformin, a well-known antidiabetes drug, reduces insulin levels improving insulin sensitivity, through an increase of glucose cell uptake. It is frequently administered to hyperinsulinemic PCOS women during fertile age. Also myo-inositol, alone or in combination with chiro-inositol or alpha-lipoic acid, administration can enhance insulin sensibility through an improvement of post-receptorial pathways' functions. On the contrary, orlistat represents a specific anti-obesity treatment since it reduces the absorption of dietary fats, promoting their faecal elimination.

Overweight, obesity and metabolic syndrome are tightly linked with the changing of the hormonal pattern during the menopausal transition. In fact, as previously mentioned, the progressive decline of oestrogens and progesterone plasma levels promotes some metabolic impairment, such as the worsening of insulin resistance or the increasing of central fat mass storage. At the same time, obesity is an important factor that affects the changes of hormonal profiles during menopausal transition since women with higher BMI were more likely to start the perimenopause earlier though moving slower towards the menopause if compared to those with a lower BMI [44]. If during fertile age, these women had PCOS and overweight/obesity, it is more likely that insulin resistance led them not only to a MS predisposition but also to mood disorders that might be more severe as soon as menopausal transition occurs. Recent findings sustain such hypothesis since it has been reported that menopausal women who suffered from PCOS have higher adiponectin and lower leptin [45] and a higher insulin response to OGTT [35] than menopausal women with no history of PCOS.

12.5 Influence of Overweight/Obesity on Menopausal Transition and on Menopausal Symptoms

Excess of body weight up to obesity has been demonstrated to alter menstrual cycle length and hormonal pattern in premenopausal women. The age of natural menopause (ANM) can be delayed in women who are not smokers, exercise a lot, not vegetarians and with higher BMI [44]. Being obese induces a later ANM since obese women show a higher oestrogenic milieu due to a higher activity of aromatase and type 1 17β-hydroxysteroid dehydrogenase [46]. Conversely, the decline of plasma oestradiol levels is more rapid in normal-weight or nonobese women.

As it can be argue there is a possible relationship between the fat deposits and menopause onset since obesity affects the magnitude of the hormonal changes observed and experienced during the menopausal transition [13]. However, the severity of the many menopausal symptoms depends on a number of factors, and among them there are not only the hormonal changes typical of the transition but also psychological factors. In fact during the menopausal transition, as weight increases so do menopausal symptoms.

In addition to the higher risks for a number of chronic diseases, overweight and obese women often show psychosocial impairments that lead to a lower self-esteem and poor general well-being. Recent review concluded that obese postmenopausal women have a lower QoL if compared to normal-weight women [47, 48], and excess of weight up to obesity during menopausal transition is an indicator of poor sexual functioning [13]. Excess of weight in peri- and postmenopause increases the intensity of sexual complaints and facilitates urinary incontinence. Moreover arousal, orgasm, lubrication and satisfaction are inversely correlated with BMI and insulin resistance and metabolic syndrome [49].

Recent data support also the fact that obesity might induce a lower bone loss during the menopausal transition than nonobese women [50]. In fact low BMI has been associated with osteopenia and osteoporosis, while obese women resulted to have a lower risk of osteoporosis and fractures [51]. However, the Global Longitudinal Study of Osteoporosis in Women [52] supported a different conclusion since it demonstrated that the fracture risks of ankle and upper leg were higher in obese women but mainly in those that have experienced early menopause and that reported two or more falls in the last 12 months [52]. Most of these women had also a higher prevalence of other diseases such as diabetes, CVD, asthma and emphysema, thus suggesting that obesity in menopausal women might be in general less protective than in normal-weight women [13, 52].

12.6 How to Prevent Weight Gain

When dealing with prevention of weight gain, the only logical solutions include physical activity, caloric-restricted diet and, eventually, specific antiobesity drugs or bariatric surgery.

As previously mentioned, physical activity is relevant to counteract the body weight increase, independently from age and menopausal condition [53]. It is important to point out that physical activity cannot block or prevent weight gain related to ageing, but it can protect against the development of obesity. An activity of 45 min at least three times in a week really improves the control of body weight and maintains elasticity and lean mass despite the decrease of fat mass [13].

It is obvious that calorie restriction induces reduction of body weight and fat similarly to physical exercise. If the body weight is reduced to 5% or more, this reduces the risk factors for CVD, that is, hypertension and dyslipidemia, and diabetes [54]. When being obese during menopause, the diet should provide a low amount of calories but not below 800 Kcal/day [55]. Whatever the diet is, the adherence to the diet is the most important factor for the success, independently from the nutrient composition. Ideally the diet should try to avoid the loss of proteins, promoting the use of fat as source of energy. If the diet is low in carbohydrate, mono- and polyunsaturated fat and protein from fish, nuts and legumes should be suggested.

Regarding antiobesity drugs, these compounds are substances that suppress appetite and give the sense of satiety, increasing the metabolism but mainly interfering on the absorption of the nutrients of the food [56]. Among these substances, there are orlistat, sibutramine and rimonabant. All of them have been demonstrated to improve body weight, but only one (orlistat) is now available, being sibutramine and rimonabant withdrawn due to severe side effects [13, 57]. Obviously natural remedies can be helpful such as herbal preparations and can be used as supplements to aid weight loss [13]. Last but not least important to mention is metformin. This drug has been approved for the treatment of diabetes, and a great use has been done to control weight gain in young women with obesity and PCOS [29], but only when compensatory hyperinsulinism is present, metformin administration is highly effective on metabolism [58]. Though it cannot be considered as a drug to induce weight loss, metformin is relevant to counteract the risk of diabetes and maintain a lower level of insulinemia [13, 29].

Bariatric surgery should be considered as the last attempt to reduce body weight since it is cost-effective, and it should be proposed only for very obese women. There are various surgical procedures such as the gastric bypass, the vertical banded gastroplasty, the adjustable gastric banding and the laparoscopic sleeve gastrectomy [13]. When compared, gastric bypass was reported to be more effective than the others [13].

Conclusions

Weight gain and obesity have been improving during the last decade so much that 20% of the world population is almost obese and women are slightly more interested by this event than men. Nevertheless it has been observed that weight gain is highly related to ageing rather than to menopausal transition though hormonal changes during the menopausal transition contribute to increase the abdominal fat and abdominal obesity [13]. Any excess in abdominal fat means a higher risk for CVD, diabetes, cancer and poor QoL.

Weight control is then essential during the perimenopause and later during menopause, but it is clear that the most important event is a specific and constant control of the diet and of the physical exercise far before the perimenopause. This control has to be adopted for a lifetime, and a specific lifestyle and an investment for the future health have to be considered, especially when ageing affects and impairs organ and system functions. Hormone replacement therapy is not associated with weight gain and certainly improves QoL and symptoms and counteracts accumulation of abdominal fat in peri- and postmenopausal women.

References

1. Innes KE, Selfe TK, Taylor AG (2008) Menopause, the metabolic syndrome and mind-body therapies. Menopause 15:1005–1013
2. Baker L, Meldrum KK, Wang M et al (2003) The role of estrogen in cardiovascular disease. J Surg Res 115:325–344
3. Spencer CP, Godsland IF, Stevenson JC (1997) Is there a menopausal metabolic syndrome? Gynecol Endocrinol 11:341–355
4. Carr MC (2003) The emergence of the metabolic syndrome with menopause. J Clin Endocrinol Metab 88:2404–2411
5. Sites CK, Toth MJ, Cushman M, L'Hommedieu GD, Tchernof A, Tracy RP, Poehlman ET (2002) Menopause-related differences in inflammation markers and their relationship to body fat distribution and insulin-stimulated glucose disposal. Fertil Steril 77:128–135
6. Kawano H, Yasue H, Hirai N, Yoshida T, Fukushima H, Miyamoto S, Kojima S, Hokamaki J, Nakamura H, Yodoi J, Ogawa H (2003) Effects of transdermal and oral estrogen supplementation on endothelial function, inflammation and cellular redox state. Int J Clin Pharmacol Ther 41:346–353
7. Ross LA, Polotsky AJ (2012) Metabolic correlates of menopause: an update. Curr Opin Obstet Gynecol 24:402–407
8. Flegal KM, Carroll MD, Ogden CL, Curtin LR (2010) Prevalence and trends in obesity among US adults, 1999–2008. JAMA 303(3):235–241
9. Genazzani AD, Vito G, Lanzoni C, Strucchi C, Mehmeti H, Ricchieri F, Mbusnum MN (2005) La Sindrome Metabolica menopausale. Giorn It Ost Gin 11/12:487–493
10. Ibrahim M (2010) Subcutaneous and visceral adipose tissue: structural and functional differences. Obes Rev 11:11–18
11. Balkau B, Deanfield JE, Després JP, Bassand JP, Fox KA, Smith SC Jr, Barter P, Tan CE, Van Gaal L, Wittchen HU, Massien C, Haffner SM (2007) International Day for the Evaluation of Abdominal Obesity (IDEA): a study of waist circumference, cardiovascular disease, and diabetes mellitus in 168,000 primary care patients in 63 countries. Circulation 116(17):1942–1951
12. Carmina E (2013) Obesity, adipokines and metabolic syndrome in polycystic ovary syndrome. Front Horm Res 40:40–50
13. Davis SR, Castelo-Branco C, Chedraui P, Lumsden MA, Nappi RE, Shah D, Villaseca P (2012) Writing Group of the International Menopause Society for World Menopause Day 2012. Understanding weight gain at menopause. Climacteric 15(5):419–429
14. Lovejoy JC, Champagne CM, De Longe L, Xie H, Smith SR (2008) Increased visceral fat and decreased energy expenditure during the menopausal transition. Int J Obes 32(6):949–958
15. Cagnacci A, Volpe A, Paoletti AM, Melis GB (1997) Regulation of the 24-hour rhythm of body temperature in menstrual cycles with spontaneous and gonadotropin-induced ovulation. Fertil Steril 68(3):421
16. Webb P (1986) 24-hour energy expenditure and the menstrual cycle. Am J Clin Nutr 44:14
17. Gambacciani M, Ciaponi M, Cappagli B, Benussi C, DeSimone L, Genazzani AR (1999) Climacteric modifications in body weight and fat tissue distribution. Climateric 2(1):37–44
18. Roubenoff R, Hughes VA, Dallal GE, Nelson ME, Morganti C, Kehayias JJ, Singh MA, Roberts S (2000) The effect of gender and body composition method on the apparent decline in lean mass-adjusted resting metabolic rate with age. J Gerontol A Biol Sci Med Sci 55(12):M757–M760
19. Ravussin E, Lillioja S, Knowler WC, Christin L, Freymond D, Abbott WG, Boyce V, Howard BV, Bogardus C (1988) Reduced rate of energy expenditure as a risk factor for body-weight gain. N Engl J Med 318(8):467–472
20. Veldhuis JD, Bowers CY (2003) Sex-steroid modulation of growth hormone (GH) secretory control: three-peptide ensemble regulation under dual feedback restraint by GH and IGF-I. Endocrine 22(1):25–40
21. Walenkamp JD, Wit JM (2006) Genetic disorders in the growth hormone-insulin-like growth factor-I axis. Horm Res 66(5):221–230

22. Peppa M, Koliacki C, Dimitriadis G (2012) Body composition as an important determinant of metabolic syndrome in postmenopausal women. Endocrinol Metabol Syndr 2:1. doi:10.4172/2161-1017.S1-009
23. Krotkiewski M, Bjorntorp P, Sjostrom L, Smith U (1983) Impact of obesity on metabolism in men and women. Importance of regional adipose tissue distribution. J Clin Invest 72:1150–1162
24. D'Eont M, Souza SC, Aronovitz M, Obin MS, Fried SK, Greenberg AS (2005) Estrogen regulation of adiposity and fuel partitioning: evidence of genomic and non-genomic regulation of lipogenic and oxidative pathways. J Biol Chem 280:35983–35991
25. Messina G, Viggiano A, DeLuca V, Messina A, Chieffi S, Monda M (2013) Hormonal changes in menopause and Orexin-A action. Obst Gynecol Int 2013:1–5
26. Willie JT, Chemelli RM, Sinton CM, Yanagisawa M (2001) To eat or to sleep? Orexin in the regulation of feeding and wakefulness. Ann Rev Neurosci 24:429–458
27. Kukkonen JP, Holmqvist T, Ammoun S, Akerman KEO (2002) Functions of the orexinergic/hypocretinergic system. Am J Physiol 283(6):C1567–C1591
28. El-Sedeek M, Korish AA, Deef MM (2010) Plasma orexin-A levels in postmenopausal women: possible interaction with estrogen and correlation with cardiovascular risk status. BJOG 117(4):488–492
29. Genazzani AD, Ricchieri F, Lanzoni C (2010) Use of metformin in the treatment of polycystic ovary syndrome. Womens Health 6(4):577–593
30. Monteleone P, Luisi S, Tonetti A, Bernardi F, Genazzani AD, Luisi M, Petraglia F, Genazzani AR (2000) Allopregnanolone concentrations and premenstrual syndrome. Eur J Endocrinol 142(3):269–273
31. Genazzani D, Chierchia E, Rattighieri E, Santagni S, Casarosa E, Luisi M, Genazzani AR (2010) Metformin administration restores allopregnanolone response to adrenocorticotropic hormone (ACTH) stimulation in overweight hyperinsulinemic patients with PCOS. Gynecol Endocrinol 26(9):684–689
32. Kerchner A, Lester W, Stuart SP, Dokras A (2009) Risk of depression and other mental health disorders in women with polycystic ovary syndrome: a longitudinal study. Fertil Steril 91:207–212
33. Genazzani AD, Strucchi C, Luisi M, Casarosa E, Lanzoni C, Baraldi E, Ricchieri F, Mehmeti H, Genazzani AR (2006) Metformin administration modulates neurosteroids secretion in non-obese amenorrhoic patients with polycystic ovary syndrome. Gynecol Endocrinol 22(1):36–43
34. Genazzani AD, Lanzoni C, Ricchieri F, Jasonni VM (2008) Myo-inositol administration positively affects hyperinsulinemia and hormonal parameters in overweight patients with polycystic ovary syndrome. Gynecol Endocrinol 24(3):139–144
35. Puurunen J, Piltonen T, Morin-Papunen L, Perheentupa A, Järvelä I, Ruokonen A, Tapanainen JS (2011) Unfavorable hormonal, metabolic, and inflammatory alterations persist after menopause in women with PCOS. J Clin Endocrinol Metab 96(6):1827–1834
36. Roussel M, Garnier S, Lemoine S, Gaubert I, Charbonnier L, Auneau G, Mauriège P (2009) Influence of a walking program on the metabolic risk profile of obese postmenopausal women. Menopause 16(3):566–575
37. Martins C, Kulseng B, King NA, Holst JJ, Blundell JE (2010) The effects of exercise-induced weight loss on appetite-related peptides and motivation to eat. J Clin Endocrinol Metab 95:1609–1616
38. Genazzani AR, Gambacciani M (2006) Effect of climacteric transition and hormone replacement therapy on body weight and body fat distribution. Gynecol Endocrinol 22(3):145–150
39. Tommaselli GA, DiCarlo C, Di Spiezio SA, Bifulco CG, Cirillo D, Guida M, Papasso R, Nappi C (2006) Serum leptin levels and body composition in postmenopausal women treated with tibolone and raloxifene. Menopause 13:660–668
40. Di Carlo C, Tommaselli GA, Sammartino A, Bifulco G, Nasti A, Nappi C (2004) Serum leptin levels and body composition in postmenopausal women: effects of hormone therapy. Menopause 11:466–473
41. Meli R, Pacilio M, Mattace Raso G, Esposito E, Coppola A, Nasti A, Di Carlo C, Nappi C, Di Carlo C (2004) Estrogen and raloxifene modulate leptin and its receptor in hypothalamus and adipose tissue from ovariectomized rats. Endocrinology 145:3115–3121

42. Sammel MD, Freeman EW, Liu Z, Lin H, Guo W (2009) Factors that influence entry into stages of the menopausal transition. Menopause 16(6):1218–1227
43. dos Reis CM, de Melo NR, Meirelles ES, Vezozzo DP, Halpern A (2003) Body composition, visceral fat distribution and fat oxidation in postmenopausal women using oral or transdermal oestrogen. Maturitas 46:59–68
44. Morris DH, Jones ME, Schoemaker MJ, McFadden E, Ashworth A, Swerdlow AJ (2012) Body mass index, exercise, and other lifestyle factors in relation to age at natural menopause: analyses from the Breakthrough Generations Study. Am J Epidemiol 175:998–1005
45. Krents AJ, von Muhlen D, Barret-Connor E (2012) Adipocytokine profiles in a putative novel postmenopausal polycystic ovary syndrome (PCOS) phenotype parallel those in premenopausal PCOS: the Rancho Bernardo Study. Metabolism 61:1238–1241
46. Sowers MR, Randolph JF, Zheng H et al (2011) Genetic polymorphisms and obesity infl uence estradiol decline during the menopause. Clin Endocrinol 74:618–623
47. Jones GL, Sutton A (2008) Quality of life in obese postmenopausal women. Menopause Int 14:26–32
48. Nappi RE, Verde JB, Polatti F, Genazzani AR, Zara C (2002) Self-reported sexual symptoms in women attending menopause clinics. Gynecol Obstet Investig 53:181–187
49. Llaneza P, Gonzalez C, Fernandez-Inarrea J, Alonso A, Arnott I, Ferrer-Barriendos J (2009) Insulin resistance and health-related quality of life in postmenopausal women. Fertil Steril 91(Suppl 4):1370–1373
50. Sowers MR, Zheng H, Jannausch ML, McConnell D, Nan B, Harlow S, Randolph JF Jr (2010) Amount of bone loss in relation to time around the final menstrual period and follicle-stimulating hormone staging of the transmenopause. J Clin Endocrinol Metab 95:2155–2162
51. Van der Voort DJ, Geusens PP, Dinant GJ (2001) Risk factors for osteoporosis related to their outcome: fractures. Osteoporos Int 12:630–638
52. Compston JE, Watts NB, Chapurlat R, Cooper C, Boonen S, Greenspan S, Pfeilschifter J, Silverman S, Díez-Pérez A, Lindsay R, Saag KG, Netelenbos JC, Gehlbach S, Hooven FH, Flahive J, Adachi JD, Rossini M, Lacroix AZ, Roux C, Sambrook PN, Siris ES, Investigators G (2011) Obesity is not protective against fracture in postmenopausal women: GLOW. Am J Med 124:1043–1050
53. Poehlman E, Toth MJ, Gardner A (1995) Changes in energy balance and body composition at menopause: a controlled longitudinal study. Ann Intern Med 123:673–678
54. Douketis JD, Macie C, Thabane L, Williamson DF (2005) Systematic review of long-term weight loss studies in obese adults: clinical significance and applicability to clinical practice. Int J Obes 29:1153–1167
55. Freedman MR, King J, Kennedy E (2001) Popular diets: a scientific review. Obes Rev 9(Suppl 1):1–40S
56. National Institute for Health and Clinical Excellence (2006) Clinical guideline CG43. Obesity: the prevention, identification, assessment and management of overweight and obesity in adults and children, London. http://guidance.nice.org.uk/CG43/NICEGuidance/pdf/English
57. Ioannides-Demos LL, Piccenna L, McNeil JJ (2011) Pharmacotherapies for obesity: past, current, and future therapies. J Obes 2011:179674
58. Genazzani AD, Lanzoni C, Ricchieri F, Baraldi E, Casarosa E, Jasonni VM (2007) Metformin administration is more effective when non-obese patients with polycystic ovary syndrome show both hyperandrogenism and hyperinsulinemia. Gynecol Endocrinol 23:146–152

Weight and Body Composition Management After Menopause: The Effect of Lifestyle Modifications

13

Irene Lambrinoudaki, Eleni Armeni, and Nikolaos Tsoltos

13.1 Definition and Prevalence of Obesity

Obesity is characterized by excessive accumulation of fat in the adipose tissue, which is attributed to a positive energy balance and subsequent weight gain [1]. The definition of obesity is based on the body mass index (BMI), calculated using the following equation: BMI = weight (kg)/height^2 (m^2) [2]. Classification of obesity according to BMI is presented in Table 13.1. However, similar values of BMI correspond to varying body fat and body composition in different individuals and populations [1, 2]. According to the World Health Organization (WHO), obesity is associated with many chronic diseases, including coronary heart disease and stroke, type 2 diabetes mellitus, as well as musculoskeletal disorders, respiratory symptoms, and several types of cancer [1].

Accumulation of body fat in the intra-abdominal region is associated with an increased metabolic risk, especially in women. Central obesity is reflected by an elevated waist to hip ratio (WHR), defined as >0.85 in women, or simply by an increased waist circumference [1, 2]. The predictive ability of waist circumference with respect to the risk of metabolic complications and cardiovascular disease is more pronounced in women compared to men [1]. As reported by the WHO, an increased risk of metabolic complications can be expected in women with a waist circumference ≥80 cm and a substantially increased risk in women with a waist circumference ≥88 cm [1].

The prevalence of overweight and obesity is highest in the region of North America and lowest in the region of Southeast Asia, according to WHO data in the year 2014 [3]. Women are far more likely to be obese compared to men [3]. In many

I. Lambrinoudaki (✉) • E. Armeni • N. Tsoltos
Second Department of Obstetrics and Gynecology, National and Kapodistrian University of Athens, Aretaieio Hospital, 76 Vas. Sofias Ave., 11528 Athens, Greece
e-mail: ilambrinoudaki@med.uoa.gr

M. Birkhaeuser, A.R. Genazzani (eds.), *Pre-Menopause, Menopause and Beyond*, ISGE Series, https://doi.org/10.1007/978-3-319-63540-8_13

Table 13.1 Classification of body mass index values (Adapted from [1, 2])

Body Mass Index					
<18.5kg/m^2	18.5 – 24.99kg/m^2	≥25kg/m^2			
UNDERWEIGHT	NORMAL RANGE	OVERWEIGHT			
		pre-obese: 25.0kg/m^2 to 29.99kg/m^2	**obese class I:** 30kg/m^2 to 34.99kg/m^2	**obese class II:** 35.0kg/m^2 to 39.99kg/m^2	**obese class III:** ≥40.0kg/m^2

European countries and in the United States of America, more than half of women are overweight [3]. Aging represents a major determinant of this problem, since the prevalence of obesity has been shown to increase steeply with advancing age [4].

13.2 Obesity and the Menopausal Transition

The menopausal transition is closely related with alterations in body composition [5]. Aging increases physical inactivity and mood instability, factors associated with sarcopenia and obesity [5]. In addition, estrogen deprivation inflicts various adverse metabolic changes with respect to energy regulation, food consumption, body weight homeostasis, as well as the secretion of adipokines [6]. Overall, the effect of aging in combination with the postmenopausal estrogen decline leads to central body fat accumulation and visceral adiposity [5, 7]. The latter is a major determinant of insulin resistance and hyperinsulinemia, conditions that further decrease energy expenditure [5, 8–10].

13.3 Management of Adiposity in Menopause

Management of obesity and body composition in postmenopausal women consists of:

- Lifestyle modification, including healthy eating and physical activity
- Medical treatment
- Bariatric surgery

This review will address the effect of lifestyle modification in the prevention and treatment of postmenopausal obesity and sarcopenia.

13.4 Healthy Diet

13.4.1 Eating Patterns

The pattern of food intake is directly related with metabolic pathways which affect body weight and fat accumulation [11, 12]. Beneficial eating patterns include the "DASH" (Dietary Approaches to Stop Hypertension) diet and the "Mediterranean" diet, whereas "Western" diets are considered as harmful [13–15]. The main characteristics of each diet are presented in Table 13.2.

The impact of the DASH diet on weight loss is still under investigation; however, available studies have shown beneficial effects on weight maintenance [16]. The National Heart, Lung, and Blood Institute and the American Heart Association recommend adherence to the DASH diet to manage elevated blood pressure and to reduce the risk of coronary heart disease [17, 18].

The effect of the Mediterranean diet on long-term weight loss has been extensively studied. A recent systematic review [19] analyzed five randomized controlled trials (RCTs) with a total sample of 998 overweight or obese adults trying to lose weight, who were followed up for at least 12 months. The results of this review showed that the Mediterranean diet is superior to low-fat diets concerning weight loss and comparable to low-carbohydrate diets [19]. A large prospective cohort study [15] showed that adherence to the Mediterranean diet was associated with a moderate reduction of weight, during a follow-up period of up to 5 years. In addition, up to 10% risk reduction to develop obesity was observed in individuals with a high vs lower adherence to the Mediterranean diet [15].

"Western"-type diets are considered unhealthy. A higher risk of cardiovascular disease has been observed in individuals adhering to a dietary pattern that consists mainly of fats and processed meat compared to individuals consuming mainly whole-grain products and fruits [14]. Higher consumption of less healthful foods (e.g., low-fiber bread and cereals, red and processed meat, cottage cheese, tomato foods, regular soft drinks, and sweetened beverages) has been positively associated with a higher rate of carotid artery atherosclerosis progression, independently of traditional cardiovascular risk factors, over a follow-up period of 5 years [12].

Table 13.2 Main characteristics of common eating patterns (Adapted from [13–15])

Beneficial eating patterns	Harmful eating pattern
• **DASH (Dietary Approaches to Stop Hypertension) diet** – Rich in fiber (whole-grain cereals) – Rich in fruits, vegetables, and low-fat dairy – Low in saturated and *trans* fat, cholesterol • **Mediterranean diet** – Rich in vegetables, beans, legumes, nuts, fruits, whole grains, and seeds – Olive oil is the main source of monounsaturated fat – Low to moderate wine consumption – Low to moderate amount of dairy products, poultry, and fish – Reduced intake of red meat	**"Western" diet** – Rich in red and processed meat – Rich in saturated fat – Rich in sugar and salt

13.4.2 Eating Patterns and Adiposity After the Menopause

Alterations in diet quality have been associated with changes in central body fat accumulation in postmenopausal women. The Women's Health Initiative Observational Study [20], including a total of 67,175 participants who were followed up for 3 years, evaluated the association between quality of food intake and adiposity, using a food frequency questionnaire and waist circumference measures, respectively. This study concluded that 10% improvement in diet quality prevented the increase in central adiposity usually seen in the menopausal transition [20]. Vitamin D3 may also play a role in weight loss after menopause. In an RCT evaluating 218 overweight/obese women 50–75 years old participating in a weight loss program, women randomized to vitamin D3 supplementation who managed to become D3 replete showed greater reductions in BMI and abdominal circumference compared to vitamin D3-deficient women [21].

13.4.3 Diet to Prevent Sarcopenia After the Menopause

Sarcopenic obesity occurs in up to 20% of older populations and is defined as obesity in individuals with reduced muscle mass [22]. This condition is increasingly prevalent and results to a higher risk for disability and mortality in the aging population [22, 23]. In this context, dietary advice aiming at weight loss should ensure the consumption of an adequate amount of protein to avoid loss of muscle mass [22, 23].

A growing body of evidence has analyzed the effect of dietary interventions on muscle cell regeneration. Nutrients shown to prevent sarcopenia and their respective food sources are presented in Table 13.3. A muscle preserving eating pattern should include high-quality protein, derived from fish (e.g., codfish protein), dairy products (e.g., whey protein), and eggs, in quantities of approximately 25–30 g/meal. Protein should be combined with a relatively low proportion of carbohydrates, as co-ingestion of carbohydrates has been shown to exert a negative effect on protein turnover [22–24].

Table 13.3 Nutrients and food sources which promote muscle cell regeneration (Adapted from [24])

Nutrients and food sources
N-3 polyunsaturated fatty acids (n-3 PUFAs): → Fish, egg, dairy products
Polyphenols → green tea
Vitamin D3 → fish / fortified dairy products / supplements

13.4.4 Diet Recommendations for a Healthy Body Composition

A healthy diet is of paramount importance for the middle-aged woman, since it controls body weight and prevents central obesity, sarcopenia, and chronic diseases in later life [25]. Dietary recommendations for a healthy body composition include the following [25]:

- High consumption of fruits, vegetables, and fiber
- Limited consumption of saturated fats, red meat, refined carbohydrates, energy-dense food, and salt
- Consumption of at least 25–30 g protein per meal derived mainly from fish, eggs, and dairy products
- Vitamin D repletion

13.5 Physical Activity

13.5.1 Physical Activity and Aging

Regular physical activity increases longevity and quality of life and contributes to the prevention and management of chronic diseases [26]. Regular exercise has positive effects on overall health, by improving well-being, functional reserve, and performance [26]. Physical inactivity, on the other hand, leads to muscle wasting, cardiovascular deconditioning, and perception of performance loss, which further decrease physical activity and complete the "vicious circle" [26]. Unfortunately, physical inactivity is very prevalent among Europeans, with women being more inactive than men [27].

13.5.2 Physical Activity and Cardiovascular Benefits

Exercise improves various cardiovascular physiological pathways. The most important effects of exercise include a reduction of systemic inflammation, which is combined with an improvement of endothelial function and atherosclerotic plaque passivation [26]. Moreover, exercise promotes ischemic preconditioning, which prevents ischemia-induced damage. Finally, regular physical activity increases maximal oxygen uptake, which is associated with enhanced muscle metabolism, pulmonary function, functional capacity, cardiac output and stroke volume, and lower cardiovascular and all-cause mortality [26].

An increasing body of evidence has documented the cardiovascular benefit of exercise in the middle-aged female population. A recent intervention study evaluated the effect of exercise on adiposity indices and cardiovascular risk factors after the menopausal transition, in 100 healthy perimenopausal women, throughout a period of 12 months [28]. According to the findings of this study [28], women in the intervention group showed a significant decrease in waist circumference measures (changes at 6 months, intervention vs control, −0.73 ± 3.39 cm vs 1.02 ± 3.50 cm; p-value = 0.012), WHR values (changes at 6 months, intervention vs control, −0.02 ± 0.04 vs −0.003 ± 0.04; p-value = 0.020), as well as levels of systolic blood pressure (changes at 6 months, intervention vs control, −7.52 ± 13.0 mmHg vs −0.63 ± 11.69 mmHg; p-value = 0.012) compared with women in the control group. Moreover, higher physical activity has been related to a decrease in the risk of atrial fibrillation conferred by obesity, as reported in a recent sub-analysis of the Women's Health Initiative database [29]. In addition, physical activity of vigorous intensity during leisure time has been associated with a lower mortality (HR = 0.54, 95% CI 0.34–0.86) compared with exercise of low-moderate intensity (HR = 0.72, 95% CI 0.48–1.08) in middle-aged individuals [30].

13.5.3 Physical Activity, Body Weight, and Adiposity

The effect of lifestyle interventions in postmenopausal women for the prevention and management of obesity has been evaluated by various studies. The long-term effects of dietary changes combined with physical activity to induce weight loss have been assessed in the participants of the WOMAN study (The Women on the Move through Activity and Nutrition study) [31]. Lifestyle change was associated with a significant reduction in waist circumference and more weight loss compared to women receiving only health education at 30 months (lifestyle change vs health education: waist circumference, −8.3 ± 8.3 cm vs −2.8 ± 6.0 cm, p-value < 0.05; ≥10% weight loss, 31% vs 9%) [31]. Interestingly, the positive effects of lifestyle alterations on adiposity measures remained significant at 18 months after the termination of the intervention [31]. A recent systematic review [32] of five RCTs aimed to assess the effectiveness of long-term physical activity interventions among postmenopausal women with excess body weight. All five RCTs analyzed in this review concluded that simple and easy to implement exercise programs like walking or cycling improved adiposity measures, such as body weight, waist circumference, as well as percent of body fat, lean mass, subcutaneous and intra-abdominal fat, and physical functioning, e.g., peak power output, peak maximal fitness, peak relative fitness, pedometer steps, and the maximum rate of oxygen consumption [32].

13.5.4 Physical Activity and Sarcopenia

Sarcopenia, the reduction of muscle mass and strength, is a consequence of aging, physical inactivity, unhealthy low-protein diet, vitamin deficiency, and steroid hormone decline [33].

Aging leads to mitochondrial dysfunction, due to increased production of reactive oxygen species which damage mitochondrial DNA, lipids, and proteins [33]. Physical activity, on the other hand, exerts positive effects on mitochondrial function, which is mediated by the following pathways [33]:

- Improved mitochondrial protein synthesis and efficient ATP synthesis
- Reduced generation of reactive oxygen species

- Increased mitochondrial turnover
- Improved clearance of damaged mitochondria
- Decreased apoptosis

The effect of exercise on sarcopenia has been addressed by many studies. A resistance training program for 4 months resulted in a significant reduction of body fat percentage and fat body mass as well as an increase in lean body mass and muscle strength in a group of healthy postmenopausal women [34]. Similarly, combined resistance and endurance training of moderate intensity for 12 weeks improved dynamic and isometric muscle strength and decreased arterial stiffness, heart rate, and mean arterial pressure in previously inactive postmenopausal women [35].

13.5.5 Physical Activity Recommendations

The benefits of physical activity in the management of postmenopausal adiposity consist of the following:

- Increased energy expenditure
- Improved cardiorespiratory fitness, which further reduces inactivity
- Increase in muscle mass and strength which prevents sarcopenia and frailty

Recommendations regarding physical activity are summarized in Table 13.4. Physical activity should consist of at least 150 min/week of moderate intensity exercise, like walking, or at least 75 min/week of vigorous intensity exercise, like running. Table 13.5 presents examples of beneficial exercise programs which can improve cardiovascular conditioning and body composition in menopause.

Table 13.4 Recommended amount of physical exercise in the postmenopausal population (Adapted from [36])

Physical activity recommendations
At least 150 min of moderate-intensity aerobic physical activity or at least 75 min of vigorous-intensity aerobic physical activity throughout the week
Aerobic activity should be performed in bouts of at least 10 min duration
Muscle-strengthening activities should be done involving major muscle groups on 2 or more days a week

Table 13.5 Beneficial exercise programs for cardiovascular conditioning and body composition improvement in menopause

Type of exercise	Frequency	Intensity	Duration (min)	Reference
Walking	Daily	40–60% maximal heart rate	45–60	Ma et al. [37]
Swimming	3–4 times/week	Mild	30–60	Nualnum et al. [38]
Running	3–4 times/week	40–60% maximal heart rate	20–40	Williams [39]
Resistance training	3–4 times/week	50% maximal heart rate	45–60	Conceicao et al. [34]

Conclusion

Menopause and aging are independently associated with weight gain, central adiposity, and sarcopenia, conditions which increase the risk for chronic disease and disability. This risk can be dramatically reduced by appropriate lifestyle modifications, which consist of:

- Consumption of whole-grain products, fruits, and vegetables combined with enough protein intake from fish, egg, and dairy products
- Physical activity incorporated in the routine of an individual which consists of at least 150-min moderate activity or 75-min vigorous activity exercise per week

References

1. WHO (2000) Obesity: preventing and managing the global epidemic. Report of a WHO Consultation, in WHO Technical Report Series, Geneva
2. WHO (1995) Physical status: the use and interpretation of anthropometry. Report of a WHO Expert Committee1995. World Health Organ Tech Rep Ser 854:1–452
3. WHO (2014) Global status report on noncommunicable diseases, World Health Organization, Geneva 2015:p 298
4. World map of obesity. Available from: http:/www.worldobesity.org/resources/world-map-obesity/
5. Davis SR et al (2015) Menopause. Nat Rev Dis Primers 1(15004):4
6. Lizcano F, Guzmán G (2014) Estrogen deficiency and the origin of obesity during menopause. Biomed Res Int 2014:757461
7. Auro K et al (2014) A metabolic view on menopause and ageing. Nat Commun 5:4708
8. Colpani V, Oppermann K, Spritzer PM (2013) Association between habitual physical activity and lower cardiovascular risk in premenopausal, perimenopausal, and postmenopausal women: a population-based study. Menopause 20(5):525–531
9. Tchernof A, Despres JP (2013) Pathophysiology of human visceral obesity: an update. Physiol Rev 93(1):359–404
10. Davis SR et al (2012) Understanding weight gain at menopause. Climacteric 15(5):419–429
11. Nettleton JA et al (2006) Dietary patterns are associated with biochemical markers of inflammation and endothelial activation in the Multi-Ethnic Study of Atherosclerosis (MESA). Am J Clin Nutr 83(6):1369–1379
12. Liese AD et al (2010) Food intake patterns associated with carotid artery atherosclerosis in the Insulin Resistance Atherosclerosis Study. Br J Nutr 103(10):1471–1479
13. Guallar-Castillón P et al (2012) Major dietary patterns and risk of coronary heart disease in middle-aged persons from a Mediterranean country: the EPIC-Spain cohort study. Nutr Metab Cardiovasc Dis 22(3):192–199
14. Nettleton JA et al (2009) Dietary patterns and incident cardiovascular disease in the Multi-Ethnic Study of Atherosclerosis. Am J Clin Nutr 90(3):647–654
15. Romaguera D et al (2010) Mediterranean dietary patterns and prospective weight change in participants of the EPIC-PANACEA project. Am J Clin Nutr 92(4):912–921
16. Soeliman FA, Azadbakht L (2014) Weight loss maintenance: a review on dietary related strategies. J Res Med Sci 19(3):268–275
17. National Heart, Lung, and Blood Institute (2006). Your Guide to Lowering Your Blood Pressure With DASH (NIH Publication No. 06–4082)
18. Lichtenstein AH et al (2006) Diet and lifestyle recommendations revision 2006: a scientific statement from the American Heart Association Nutrition Committee. Circulation 114(1):82–96

19. Mancini JG et al (2016) Systematic review of the Mediterranean diet for long-term weight loss. Am J Med 129(4):407–415.e4
20. Cespedes Feliciano EM et al (2016) Change in dietary patterns and change in waist circumference and DXA trunk fat among postmenopausal women. Obesity 24(10):2176–2184
21. Mason C et al (2014) Vitamin D3 supplementation during weight loss: a double-blind randomized controlled trial. Am J Clin Nutr 99(5):1015–1025
22. Bouchonville MF, Villareal DT (2013) Sarcopenic obesity—how do we treat it? Curr Opin Endocrinol Diabetes Obes 20(5):412–419
23. Li Z, Heber D (2012) Sarcopenic obesity in the elderly and strategies for weight management. Nutr Rev 70(1):57–64
24. Domingues-Faria C et al (2016) Skeletal muscle regeneration and impact of aging and nutrition. Ageing Res Rev 26:22–36
25. Lambrinoudaki I et al (2012) EMAS position statement: diet and health in midlife and beyond. Maturitas 74(1):99–104
26. Gremeaux V et al (2012) Exercise and longevity. Maturitas 73(4):312–317
27. Ekelund U et al (2015) Physical activity and all-cause mortality across levels of overall and abdominal adiposity in European men and women: the European Prospective Investigation into Cancer and Nutrition Study (EPIC). Am J Clin Nutr 101(3):613–621
28. Wu L et al (2014) Effects of lifestyle intervention improve cardiovascular disease risk factors in community-based menopausal transition and early postmenopausal women in China. Menopause 21(12):1263–1268
29. Azarbal F et al (2014) Obesity, physical activity, and their interaction in incident atrial fibrillation in postmenopausal women. J Am Heart Assoc 3(4):001127
30. Lahti J et al (2014) Leisure-time physical activity and all-cause mortality. PLoS One 9(7):e101548
31. Kuller LH et al (2012) The Women on the Move Through Activity and Nutrition (WOMAN) study: final 48-month results. Obesity 20(3):636–643
32. Baker A, Sirois-Leclerc H, Tulloch H (2016) The impact of long-term physical activity interventions for overweight/obese postmenopausal women on adiposity indicators, physical capacity, and mental health outcomes: a systematic review. J Obes 2016:6169890
33. Joseph AM, Adhihetty PJ, Leeuwenburgh C (2016) Beneficial effects of exercise on age-related mitochondrial dysfunction and oxidative stress in skeletal muscle. J Physiol 594(18):5105–5123
34. Conceição MS et al (2013) Sixteen weeks of resistance training can decrease the risk of metabolic syndrome in healthy postmenopausal women. Clin Interv Aging 8:1221–1228
35. Figueroa A et al (2011) Combined resistance and endurance exercise training improves arterial stiffness, blood pressure, and muscle strength in postmenopausal women. Menopause 18(9):980–984
36. WHO. Available from: http://www.who.int/dietphysicalactivity/factsheet_adults/en/
37. Ma D, Wu L, He Z (2013) Effects of walking on the preservation of bone mineral density in perimenopausal and postmenopausal women: a systematic review and meta-analysis. Menopause 20(11):1216–1226
38. Nualnim N et al (2012) Effects of swimming training on blood pressure and vascular function in adults >50 years of age. Am J Cardiol 109(7):1005–1010
39. Williams PT (2013) Greater weight loss from running than walking during a 6.2-yr prospective follow-up. Med Sci Sports Exerc 45(4):706–713

Part IV

Bone and Cardiovascular Impact

Healthy Bones After Menopause: What Has to Be Done?

14

Martin Birkhaeuser

14.1 Introduction

Osteoporosis is one of the most frequent and most devastating diseases. Fragility fractures (minimal trauma fractures) belong to the most important morbidity and mortality causes in the elderly. Usually they occur as a result of a fall from standing height. In women, the incidence of vertebral fractures starts to rise steeply in the first years after menopause, whereas the incidence of hip fractures rises sharply around the age of 70. Globally, during the year 2000, there were an estimated 9 million new fragility fractures, of which 1.6 million were at the hip, 1.7 million at the wrist, 0.7 million at the humerus and 1.4 million symptomatic vertebral fractures [1]. In the age group of 50–80 years corresponding to the life period after menopause, around 36% of classical fragility fractures occur in those below age 65 years [2, 3]. In the UK, this amounts to more than 100,000 fractures per year in women aged 50–65 years, over 9000 of which are hip fractures ([2, 3]; www.uk2u.net). Nonetheless the importance of osteoporosis is still largely underestimated by lay people and by doctors. Prevention of osteoporotic fractures should be one of the major goals of menopause specialists.

14.1.1 Definition of Osteoporosis

Osteoporosis leads to weakness of the skeleton and increased risk of fracture. The World Health Organization (WHO) has defined osteoporosis as a systemic skeletal disease characterised by low bone mass and micro-architectural deterioration of bone tissue, with a consequent increase in bone fragility and susceptibility to fracture.

M. Birkhaeuser
Professor emeritus for Gynaecological Endocrinology and Reproductive Medicine, University of Bern, Bern, Switzerland

Postal correspondence/address: Gartenstrasse 67, CH-4052, Basel, Switzerland
e-mail: martin.birkhaeuser@balcab.ch

M. Birkhaeuser, A.R. Genazzani (eds.), *Pre-Menopause, Menopause and Beyond*, ISGE Series, https://doi.org/10.1007/978-3-319-63540-8_14

14.1.2 Epidemiology

In developed countries, lifetime risk for a normal woman aged 50 years to suffer an osteoporotic fracture at any place is 52.3% [1, 4–8], and the likelihood of a fracture at any of the four major sites (spine, femoral neck, wrist, proximal humerus) is 40% or more. Forty per cent is close to the probability of coronary heart disease. In a woman at the menopause, the remaining lifetime probability after a major fracture is less favourable than the one after breast cancer.

14.1.2.1 Vertebral Fractures

Vertebral fractures remain most of the time ignored, even if they cause pain. Less than 10% result in hospitalisation [9, 10]. They may cause acute pain, loss of function and loss of quality of life but may also occur without serious symptoms. They occur typically in the mid-thoracic or thoracolumbar regions of the spine [9]. In Europe, the prevalence defined by radiological criteria increases with age and is 12% in females (range 6–21%). The age-standardised incidence of morphometric fracture is 10.7 per 1000 person-years in women [11], increasing markedly with age. Vertebral fractures often recur. New fractures are most likely in nearby vertebrae. The consequent disability increases with the number of fractures.

14.1.2.2 Distal Forearm (Wrist) Fractures

In Europe, the annual incidences of distal forearm fractures in female were 7.3 per 1000 person-years in 2002 [12]. Wrist fractures are most likely to occur in women over 65 years old. There is an increase in age adjusted between 45 and 60 years of age. Then the trend stabilises or slightly increases. Functional recovery of distal radial fractures is usually good or excellent [12].

14.1.2.3 Humerus Fractures

No reliable figures are available.

14.1.2.4 Hip Fractures

The worldwide annual incidence of hip fracture is approximately 1.7 million [13]. They are more common in northern than in southern countries. This might be due to a different duration, intensity and efficiency of sunlight in stimulating vitamin D production in the skin. The sex ratio of hip fractures F/M is 4/5. 90% of the hip fractures occur in people over 50 years old [14]. Hip fracture is associated with serious disability and excess mortality. Women who have sustained a hip fracture have a 10–20% higher mortality than would be expected for their age [15]. Recovery is slow and rehabilitation is often incomplete, with many patients permanently institutionalised in nursing homes.

14.2 General Prevention of Fragility Fractures

General prevention of osteoporosis and fragility fractures is not restricted to women at risk. It is of utmost importance that general preventive measures are undertaken even without diagnostic investigations to reduce the incidence of osteoporosis and of fragility fractures.

Primary prevention of osteoporosis includes all measures preventing the occurrence of osteoporosis. Primary prevention starts in adolescence. Its target is to obtain an optimal peak bone mass in adolescence and young adulthood, to slow down the physiological decrease of bone mineral density (BMD) after menopause up to the advanced age and to avoid a pathological loss of bone mass leading to osteoporosis.

Secondary prevention aims at the hindrance of fracture occurrence manifestation in already osteoporotic women. In contrast to primary prevention, secondary prevention usually demands a complete investigation before preventive measures can be started. Often a specific treatment has to be initiated being beyond the scope of the field of postmenopausal osteoporosis.

General prevention ensuring a normal bone metabolism includes [16–18]:

14.2.1 Supplementation with Vitamin D

- 50–70% of adults living in developed countries are undersupplied with vitamin D [19]. In elderly patients suffering from an acute hip fracture, more than 50% display a severe vitamin D deficiency (25-hydroxy-vitamin D = 25-OHD < 30 nmol/l). Less than 5% reach the actually recommended target for an optimal prevention of fractures and falls of 75 nmol/l (30 ng/ml) [20].
- In postmenopausal women, 800–1000 IU vit D/day is needed, in the elderly up to 2000 IU/day. 25(OH)D values should be maintained above the required serum level of 75 nmol/l (30 ng/ml). Vitamin D supplementation improves also muscle strength in the lower limbs, reducing the risk of falls by 20% [21–23]. In addition, vitamin D reduces the incidence of all cancers by 17% and cancer mortality by 29% [24, 25]. It may reduce the incidence of arterial hypertension to about 30% [26], the risk of myocardial infarction to about 50% and cardiovascular mortality to less than 50% [27, 28]. However, RCT confirming these preliminary findings are still missing.
- The safe upper limit for the daily intake of vitamin D is 4000 IU for adults and for children above the age of 9 years [29]. Therefore, all dosages recommended by the various guidelines available today are within the safe range.

14.2.2 Total Calcium Intake

Calcium intake should reach 1000–1200 mg/day. Mostly this target can be reached by a balanced nutrition and by the use of drinking water rich in calcium. An additional calcium supplementation should only be prescribed if an adequate calcium intake cannot be reached by nutrition. An excessive calcium intake >1500 mg/day may lead to an increased cardiovascular risk, particularly in the presence of renal insufficiency [30–34].

14.2.3 Protein Intake

A minimal protein intake of 1 g/kg body weight per day should be guaranteed for the maintenance of the musculoskeletal function. Protein deficiency and underweight (body mass index < 20 kg/m^2) due to an inadequate nutrition are risk factors for osteoporotic fractures [16, 17, 35, 36]. Weight increase leads to a risk reduction. After an osteoporotic fracture, a protein supply of at least 1 g protein/kg body weight per day reduces the rate of complications such as decubitus, severe anaemia and infections of the lung and the kidney and thus the days of hospitalisation [37].

14.2.4 Physical Activity, Prevention of Falls, Healthy Lifestyle

Regular physical activity and prevention of falls are indispensable in the elderly. The goal is the stimulation of muscle strength and the coordination of movements [16, 17, 35, 38]. Immobilisation should be avoided if ever possible. After the age of 70 years, a history of falls should be taken every year. In case of an increased risk, the causes have to be investigated. Trip hazards at home have to be eliminated, and the use of psychotropic substances and the abuse of alcohol and nicotine avoided.

14.3 How to Recognise Postmenopausal Women at Increased Risk

14.3.1 Medical History and Clinical Findings

The most relevant fracture risk factors [16, 17] are based on family and personal history as well as on the presence of other diseases (secondary causes of osteoporosis). Their clinical importance, in function of the available evidence (grading A–D), is presented in Table 14.1 [16].

The *specific questions* to be asked concern the following domains:

- General well-being and alimentation (including vitamin D and calcium deficiency, alcohol and drug addiction). Sleeping pills and tranquillisers are both increasing the risk of falls.
- History of fractures and of falls, subjective complaints and sudden back pain.
- Diseases and intake of drugs known to have an impact on bone metabolism and/or equilibrium, such as seizure medication, immunosuppressive drugs, glucocorticoids, heparin, lithium and excess thyroxine (thyroid replacement).

The *clinical examination* has to be targeted at signs of osteoporosis and of increased risk of falls:

- Body height and weight (BMI): is there a decrease of body height > 3 cm?
- Deformities of the spine and other signs for a vertebral compression fracture. This often results in the curvature of the spine at the shoulders. In older people, this is sometimes called a 'widow's hump' or a 'dowager's hump'.
- Indications for other fractures.
- Signs pointing to a secondary osteoporosis or a malignancy.
- Signs pointing to an increased risk of falls, such as poor sight, muscle weakness, poor equilibrium and coordination and neurological affections.

Table 14.1 Clinical risk factors associated with an increased fracture risk in women [16]

Women, age	<50 years	50–60 years	>60 years
Vertebral fractures	+ (D)	+ (A)	+ (A)
Oral glucocorticoids >5.0 mg/d Prednisolon equivalents >3 months	+ (A)	+ (A)	+ (A)
Cushing syndrome	+ (B)	+ (B)	+ (A)
Primary hyperparathyroidism (pHPT)	+ (B)	+ (B)	+ (B)
Hypogonadismus (incl. premature menopause)	+ (D)	+ (B)	+ (B)
Therapy with glitazones	+ (D)	+ (A)	
Non-vertebral fracture(s) after the age of 50	**	+ (A)	
Therapy with aromatase inhibitors		**	+ (A)
Anti-androgen therapy		**	+ (A)
Rheumatoid arthritis		**	+ (A)
Proximal fracture of the hip in one parent			+ (A)
Low body weight (BMI < 20)			+ (A)
Current cigarette smoking			+ (A)
High alcohol intake (>2 units/day)		+ (A)	+ (A)
Multiple falls (more than 1 within the last 12 months)			+ (A)
Immobility (cannot leave the house without help by someone else)			+ (A–B)
Diabetes mellitus type 1			+ (A)
TSH levels <0.3 mU/l			+ (B)

**To be decided case by case, see www.SVGO.ch [16]+Indication for diagnostic intervention (DXA, poss. additional laboratory investigation)A–D: evidence grading:A: At least one study of evidence 1a, or several concordant studies of evidence 1bB: At least one study of evidence 2a or 3a, or several concordant studies of evidence 2b, 2c or 3bC: At least one study of evidence 3b, or several concordant studies of evidence 4D: No study of evidence 4 or better, only studies of evidence 5

14.3.2 Additional Diagnostic Steps and Diagnosis of Osteoporosis

In all women with the suspicion of an increased fracture risk on the basis of their medical history or of clinical signs, additional diagnostic steps are recommended [16, 17, 35]. The diagnosis of osteoporosis is based on the presence of fragility fractures or (in women without prevalent fractures) on the results of the measurement of bone mineral density (BMD).

14.3.2.1 Conventional X-Ray (Fracture Detection)

Traditional X-rays can identify suspected spine fractures. Assessment of vertebral fractures is recommended in case of acute newly developed back pain, if strong and/or unchanged for several days, and in unexplained chronic back pain. To diagnose, X-rays of the thoracic and lumbar spine (a/p and lateral image, depending on clinical examination and fracture evaluation) are done, for follow-up usually lateral image only. Today, vertebral fracture assessment by DXA (VFA) is also regarded as adequate. VFA has a lower radiation exposure (3 μSV only) than X-ray, but its image quality is lower.

14.3.2.2 Densitometry by Dual-Energy X-Ray Absorptiometry (DXA) for the Measurement of BMD

Without a suspicion of vertebral fracture, the first diagnostic step is the determination of BMD by DXA. According to the WHO, DXA (dual-energy X-ray absorptiometry) is still the gold standard for the measurement of bone mineral density (BMD) and for the diagnosis of osteoporosis [16, 17, 35, 39]. DXA is usually performed at the lumbar spine and the hip. It is recommended in the presence of vertebral fracture(s), peripheral fracture(s) and secondary causes and risk factors. At the lumbar spine, the average *T*-score is determined by a measurement of those vertebrae of L1–L4 on which it is possible to make an evaluation. At least two vertebrae must be assessable. Assessment is impaired in spondylophytes, vertebral fractures, severe degenerative changes (>grade 2 according to Kellgren), significant scoliosis and torsion scoliosis as well as atherosclerosis.

The results of DXA measurements are express as *T*-score (Table 14.2). The recommended reference range (IOF) is the NHANES III reference database [39–41]. For diagnostic purposes, the *Z*-score is only used in premenopausal women.

The prevalence of low BMD and of osteoporosis rises with increasing age. At the age of 80 years, 50% of all healthy women have a *T*-score of ≤2.5 and are therefore osteoporotic. There is a significant correlation between age and *T*-score at the femoral neck and the absolute 10-year fracture risk. But normal BMD or osteopenia do not protect against hip fractures [8, 17, 35, 42, 43] (Table 14.3).

Table 14.2 Densitometric classification at the spine or at the hip of osteoporosis by DXA measurement

Status	Hip BMD
Normal	*T*-score of −1 or above
Osteopenia	*T*-score lower than −1 and greater than −2.5
Osteoporosis	*T*-score of −2.5 or lower
Severe (established) osteoporosis	*T*-score of −2.5 or lower, and the presence of at least one fragility fracture

The World Health Organization has defined a number of threshold values (measurements) for osteoporosis. The reference measurement is derived from bone density measurements in a population of healthy young adults (called a *T*-score). Osteoporosis is diagnosed when a person's BMD is equal to or more than 2.5 standard deviations below this reference measurement [16, 17] Osteopenia is diagnosed when the measurement is between 1 and 2.5 standard deviations below the young adult reference measurement

Table 14.3 Relation between bone mineral density (BMD) and fracture risk

BMD	*N* (total)	10 years fracture incidence	Number of women with fractures (%)
Normal	204	7%	15 (11%)
Osteopenia	322	21%	67 (50%)
Osteoporosis	142	37%	52 (39%)
All women	668	20%	134 (100%)

Data from: OFELY study [42]

Limitation to the Use of DXA Osteodensitometry by DXA is not a cost-effective screening method. It should be used selectively in function of age and other relevant risk factors.

14.3.2.3 Alternative Procedures to Evaluate Bone Density

Quantitative ultrasound measurements and peripheral BMD can also provide information about the fracture risk [16, 17, 35]. However, before starting osteoporosis treatment, a measurement of BMD by DXA cannot be replaced by ultrasound measurements.

14.3.2.4 Scintigraphy

In case of suspicion of a malignancy, *scintigraphy of the skeleton* is recommended (exception: the first step in a suspicion for multiple myeloma is a MRI).

14.3.3 Evaluation of Fracture Risk by FRAX©

The individual 10-year risk of osteoporotic fractures can be evaluated by a computer-based algorithm, the Fracture Risk Assessment Tool (FRAX©, www.sheffield.ac.uk/FRAX/; 38, 44, 45). FRAX© is a scientifically validated risk assessment tool, endorsed by the World Health Organization. It exists in specific versions for most countries, established by using local epidemiological data. FRAX© is based on age and on individual risk factors. It can be calculated with or without BMD value at the femoral neck. Use of FRAX© without BMD is appropriate when BMD is not available or if individuals should be identified who may benefit from a BMD measurement [16, 17, 35, 38, 44, 45]. Where DXA is available, BMD testing can be performed alongside the assessment of fracture probability using clinical risk factors. Measurements other than BMD or *T*-score at the femoral neck by DXA are not recommended for use in FRAX©. FRAX© with BMD predicts fracture risk better than clinical risk factors or BMD alone.

However, there are three important limitations to the use of FRAX®: FRAX® can only be used in women ≥40 years of age and without a treatment of osteoporosis; it is not appropriate to use FRAX© to monitor treatment response; fracture severity cannot be quantified in FRAX© (for additional clinically relevant limitations, see ref. 38, 44, 46).

The *intervention level* based on the 10-year fracture probability (%) calculated by FRAX is increasing from the age of 50 to the age of 85 [17, 38, 44, 45]. Figure 14.1 shows the intervention threshold set at a fracture probability equivalent to a woman with a previous fragility fracture. If DXA has not yet been done, BMD testing is recommended in individuals in whom fracture probabilities (assessed from clinical risk factors alone) are close to the intervention threshold (left-hand panel). This minimises the risk of misclassifying a high-risk patient as low risk and vice versa.

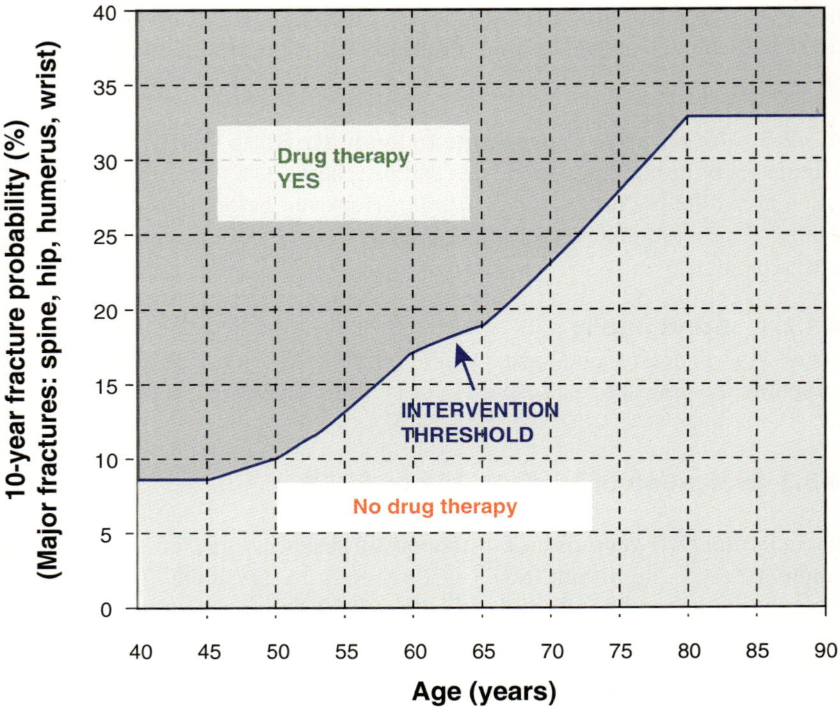

10-year fracture probability (FRAX®; %
(Major fractures: spine, hip, humerus, wrist)

Age			
50 years	≥ 10%	**55 years**	≥ 13%
60 years	≥ 17%	**65 years**	≥ 20%
70 years	≥ 23%	**75 years**	≥ 28%
≥ 80 years	≥ 33%		

Fig. 14.1 Intervention in women without fractures [16]

14.3.4 Other Diagnostic Steps

Biochemical analysis should be done in the presence of fractures combined with indications from medical history and/or clinical examinations for particular fracture risks due for secondary osteoporosis. In this review, the further diagnostic steps in secondary osteoporosis are not discussed (see [16, 17, 35]).

Bone Turnover Markers Although bone turnover markers (BTMs) may predict fracture risk independently from BMD in postmenopausal women, they are not used for screening purposes [16, 17, 35]. BTMs are used for monitoring treatment in the individual. As adherence is an important issue of long-term therapy in chronic disease, some BTM (mainly s-CTX and s-PINP) may be used in clinical practice to assess the patient's adherence to treatment [17, 47, 48].

Clinical Diagnostic Tests The evaluation of muscle strength and coordination is important in elderly women prone to falls. The risk of falls can be effectively evaluated by examinations such as the 'timed up and go test' or the 'chair-rising test' in combination with the 'tandem stance test' (for further information, see DVO (www.dv-osteologie.org; [16, 17, 35])).

14.4 Menopausal Hormone Therapy (MHT) Including Tibolone for Fracture Prevention

14.4.1 Oestrogen and Oestrogen + Progestin

14.4.1.1 Efficacy

Bone architecture and quality has to be maintained as early as in the peri- and early postmenopause. Prescription of MHT for primary prevention of fragility fractures should be part of an overall preventive strategy including general preventive measures and lifestyle recommendations (see above). In peri- and postmenopausal women at risk of fracture and younger than 60 years or within 10 years of menopause ('window of opportunity'), the International Menopause Society (IMS) recommendations on MHT and preventive strategies for midlife health, updated in 2016 [49], consider *MHT as one of the first-line therapies for the prevention and treatment of osteoporosis-related fractures*, because a first vertebral fracture should be avoided. Although treatment of osteoporosis can reduce the increased risk for a subsequent fracture, it cannot eliminate the excess risk of a first fracture.

Oestrogen deficiency leads to a rapid loss of BMD. Already before 2002, some RCTs, many observational studies and several meta-analyses documented that MHT prevents menopausal bone loss when begun around or early after menopause [50–53]. In contrast to all trials done with selective oestrogen receptor modulators (SERMs), bisphosphonates, denosumab or strontium ranelate, the WHI trial using MHT is the first RCT demonstrating that a therapeutic intervention reduces the risk of fractures in women without increased fracture risk at the hip, vertebrae and wrist and with mean *T*-scores in the normal to osteopenic range [49, 54–59]. These data are consistent with the earlier observational data and meta-analyses mentioned above [50–53]. In the CEE + MPA study, active therapy reduced (in the global analyses) all fractures significantly by 24% (RR, 0.76; 95% CI, 0.69–0.83) and hip fractures by 33% (95% CI, 0.47–0.96). In the CEE-alone study, CEE reduced all fractures by 29% (RR, 0.71; 95% CI, 0.45–0.94) and hip fractures by 29% (RR, 0.71; 95% CI, 0.64–0.80) (see Table 14.4; [54, 56]). Regarding the effect of therapy on all fractures, a beneficial effect was seen in all groups categorised by decade after menopause. If the fracture data are analysed both by decade of age and by decade after menopause, the MHT effect on hip fractures (but not on vertebral fractures)

Table 14.4 WHI: Effect of CEE + MPA and CEE alone on fracture risk

	CEE + MPA [54] HR (95% CI)[a]	CEE alone [57] HR (95% CI)[a]
Hip	0.67 (0.47–0.96)	0.65 (0.45–0.94)
Spine	0.65 (0.46–0.92)	0.64 (0.44–0.93)
Forearm/Wrist	0.71 (0.59–0.85)	0.58 (0.47–0.72)
Total	0.76 (0.69–0.83)	0.71 (0.64–0.80)

[a]Hazard ratio (nominal 95% confidence interval)

Table 14.5 Terminologies for dosing of different oestrogens in hormone replacement preparations. Available doses may vary in different countries. Bioequivalence not tested (modified from [60])

	High	Moderate	Low	Ultra-low
Conjugated equine estrogens (mg)	1.25/0.9[a]	0.625	0.3/0.45	
Micronized 17β-estradiol (mg)	4.0	2.0	1.0	0.5
Estradiol valerate (mg)		2.0	1.0	
Transdermal 17β-estradiol (µg)	100	50	25	14[a]

[a]Just one per oral (0.9 mg conjugated equine oestrogens) and one transdermal (14 µg 17β-oestradiol) product available in the USA only. 14 µg 17β-oestradiol is indicated only for prevention of osteoporosis

was only apparent in women older than age 70 years or more than 20 years after menopause, consistent with the epidemiological data concerning hip fracture.

14.4.1.2 Low-Dose and Ultra-low-Dose Administration of MHT

Low-dose and ultra-low-dose oestrogen administration (Table 14.5) has been shown to be effective for the treatment of climacteric symptoms, particularly hot flushes [49, 50, 59–61]. It has been postulated that lower than moderate doses might be effective also for the prevention of osteoporosis [62–68]. An ultra-low-dose oestrogen patch (14 µg oestradiol transdermally per day) has been licensed for osteoporosis prevention by the US Food and Drugs Administration, but not in Europe. However, the percentage of so-called non-responders (>2% of bone loss at the lumbar spine within 26 lunar months) is increasing in parallel to dose reduction [69]. It reaches 3% in the moderate, 8% in the low-dose, 13–22% in the ultra-low-dose regimen and 51% in the placebo group [69]. Furthermore, there is no evidence for fracture reduction with lower than standard dosages. In addition, for low- and ultra-low-dose regimens, no long-term data are available concerning cardiovascular and oncological risks.

Therefore, the efficacy of lower than standard oestrogen administration on bone has to be controlled by the determination of serum bone markers (approx. at 3 months) and later by DXA measurements of BMD (at 2 years after initiating MHT) if MHT has been given for prevention of bone loss.

14.4.1.3 Cost-Effectiveness

The numbers of women on CEE alone or CEE + MPA in the WHI trials can be expressed as the number of women whose fractures were prevented over a 5-year period of use. For CEE alone, this represents 27.1 women per 1000 per 5 years, and for CEE + MPA, 21.8. women per 1000 per 5 years. Therefore, MHT use for osteoporosis prevention and primary prevention of fragility fractures is cost-effective [70]. MHT is a first-line treatment for fracture prevention in younger postmenopausal women, with or without increased risk.

14.4.1.4 Continuation of MHT After the Age of 60 Years

The evidence does not support any restrictions imposed on MHT when given as a bone-specific drug. Continuation of MHT for the indication offracture prevention is fully justified: there are no reasons to place arbitrary limitations on the duration of MHT [49, 59] provided that MHT is individualised and tailored according to symptoms and the needs of the patient. Whether or not to continue therapy should be decided at the discretion of the well-informed woman and her health professional.

14.4.1.5 Consequence of Oestrogen Discontinuation on Bone

Discontinuation of oestrogens results in bone loss at a rate similar to that seen in early menopause [71–75], but the once gained preventive effect is maintained. The PERF study [75] demonstrated at 5, 11 and 15 years after stopping MHT that administration of oestrogens in early postmenopause offers a significant long-lasting benefit for the prevention of postmenopausal bone loss and osteoporotic fracture. In PERF, odds ratio (OR) for fractures at 15 years is 0.48 (CI 0.26–0.88) in former oestrogen users. In PERF, the number needed to treat to prevent any fracture is 7 [75]. PERF has been confirmed by the WHI study [76, 77]. In the CEE + MPA arm, fracture reduction continues significantly for 13 years after the end of the intervention phase (OR 0.81; 95% CI, 0.68–0.97), in the CEE-only arm non-significantly (OR 0.91; 95% CI, 0.72–1.15). This risk reduction corresponds to −5 and −2 cases, respectively, per 10,000 women-years [76].

In contrast to the restart of bone loss after discontinuation of MHT, gains in bone mass induced by alendronate (with or without oestrogen) are sustained for at least 1 year after all therapy was discontinued [102]. These data underscore the different mechanisms by which bisphosphonates and oestrogens affect bone remodelling.

14.4.1.6 Initiation of MHT for Bone Protection After the Age of 60 Years

Initiation of MHT after the age of 60 years for the indication of fracture prevention is considered second-line therapy and requires individually calculated benefit/risk, compared to other approved drugs. If MHT is elected, the lowest effective dose should be used.

14.4.1.7 Safety Concerns

Healthy women younger than 60 years should not be unduly concerned about the safety profile of MHT where there are indications for its use. The available evidence suggests that there is a probable therapeutic window of benefit for long-term fracture prevention as well as cardioprotection and possibly for aspects of long-term neuroprotection if MHT is prescribed in midlife and continued for several years. Initiated within this 'window of opportunity', the benefits of MHT outbalance the risks [49, 50, 59].

14.4.2 Tibolone

Tibolone is a synthetic steroid belonging to the progestogen family of 19-nortestosterone derivatives. Tibolone is a prodrug. Its three active metabolites 3-alpha-hydroxy-tibolone, 3-beta-hydroxy-tibolone and delta^4-isomer metabolite possess an affinity to oestrogen, progesterone and androgen receptors [78]. Tibolone has properties of E + P as well as of a SERM [78]. The International Menopause Society (IMS) classes tibolone among the substances suitable for menopausal hormonal therapy [49, 50]. The effects of Tibolone on breast are discussed in chapter 4.

Tibolone is given per orally and is effective for the prevention of osteoporosis and fractures. There is evidence in elderly women for its significant reduction of the incidence of vertebral and non-vertebral fractures [78–81]. In the LIFT trial, a RCT in older women (mean age 68.3; range 60–85 years) having an increased fracture risk (*T*-score of −2.5 or less at the hip or spine or a *T*-score of −2.0 or less and radiological evidence of a vertebral fracture), the effect of a low-dose treatment by tibolone 1.25 mg/day (half of the usual dosage) has been compared to placebo [79]. After 34 months (mean) of tibolone administration, a significant reduction of the risk of vertebral (RR, 0.55; 95% CI, 0.41–0.74; $p < 0.001$) and non-vertebral (RR, 0.74; 95% CI, 0.58–0.93; $p = 0.01$) fractures was observed.

14.5 Fracture Prevention with SERMs

Selective oestrogen receptor modulators (SERMs) are not steroid hormones such as oestradiol, but their non-steroidal structure is such that they are able to bind to the oestrogen receptor where they possess agonistic as well as antagonistic properties [18, 50]. In 1998, the first modern SERM, raloxifene, has been registered for prevention and treatment of osteoporosis, followed in 2009 by lasofoxifene and in 2011 by bazedoxifene. In Europe, only raloxifene and bazedoxifene are available on the market for osteoporosis prevention.

14.5.1 Raloxifene

In postmenopausal women with osteoporosis, raloxifene at a dose of 60 mg per day was associated with reduced risks of vertebral fractures and ER-positive breast cancer, an adequate endometrium protection, but an increased risk of venous thromboembolic events and no detectable effect on the endometrium. In a meta-analysis of seven clinical trials [82], raloxifene (60 mg/day) reduced the risk for vertebral fractures at the average significantly by 40% (RR 0.60; 95% CI 0.49–0.74). Raloxifene reduced vertebral fracture risk in the presence of osteoporosis as well as of osteopenia [83]. Another more recent meta-analysis concluded that the effect on the risk for vertebral fractures calculated by FRAX® is greater in younger than in older women [84]. There is evidence that the preventive effect of raloxifene at the spine still continues at 8 years after treatment initiation [50, 82–84]. On the other hand, for raloxifene, there is no direct evidence that it decreases hip fracture risk. A reduction of the risk for non-vertebral fractures and hip fractures has only been shown in post hoc analyses in women with prevalent vertebral fractures [50, 82–84]. An important beneficial side effect of raloxifene treatment is the reduction of oestrogen receptor (ER)-positive breast cancer. In the USA (but not in Europe), raloxifene is also licensed for prevention of breast cancer.

14.5.2 Bazedoxifene

Bazedoxifene was associated with a significant 39% decrease in incident morphometric vertebral fractures (hazard ratio HR = 0.61; 95% CI = 0.43–0.86; $\boldsymbol{p} = 0.005$) and a non-statistically significant 16% decrease in all clinical fractures (hazard ratio HR = 0.84; 95% CI = 0.67–1.06; $\boldsymbol{p} = 0.14$) compared to placebo [85–87]. In a 2-year extension of the 3-year study [88], bazedoxifene showed sustained efficacy in preventing new vertebral fractures in postmenopausal women with osteoporosis and in preventing non-vertebral fractures in higher-risk women. At 5 years, the incidence of new vertebral fractures in the intent-to-treat population was significantly lower with bazedoxifene 20 mg (4.5%) and 40/20 mg (3.9%) versus placebo (6.8%; $p < 0.05$), with relative risk reductions of 35% and 40%, respectively.

Non-vertebral fracture incidence was similar among groups. In a subgroup of higher-risk women ($n = 1324$; femoral neck T-score ≤ -3.0 and/or ≥ 1 moderate or severe or ≥ 2 mild vertebral fracture(s)), bazedoxifene 20 mg reduced non-vertebral fracture risk versus placebo (37%; $p = 0.06$); combined data for bazedoxifene 20 and 40/20 mg reached statistical significance (34% reduction; $p < 0.05$).

14.5.3 Bazedoxifene + CEE

In women with a uterus, bazedoxifene can be used to oppose the stimulatory effects of conjugated equine oestrogens (CEE) on the endometrium. This combination not yet available in Europe, also known as tissue-selective oestrogen complex, has been shown to prevent the bone loss associated with menopause, but the effect on fracture reduction has not been explored [89].

14.6 Non-hormonal Anti-resorptive Therapies and Osteo-anabolic Treatment

Initiation of MHT in the age group 60–70 years requires an individually calculated benefit/risk ratio and the consideration of other available drugs. MHT should not be initiated after age 70 years. Therefore, in elderly women non-hormonal anti-resorptive substances are becoming the first-line therapeutic methods.

14.6.1 Bisphoshonates

Nitrogen-containing bisphosphonates are potent inhibitors of bone resorption. They have been proven in numerous randomised controlled outcome trials (RCTs) in postmenopausal osteoporosis to reduce significantly the incidence of fragility fractures [90–92]. They are suitable first-line treatments for women with postmenopausal osteoporosis. After the age of 60 years, alendronate, risedronate, ibandronate and zoledronic acid all provide fracture protection for patients with postmenopausal osteoporosis [93–96]. Ibandronate and zoledronic acid have the most persistent anti-fracture effect.

For *alendronate*, a meta-analysis of 11 RCTs [93] confirmed the significant reduction of vertebral fractures observed in the FIT trial. For vertebral fractures, the pooled estimate for prevention trials ($n = 1355$; RR, 95% CI) was 0.45 (0.06–3.15), the pooled estimate for treatment trial ($n = 8005$; RR, 95% CI) 0.53 (0.43–0.65) and the global pooled estimate ($n = 9360$; RR, 95% CI) 0.52 (0.43–0.65). The risk ratios for non-vertebral fractures with alendronate (10 mg and greater) decreased significantly for the global pooled estimate (RR 0.51; 95% CI 0.38–0.69).

In osteoporotic postmenopausal women, per oral *risedronate* 5 mg daily, oral risedronate (delayed-release 35 mg) once weekly or 75 mg risedronate monthly has been shown to possess a high efficacy in preventing vertebral, non-vertebral and hip fractures in osteoporotic women, along with increased safety and tolerability [94]. In osteopenia, risedronate increases significantly BMD and, as shown by a post hoc analysis, reduces significantly fragility fractures (combined morphometric vertebral and non-vertebral fractures) [94].

Ibandronate reduces the risk of vertebral fractures by 50–60% [95]. For ibandronate, an effect on non-vertebral fractures was only demonstrated in a post hoc analysis of women with a baseline of BMD *T*-score below −3 SD. There are no adequate data showing a significant reduction of hip fractures [95].

Zoledronic acid [96] is a long-acting bisphoshonate. A once-yearly infusion of zoledronic acid during a 3-year period is associated with a significant and sustained decrease in the risk of vertebral, non-vertebral and hip fractures. In postmenopausal women with osteoporosis, zoledronic acid reduces over 3 years the risk of vertebral and hip fracture by 70% and 41%, respectively, versus placebo. The 70% reduction in the vertebral fracture rate was greater than the 3-year reduction previously observed for oral bisphosphonates (40–50%). Intravenous zoledronic acid decreases the risk of fracture and of mortality when given shortly after a first hip fracture. Zoledronic acid has a favourable safety profile. Most side effects are the well-documented association between oral bisphosphonates and gastrointestinal adverse events, as well as between acute phase reactions and intravenous administration. Serious adverse effects such as atypical subtrochanteric fracture and osteonecrosis of the jaw are very rare in women receiving bisphosphonates for fracture prevention in the presence of postmenopausal osteoporosis, and not for oncological indications [97, 98].

14.6.2 Adherence, Drug Holiday

Adherence may be insufficient in some patients treated by oral drugs. In these patients, the administration of non-oral bisphosphonates or denosumab is recommended.

In women with low fracture risk, a 'drug holiday' after 5–10 years of bisphosphonate treatment has been recommended. Limited data suggest that patients at lower risk can start a drug holiday after 5 years of oral or 3 years of intravenous bisphosphonate treatment, whereas patients at higher risk should continue oral treatment for 10 years or intravenous treatment for at least 6 years [99]. Patients at low risk may remain off treatment as long as bone mineral density is stable and no fractures occur, whereas women at very high risk of clinical vertebral fractures may benefit by continuing bisphosphonates beyond 5 years.

14.6.3 Denosumab

Denosumab [100–103] is a humanised monoclonal antibody that works by decreasing the activity of the receptor activator of nuclear factor kappa-B ligand. In contrast to bisphosphonates, denosumab has a short half-life so that its anti-resorptive effects as well as its adverse effects are rapidly reversible. Denosumab is given as a subcutaneous injection in a physician's office (60 mg every 6 months). This might lead to a better adherence to therapy. Denosumab reduces median bone formation rate to zero after 2–3 years use. In postmenopausal women, denosumab increased BMD at 3 years in the spine, the hip and the distal third of the radius and decreased vertebral, non-vertebral and hip fractures. Over 8 years, mean BMD continued to increase significantly at each time point measured, for cumulative 8-year gains of 18.4 and 8.3% at the lumbar spine and total hip, respectively. Continuous use of denosumab to 8 years maintains the reduced fracture rates and appears to be safe [100]. The relative risk of serious adverse events is low. Osteonecrosis of the jaw has only been seen in cancer patients receiving very high doses of denosumab.

The effects of denosumab are not sustained when treatment is stopped, so there is no drug holiday with this medication [104]. There are reports showing that BMD may decrease very rapidly after stopping Denosumab, leading to early fractures.

14.6.4 Strontium Ranelate

Strontium ranelate [105, 106] has both a mild anabolic effect and a mild anti-resorptive effect on bone tissue. Administered for 5 years, it produces significant reductions in the incidence of non-vertebral, hip and vertebral fractures in postmenopausal women with osteoporosis. Long-term treatment with strontium ranelate is associated with sustained increases in BMD over 10 years. During post-marketing surveillance, some rare but serious side effects have been reported. Because of the increased risk for myocardial infarction and venous thromboembolic events observed in post-marketing surveillance, EMA recommended in 2014 that strontium ranelate should only be used for the treatment of severe osteoporosis in postmenopausal women at high risk of fracture [107].

14.6.5 Parathyroid Hormone

Parathyroid hormone (PTH [1–84]) and human recombinant PTH [1–34] (teriparatide) [108, 109] are the only anabolic agents available today. They work by promoting bone formation (osteo-anabolic therapies). Teriparatide reduces efficiently the risk of new vertebral and non-vertebral fractures in postmenopausal women with and without prior fractures. The efficacy of teriparatide to prevent corticosteroid-induced osteoporosis is higher than the one of bisphosphonates. Its use is only limited by its high price. With sequential treatment, BMD gain is maintained or increased with alendronate or with raloxifene, but lost if parathyroid hormone or teriparatide is not followed by an anti-resorptive agent. These findings have clinical implications for therapeutic choices after the discontinuation of teriparatide or parathyroid hormone: sequential therapy after teriparatide or PTH is mandatory although fracture data are missing.

Conclusion

The goal of osteoporosis treatment is the prevention of fracture. DXA measurement of BMD is the gold standard for the diagnosis of osteoporosis and osteopenia (*T*-score of ≤ -2.5 osteoporosis or *T*-score of $< -1.04 > -2.5$ osteopenia).

Postmenopausal women need a dietary reference intake (DRI) of 1000–1500 mg of elemental calcium, of 800–1000 IU Vit D (in elderly women up to 2000 IU) and a minimal protein intake of 1 g/kg body weight per day. Regular physical activity, prevention of falls and a healthy lifestyle are indispensable in the elderly. Choice of therapy should be based on a balance of effectiveness, risk and cost. Intervention thresholds for therapy can be based on 10-year fracture probability but will be country specific. The individual 10-year risk of osteoporotic fractures can be evaluated by a computer-based algorithm, the Fracture Risk Assessment Tool (FRAX©). FRAX© allows to calculate the *intervention level* based on the 10-year fracture probability (%). The intervention level is increasing from the age of 50 to the age of 85.

MHT is the first choice for fracture prevention in women <60 years and/or less than 10 years from menopause [111]. In postmenopausal women with a simultaneously increased breast cancer risk, SERMs should be preferred. MHT decreases fracture risk at all vertebral and non-vertebral localisations including significantly by 25–40% [110]. The option of MHT (including tibolone) or selective oestrogen receptor modulators (SERMs) is an individual decision in terms of quality of life and health priorities as well as personal risk factors such as age or time since menopause and the risk of diseases, such as venous thromboembolism and stroke (both are not increased in transdermal MHT), ischemic heart disease and breast cancer [110, 111]. MHT has been shown to be an effective treatment for the primary prevention of fracture at all sites in healthy and in at-risk women before the age of 60 years or within 10 years after menopause [50, 90 110, 111]. Within this window of opportunity, the benefits of MHT outbalance the risks.

In women aged 60 years or more and in women with a contraindication against MHT, non-hormonal anti-resorptive therapies such as bisphosphonates or denosumab are first-choice treatments [110]. If costs are considered without taking into account adherence, some older bisphosphonates have the best cost/benefit ratio. Following the recommendation of EMA, strontium ranelate should only be used for the treatment of severe osteoporosis in postmenopausal women at high risk of fracture.

For economic reasons, the anabolic agent teriparatide is reserved for the treatment of severe osteoporosis.

References

1. Johnell O, Kanis JA (2006) An estimate of the worldwide prevalence and disability associated with osteoporotic fractures. Osteoporos Int 17(12):1726–1733
2. Singer BR, McLauchlan GJ, Robinson CM, Christie J (1998) Epidemiology of fractures in 15,000 adults: the influence of age and gender. J Bone Joint Surg Br 80:243–248
3. Kanis JA, Johnell O, Oden A, De Laet C, Malstrom D (2004) Epidemiology of osteoporosis and fracture in men. Calcif Tissue Int 75:90–99
4. Assessment of fracture risk and its application to screening for postmenopausal osteoporosis. Report of a WHO Study Group. Geneva, World Health Organization, 1994 (WHO Technical Report Series, No. 843)
5. Office of the Surgeon General (US) (2004) Bone Health and Osteoporosis: A Report of the Surgeon General. Rockville, MD
6. Schwenkglenks M, Lippuner K, Hauselmann HJ, Szucs TD (2005) A model of osteoporosis impact in Switzerland 2000–2020. Osteoporos Int 16:659–6571
7. Lippuner K, Johansson H, Kanis JA, Rizzoli R (2009) Remaining lifetime and absolute 10-year probabilities of osteoporotic fracture in Swiss men and women. Osteoporos Int 20:1131–1140
8. Kanis JA, Johnell O, Oden A, Sembo I, Redlund-Johnell I, Dawson A et al (2000) Long-term risk of osteoporotic fracture in Malmø. Osteoporosis Int 11:669–674
9. Melton LJ III, Kallmes DF (2006) Epidemiology of vertebral fractures: implications for vertebral augmentation. Acad Radiol 13:538–545
10. Nevitt MC, Ettinger B, Black DM et al (1998) The association of radiologically detected vertebral fractures with back pain and function: a prospective study. Ann Intern Med 128: 793–800
11. EPOS Group (2002) Incidence of vertebral fracture in Europe: results from the European prospective osteoporosis study (EPOS). J Bone Miner Res 17:716–724
12. EPOS Group (2002) Incidence of limb fracture across Europe: results from the European Prospective Osteoporosis Study (EPOS). Osteoporosis Int 13:565–5671
13. Cooper C, Campion G, Melton LJ III (1992) Hip fractures in the elderly: a world-wide projection. Osteoporosis Int 2:285–289
14. Sambrook P, Cooper C (2006) Osteoporosis. Lancet 367:2010–2018
15. Cummings SR, Melton JR III (2002) Epidemiology and outcomes of osteoporotic fractures. Lancet 359:1761–1767
16. Empfehlungen 2015 zur Prävention, Diagnostik und Therapie der Osteoporose. SVGO/ASCO 2015, http://www.svgo.ch/content/inhalt_deutsch/inhalt/broschueren/broschueren.html

17. Kanis JA, EV MC, Johansson H et al (2013) European guidance for the diagnosis and management of osteoporosis in postmenopausal women. Osteop Int 24:23–57
18. Birkhäuser M (2013) Präventionskonzepte und aktuelle Therapieempfehlungen in der Peri- und Postmenopause. UNI-MED Verlag AG Bremen, London, Boston
19. Lips P, Vitamin D (2007) Status and nutrition in Europe and Asia. 13th workshop on vitamin D (Victoria, British Columbia, Canada, April 2006). J Steroid Biochem Mol Biol 203:620–625
20. Bischoff-Ferrari HA, Can U, Staehelin HB et al (2008) Severe vitamin D deficiency in Swiss hip fracture patients. Bone 42(3):597–602
21. Bischoff-Ferrari HA et al (2004) Positive association between 25-hydroxy vitamin D levels and bone mineral density: a population-based study of younger and older adults. Am J Med 116(9):634–639
22. Cauley JA, Lacroix AZ, Wu L, Horwitz M, Danielson ME, Bauer DC, Lee JS, Jackson RD, Robbins JA, Wu C, Stanczyk FZ, LeBoff MS, Wactawski-Wende J, Sarto G, Ockene J, Cummings SR (2008) Serum 25-hydroxyvitamin D concentrations and risk for hip fractures. Ann Intern Med 149(4):242–250
23. Bischoff-Ferrari HA, Dawson-Hughes B, Staehelin HB et al (2009) Fall prevention with supplemental and active forms of vitamin D: a meta-analysis of randomised controlled trials. Br Med J 339:b3692
24. Grant WB, Garland CF, Gorham ED (2007) An estimate of cancer mortality rate reductions in Europe and the US with 1000 IU oral vitamin D per day. Recent Results Cancer Res 174:225–234
25. Giovannucci E, Liu Y, Rimm EB et al (2006) Prospective study of predictors of vitamin D status and cancer incidence and mortality in men. J Natl Cancer Inst 98(7):451–459
26. Forman JP, Giovannucci E, Holmes MD et al (2007) Plasma 25-Hydroxyvitamin D levels and risk of incident hypertension. Hypertension 49:1063–1069
27. Pilz S, Dobnig H, Nijpels G et al (2009) Vitamin D and mortality in older men and women. Clin Endocrinol 71:666–672
28. Giovannucci E, Liu Y, Hollis BW, Rimm EB (2008) 25-hydroxyvitamin D and risk of myocardial infarction in men: a prospective study. Arch Intern Med 168(11):1174–1180
29. Medicine Io: Dietary Reference Ranges for Calcium and Vitamin D. http://www.iom.edu/Reports/2010/Dietary-Reference-Intakes-for-Calcium-and-Vitamin-D/Report-Brief.aspx. 2010
30. Ross AC, Manson JE, Abrams SA et al (2011) The 2011 report on dietary reference intakes for calcium and vitamin D from the Institute of Medicine: what clinicians need to know. J Clin Endocrinol Metab 96:53–58
31. Holick MF, Binkley NC, Bischoff-Ferrari HA et al (2011) Evaluation, treatment, and prevention of vitamin D deficiency: an Endocrine Society clinical practice guideline. J Clin Endocrinol Metab 96:1911–1930
32. Bolland MJ, Avenell A, Baron JA et al (2010) Effect of calcium supplements on risk of myocardial infarction and cardiovascular events: meta-analysis. BMJ 341:c3691
33. Li K, Kaaks R, Linseisen J et al (2012) Associations of dietary calcium intake and calcium supplementation with myocardial infarction and stroke risk and overall cardiovascular mortality in the Heidelberg cohort of the European prospective investigation into cancer and nutrition study (EPIC-Heidelberg). Heart 98:920–925
34. Verbrugge FH, Gielen E, Milisen K, St B (2012) Who should receive calcium and vitamin D supplementation? Age Ageing 41:576–580
35. Dachverband Osteologie. DVO-Leitlinie 2014 zur Prophylaxe, Diagnostik und Therapie der Osteoporose bei Erwachsenen. http://www.dv-osteologie.org/dvo_leitlinien/osteoporose-leitlinie-2014
36. De Laet C, Kanis JA, Oden A, Johanson H, Johnell O, Delmas P, Eisman JA, Kroger H, Fujiwara S, Garnero P, McCloskey EV, Mellstrom D, Melton LJ 3rd, Meunier PJ, Pols HA, Reeve J, Silman A, Tenenhouse A (2005) Body mass index as a predictor of fracture risk: a meta-analysis. Osteoporos Int 16:1330–1338
37. Rizzoli R, Bonjour JP (2004) Dietary protein and bone health. J Bone Miner Res 19:527–531

38. Kanis JA, Hans D, Cooper C, Baim S, Bilezikian JP, Binkley N, Cauley JA, Compston JE, Dawson-Hughes B, El-Hajj Fuleihan G, Johansson H, Leslie WD, Lewiecki EM, Luckey M, Oden A, Papapoulos SE, Poiana C, Rizzoli R, Wahl DA, McCloskey EV (2011) Task force of the FRAX Initiative. Interpretation and use of FRAX in clinical practice. Osteoporos Int 22:2395–2411
39. Kanis JA, Glüer CC for the Committee of Scientific Advisors, International Osteoporosis Foundation (2000) An update on the diagnosis and assessment of osteoporosis with densitometry. Osteoporos Int 11:192–202
40. Looker AC, Orwoll ES, Johnston CC, Lindsay RL, Wahner HW, Dunn WL et al (1997) Prevalence of low femoral bone density in older US adults from NHANES III. J Bone Miner Res 12:1761–1768
41. Looker AC, Wahner HW, Dunn WL, Calvo MS, Harris TB, Heyse SP (1998) Updated data on proximal femur bone mineral levels of US adults. Osteoporos Int 8:468–486
42. Sornay-Rendu E, Munoz F, Garnero P, Duboeuf F, Delmas PD (2005) Identification of osteopenic women at high risk of fracture: the OFELY study. J Bone Miner Res 20(10):1813–1819
43. Schott AM, Cormier C, Hans D, Favier F et al (1998) How hip and whole-body bone mineral density predict hip fracture in elderly women: the EPIDOS prospective study. Osteoporos Int 8:247–254
44. Rizzoli R, Ammann P, Birkhäuser M et al (2009) Au nom de l'Association Suisse Contre l'Ostéoporose (Schweizerische Vereinigung gegen die Osteoporose) Ostéoporose: du diagnostic ostéodensitométrique à l'évaluation du risque absolu de fracture. Schweiz Med Forum 9(36):633–635
45. Trémollières FA, Pouillès JM, Drewniak N et al (2010) Fracture risk prediction using BMD and clinical risk factors in early postmenopausal women: sensitivity of the WHO FRAX tool. J Bone Miner Res 25:1002–1009
46. Leslie WD, Lix LM, Johannson H et al (2011) Spine–hip discordance and fracture risk assessment: a physician-friendly FRAX enhancement. Osteoporos Int 22:839–884
47. Vasikaran S, Eastell O, Bruyère A et al (2011) Markers of bone turnover for the prediction of fracture risk and monitoring of osteoporosis treatment: a need for international reference standards. Osteoporo Int 22:391–420
48. Delmas PD, Vrijens B, Roux C et al (2003) Reinforcement message based on bone turnover marker response influences long-term persistence with risedronate in osteoporosis: the IMPACT study. ASBMR 2003 [Poster M330]
49. Baber RJ, Panay N, Fenton A (2016) The IMS writing group 2016 IMS recommendations on Women's midlife health and menopause hormone therapy. Climacteric 19(2):109–150. doi:10.3109/13697137.2015.1129166
50. Birkhaeuser M (2014) Primary prevention of fragility fractures in postmenopausal women(part 1): general prevention and primary prevention by MHT Ref. Gynecol Obstet 16:79–110
51. Wells G, Tugwell P, Shea B et al (2002) A meta-analyses of therapies for postmenopausal osteoporosis. V. Meta-analysis of the efficacy of hormone replacement therapy in treating and preventing osteoporosis in postmenopausal women. Endocr Rev 23:529–539
52. Torgerson DJ, Bell-Syer SE (2001) Hormone replacement therapy and prevention of vertebral fractures: a meta-analysis of randomised trials. BMC Musculoskelet JAMA 2:2891–2897
53. Torgerson DJ, Bell-Syer SE (2001) Hormone replacement therapy and prevention of non-vertebral fractures: a meta-analysis of randomized trials. BMC Musculoskelet Disord 285:7–10
54. Cauley JA, Robbins J, Chen Z et al (2003) Effects of estrogen plus progestin on risk of fracture and bone mineral density: the Women's health Initiative randomized trial. JAMA 290:1729–1738
55. Women' Health Initiative Steering Committee (2004) Effects of conjugated estrogen on postmenopausal women with hysterectomy: the Women's Health Initiative randomized controlled trial. JAMA 291:1701–1712
56. Anderson GL, Hutchinson F, Limacher M, The Women's Health Initiative Steering Committee et al (2004) The Women's health initiative randomized controlled trial. Effects of conjugated

equine estrogen in postmenopausal women with hysterectomy. The Women's health initiative controlled trial. JAMA 291:1701–1712
57. Jackson RD, Wactawski-Wende J, LaCroix AZ et al (2006) Effects of conjugated equine estrogen on risk of fractures and BMD in postmenopausal women with hysterectomy: results from the women's health Initiative randomized trial. J Bone Miner Res 21:817–828
58. LaCroix AZ, Chlebowski RT, Manso JAE et al (2011) Health outcomes after stopping conjugated equine estrogens among postmenopausal women with prior hysterectomy. A randomized controlled trial. JAMA 305:1305–1314
59. de Villiers TJ, Hall JE, Pinkerton JV et al (2016) Revised global consensus Statement on menopausal hormone therapy. Climacteric 19:313–315. doi:10.1080/13697137.2016.1196047
60. Birkhäuser MH, Panay N, Archer DF et al (2008) Updated practical recommendations for hormone replacement therapy in the peri- and postmenopause. Climacteric 11:108–123
61. NAMS Position Statement (2012) The 2012 hormone therapy position statement of the North American Menopause Society. Menopause 19:257–271
62. Lindsay R, Gallagher JC, Kleerekoper M, Pickar JH (2002) Effect of lower doses of conjugated equine estrogens with and without medroxyprogesterone acetate on bone in early postmenopausal women. J Am Med Assoc 287:2668–2676
63. Lees B, Stevenson JC (2001) The prevention of osteoporosis using sequential low-dose hormone replacement therapy with estradiol-17-beta and dydrogesterone. Osteoporos Int 12:251–258
64. Ettinger B, Ensrud KE, Wallace R, Johnson KC, Cummings SR, Yankov V, Vittinghoff E, Grady D (2004) Effects of ultralowdose transdermal estradiol on bone mineral density: a randomized clinical trial. Obstet Gynecol 104:443–451
65. Greenwald MW, Gluck OS, Lang E, Rakov V (2005) Oral hormone therapy with 17beta-estradiol and 17beta-estradiol in combination with norethindrone acetate in the prevention of bone loss in early postmenopausal women: dose-dependent effects. Menopause 12:741–748
66. Prestwood KM, Kenny AM, Kleppinger A, Kulldorff M (2003) Ultra low-dose micronized 17beta-estradiol and bone density and bone metabolism in older women: a randomized controlled trial. JAMA 290:1042–1048
67. Ettinger B, Genant HK, Steiger P, Madvig P (1992) Low-dosage micronized 17 beta-estradiol prevents bone loss in postmenopausal women. Am J Obstet Gynecol 166:479–488
68. Huang AJ, Ettinger B, Vittinghoff E, Ensrud KE, Johnson KC, Cummings SR (2007) Endogenous estrogen levels and the effects of ultra-low dose transdermal estradiol therapy on bone turnover and BMD in postmenopausal women. J Bone Miner Res 22:1791–1797
69. McClung MR et al (1998) Osteoporosis prevention by low-dose regimens, presented at the ASBRM, San Francisco, PDI/II/USA 1998
70. Lamy O, Krieg MA, Burckhardt B, Wasserfallen JB (2003) An economic analysis of hormone replacement therapy for the prevention of fracture in young postmenopausal women. Expert Opin Pharmacother 4:1479–1488
71. Trémollières FA, Pouilles JM, Ribot C et al (2001) Withdrawal of hormone replacement therapy is associated with significant vertebral bone loss in postmenopausal women. Osteoporos Int 12:385–390
72. Yates J, Barrett-Connor E, Barlas S et al (2004) Rapid loss of hip fracture protection after estrogen cessation: evidence from the National Osteoporosis Risk Assessment. Obstet Gynecol 103:440–446
73. Mosekilde L, Beck-Nielsen H, Sørensen OH et al (2000) Hormonal replacement therapy reduces forearm fracture incidence in recent postmenopausal women — results of the Danish osteoporosis prevention study. Maturitas 36:181–193
74. Finkelstein JS, Brockwell SE, Mehta V, Greendale GA, Sowers MR, Ettinger B, Lo JC, Johnston JM, Cauley JA, Danielson ME, Neer RM (2008) Bone mineral density changes during the menopause transition in a multiethnic cohort of women. J Clin Endocrinol Metab 93:861–868

75. Bagger YZ, Tanko LB, Alexandersen P et al (2004) Two to three years of hormone replacement treatment in healthy women have long-term preventive effects on bone mass and osteoporotic fractures: the PERF study. Bone 34:728–735
76. Manson JA, Chlebowski RT, Stefanick ML (2013) Menopausal hormone therapy and health outcomes during the intervention and extended poststopping phases of the women's health Initiative randomized trials. JAMA 310:1353–1368
77. Watts NB, Cauley JA, Jackson RD et al, Women's Health Initiative Investigators (2016) No increase in fractures after stopping hormone therapy: results from the Women's health Initiative. J Clin Endocrinol Metab 102:302–308. doi:10.1210/jc.2016-3270
78. Kloosterboer HL (2011) Historical milestones in the development of tibolone (Livial®). Climacteric 14:609–621
79. Cummings SR, Ettinger B, Delmas PD et al (2008) The effects of tibolone in older postmenopausal women. N Engl J Med 359:697–708
80. Lippuner K, Haenggi W, Birkhaeuser MH et al (1997) Prevention of postmenopausal bone loss using tibolone or conventional peroral or transdermal hormone replacement therapy with 17beta-oestradiol and dydrogesterone. J Bone Miner Res 12:806–812
81. Delmas PD, Davis SR, Hensen S et al (2008) Effects of tibolone and raloxifene on bone mineral density in osteopenic postmenopausal women. Osteoporos Int 19:1153–1160
82. Seeman E, Crans GG, Diez-Perez A, Pinette KV, Delmas PD (2006) Anti-vertebral fracture efficacy of raloxifene: a meta-analysis. Osteoporos Int 17:313–316
83. Kanis JA, Johnell O, Black DM et al (2003) Effect of raloxifene on the risk of new vertebral fracture in postmenopausal women with osteopenia or osteoporosis: a reanalysis of the multiple outcomes of raloxifene evaluation trial. Bone 33:293–300
84. Kanis JA, Johansson H, Oden A, McCloskey EV (2010) A meta-analysis of the efficacy of raloxifene on all clinical and vertebral fractures and its dependency on FRAX. Bone 47:729–735
85. Miller P et al (2008) Effects of bazedoxifene on BMD and bone turnover in postmenopausal women: 2-yr results of a randomized, double-blind, placebo-, and active-controlled study. J Bone Miner Res 23:525–535
86. Silverman SL, Christiansen C, Genant HK, Vukicevic S, Zanchetta JR, de Villiers TJ, Constantine GD, Chines AA (2008) Efficacy of bazedoxifene in reducing new vertebral fracture risk in postmenopausal women with osteoporosis: results from a 3-year, randomized, placebo-, and active-controlled clinical trial. J Bone Miner Res 23:1923–1934
87. Kanis JA, Johansson H, Oden A, McCloskey EV (2009) Bazedoxifene reduces vertebral and clinical fractures in postmenopausal women at high risk assessed with FRAX. Bone 44:1049–1054
88. Silverman SL, Chines AA, Kendler DL et al (2012) Sustained efficacy and safety of bazedoxifene in preventing fractures in postmenopausal women with osteoporosis: results of a 5-year, randomized, placebo-controlled study. Osteoporosis Int 23:351–363
89. Lindsay R, Gallagher JC, Kagan R, Pickar JH, Constantine G (2009) Efficacy of tissue-selective estrogen complex of bazedoxifene/conjugated estrogens for osteoporosis prevention in at-risk postmenopausal women. Fertil Steril 92:1045–1052
90. Birkhaeuser M (2016) Primary prevention of fragility fractures in postmenopausal women (part 2): non-hormonal antiresorptive therapies and osteo-anabolic treatment. Ref Gynecol Obstet 17:30–73
91. Black DM, Delmas PD, Eastell R et al (2007) Once-yearly zoledronic acid for treatment of postmenopausal osteoporosis. N Engl J Med 356:1809–1822
92. Black DM, Cummings SR, Karpf DB et al (1996) Randomized trial of effect of alendronate on risk of fracture in women with existing vertebral fractures. Lancet 348:1535–1541
93. Cranney A, Wells G, Willan A et al (2002) II. Meta-analysis of alendronate for the treatment of postmenopausal women. Endocr Rev 23:508–516
94. Wells G, Cranney A, Peterson J et al (2008) Risedronate for the primary and secondary prevention of osteoporotic fractures in postmenopausal women. Cochrane Database Syst Rev 1:CD004523

95. Rossini M, Idolazzi L, Adami S (2011) Evidence of sustained vertebral and nonvertebral antifracture efficacy with ibandronate therapy: a systematic review. Ther Adv Musculoskel Dis 3:67–79
96. Rizzoli R (2010) Zoledronic acid for the treatment and prevention of primary and secondary osteoporosis. Ther Adv Musculoskel Dis 2:3–16
97. Shane E, Burr D, Abrahamsen B et al (2014) Atypical sub-trochanteric and diaphyseal femoral fractures: second report of a task force of the American Society for Bone and Mineral Research. J Bone Miner Res 29:1–23
98. Rizzoli R, Reginster J-Y, Boonen S et al (2011) Adverse reactions and drug–drug interactions in the Management of Women with postmenopausal osteoporosis. Calcif Tissue Int 89:91–104
99. Adler RA, El-Hajj Fuleihan G, Bauer DC et al (2016) Managing osteoporosis in patients on long-term bisphosphonate treatment: a report of a task force of the American Society for Bone and Mineral Research. J Bone Miner Res 31(1):16–35
100. Papapoulos S, Lippuner K, Roux C et al (2015) The effect of 8 or 5 years of denosumab treatment in postmenopausal women with osteoporosis: results from the FREEDOM extension study. Osteoporos Int 26:2773–2783. doi:10.1007/s00198-015-3234-7
101. Reid IR (2015) Denosumab after 8 years. Editorial Osteoporos Int 26:2759–2761
102. McCloskey EV, Johansson H, Oden A, Austin M, Siris E, Wang A, Lewiecki EM, Lorenc R, Libanati C, Kanis JA (2012) Denosumab reduces the risk of osteoporotic fractures in postmenopausal women, particularly in those with moderate to high fracture risk as assessed with FRAX(R). J Bone Miner Res 27:1480–1486. doi:10.1002/jbmr.1606
103. von Keyserlingk C, Hopkins R, Anastasilakis A et al (2011) Clinical efficacy and safety of denosumab in postmenopausal women with low bone mineral density and osteoporosis: a meta-analysis. Semin Arthritis Rheum 41:178–186
104. McClung MR (2016) Cancel the denosumab holiday. Osteoporos Int 27(5):1677–1682
105. Meunier PJ, Roux C, Ortolani S et al (2009) Effects of long-term strontium ranelate treatment on vertebral fracture risk in postmenopausal women with osteoporosis. Osteoporos Int 20:1663–1673
106. Reginster J-Y, Kaufman J-M, Goemare S et al (2012) Maintenance of antifracture efficacy over 10 years with strontium ranelate in postmenopausal osteoporosis. Osteoporos Int 23:1115–1122
107. European Medicine Agency (15 Apr 2014) Protelos/Osseor to remain available but with further restrictions. EMA/235924/2014
108. Meier C, Lamy O, Krieg M-A, Mellinghoff H-U, Felder M, Ferrari S, Rizzoli R (2014) The role of teriparatide in sequential and combination therapy of osteoporosis. Swiss Med Wkly 144:w13952
109. Kraenzlin ME, Meier C (2011) Parathyroid hormone analogues in the treatment of osteoporosis. Nat Rev Endocrinol 7:647–656. doi:10.1038/nrendo.2011.108
110. Expertenbrief der SGGG No 28 (2015) Aktuelle Empfehlungen zur menopausalen Hormon-Therapie (MHT) (www.sggg.ch/ im Druck, 2015)
111. Baber R.J. et al., Climacteric 2016; 19 (2): 109–150; doi:10.3109/13697137.2015.1129166

The Effect of Menopause and HRT on Coronary Heart Disease

15

John C. Stevenson

15.1 Introduction

Coronary heart disease (CHD) is a leading cause of death in women. Whilst many risk factors for CHD are common to both men and women [1], the deficiency of female gonadal steroids is an additional risk for women. Thus, menopause leads to an increase in CHD in addition to that due to ageing. This is well demonstrated by studying the effects of early menopause where it is easy to compare CHD risk with that of normal age of menopause [2]. It therefore seems logical to see if hormone replacement therapy (HRT) can reverse the effects of menopause on CHD risk. This chapter will examine the metabolic and vascular effects of menopause and HRT.

15.2 Effects of Menopause on Metabolic Parameters

Oestrogen deficiency has profound metabolic and vascular effects. It is associated with adverse changes in lipids and lipoproteins. There is an increase in total and LDL cholesterol, together with apolipoprotein B, an increase in triglycerides, and a decrease in HDL cholesterol and apolipoprotein A1 [3]. Levels of lipoprotein (a), an independent coronary risk factor, also increase. There may be increased oxidation of LDL particles which encourages atheroma formation. Glucose and insulin metabolism also changes at the menopause. Whilst there is no immediate change in circulating glucose and insulin concentrations, this masks a decrease in pancreatic insulin secretion with a simultaneous decrease in insulin clearance [4]. Following the menopause, there is a steady decrease in insulin sensitivity so that postmenopausal women become increasingly insulin resistant. There is often an increase in

J.C. Stevenson
National Heart and Lung Institute, Imperial College London,
Royal Brompton Hospital, London SW3 6NP, UK
e-mail: j.stevenson@imperial.ac.uk

M. Birkhaeuser, A.R. Genazzani (eds.), *Pre-Menopause, Menopause and Beyond*,
ISGE Series, https://doi.org/10.1007/978-3-319-63540-8_15

fat mass, but more importantly, there is a redistribution of body fat with a relative increase in central fat [5]. This results in further abnormalities of lipids, lipoproteins, glucose, and insulin metabolism due to increased fatty acid fluxes into the portal vein. It is possible that there are increases in blood pressure associated with the menopause although it is difficult to separate menopausal effects from those of ageing, but there is an increased incidence of hypertension in postmenopausal women [6]. There is also an impairment of vascular endothelial function [7]. All of these changes encourage the development of atheroma. Recently, a highly accurate epigenetic marker of ageing has been studied in large female populations to assess the effects of menopause [8]. An increased epigenetic age acceleration was associated with earlier menopause and with bilateral ovariectomy, whilst HRT use was associated with a lower epigenetic age.

15.3 Effects of HRT on Metabolic Parameters

Oestrogen replacement results in a decrease in total and LDL cholesterol and an increase in HDL cholesterol [9]. This effect is greater with oral than with transdermal oestrogen. Triglycerides are increased with oral oestrogen but decreased with transdermal oestrogen administration. These effects may be modified by progestogen administration. Androgenic progestogens such as norethisterone acetate (NETA) and medroxyprogesterone acetate (MPA) can blunt the increase in HDL but may also blunt the increase in triglycerides induced by oral oestrogens. Non-androgen progestogens such as micronised progesterone and dydrogesterone do not impede the increase in HDL [10]. Oral oestradiol improves glucose tolerance and reduces insulin resistance more than transdermal oestradiol [11]. High-dose, but not low-dose, conjugated equine oestrogens can impair glucose tolerance. The effects of progestogens can modify these oestrogen-induced effects. Androgenic progestogens increase insulin resistance [11], whilst non-androgenic progestogens are neutral in this respect [12]. HRT reduces the central deposition of body fat [13], thus reversing the menopausal effect. Oral oestrogens increase coagulation activation and are associated with a transient increase in venous thromboembolism (VTE). This is avoided with the use of transdermal oestrogen [14] and possibly reduced with very low-dose oral oestrogen.

15.4 Vascular Effects of HRT

Oestrogen induces vasodilatation by stimulating nitric oxide production and by reducing the release of the potent vasoconstrictor, endothelin-1. It also inhibits calcium channels and activates BKCa channels [15]. Oestrogen reduces angiotensin-converting enzyme activity and is usually associated with small decreases in blood pressure. The addition of drospirenone, a progestogen with antimineralocorticoid effects, results in a further decrease in blood pressure [16]. Oestrogen has a dose-dependent effect on matrix metalloproteinases which are involved with vascular remodelling [17]. Thus high-dose oestrogen could potentially destabilise atheromatous plaques but at lower doses oestrogen may normalise the remodelling processes and potentially reduce atheroma formation.

15.5 HRT and CHD Outcomes

Many observational studies have shown that postmenopausal HRT use is associated with a 40–50% reduction in cardiovascular outcomes, primarily CHD events. There is also good evidence that HRT use is associated with reduced CHD mortality. In a study of over 90,000 women, those initiating HRT below age 60 years showed a significant reduction in CHD death, whereas in those initiating HRT above age 60 years, the reduction was non-significant [18]. A recent study using national registry data examined the effects of stopping HRT on cardiovascular outcomes [19]. The study population comprised over 330,000 postmenopausal women who discontinued HRT, and the standardised mortality ratios were compared with those expected for the general population. A significant increase in mortality was seen during the first year after HRT cessation but thereafter returned to that expected. Compared with those women continuing HRT, the mortality was higher during the first year following HRT cessation and was still significantly increased beyond the first year. This probably reflects the continuing CHD benefit of HRT on those remaining on the treatment. It is not known whether the women discontinuing HRT did so abruptly or gradually. Numerous studies looking at the effects of HRT on surrogate outcomes for CHD have been conducted. A series of studies of cynomolgus macaques gave rise to the concept of the timing hypothesis or window of opportunity for CHD prevention. In the first study [20], monkeys were given a normal diet, made surgically menopausal, and then given an atherogenic diet and randomised to either conjugated equine oestrogens or placebo. At the end of the study, the amount of atheromatous plaque was reduced by 70% in the oestrogen group compared with placebo. In a second study [21], the monkeys were put on an atherogenic diet to induce atheroma formation before being made surgically menopausal. They continued on the atherogenic diet and were randomised to either conjugated equine oestrogens or placebo. At the end of this study, the oestrogen group still had 50% less atheromatous plaque than the placebo group. In a third study [22], the monkeys were made surgically menopausal and put onto an atherogenic diet, but there was then a delay of the equivalent of 6 human years before being randomised to conjugated equine oestrogens or placebo. At the end of this study, there was no difference in atheromatous plaque between the oestrogen and placebo groups. These studies suggested that early intervention with HRT after the menopause is needed to get CHD benefit. There is a support for this concept from human studies. A clinical trial of healthy women in the early postmenopausal period showed less progression of atheroma as assessed by ultrasound measurement of carotid artery intima-media thickness in those randomised to oral oestradiol compared with placebo [23]. In contrast, a study of elderly women with established CHD showed no difference in atheroma progression as measured by coronary angiography between those randomised to conjugated equine oestrogens alone, those randomised to conjugated equine oestrogens plus MPA, or those randomised to placebo [24]. In the ELITE trial comprising almost 650 healthy postmenopausal women treated for around 6 years, oral oestradiol 1 mg daily reduced carotid artery atheroma progression if initiated within 6 years of the onset of menopause, whilst no such effect was seen in those initiating treatment beyond 10 years postmenopause [25]. However, no effect was seen on coronary artery calcium scores. The KEEPS trial enrolled over 700 women within 3 years of menopause onset and randomised them to either conjugated equine oestrogens 0.45 mg daily, transdermal oestradiol 50 mcg, or placebo [26]. After 4 years, there was no difference between the groups in terms of carotid artery intima-media thickness changes and those of coronary artery calcification scores. It has been suggested that the women were too healthy to show any change in atheroma development. Irrespective of effects on atheroma development, there is also evidence that oestrogen can improve myocardial ischemia in women with CHD [27]. Several randomised clinical trials have been conducted for both primary and secondary prevention of CHD events. The Heart and Estrogen/Progestin Replacement Study (HERS) comprised over 2500 postmenopausal women, average age 67 years, with established CHD randomised to conjugated equine oestrogens 0.625 mg plus MPA or placebo [28]. After 4 years, there was no overall benefit or harm seen with the HRT group, although there was a significant trend to reducing CHD events with the HRT. It seems likely that the dose of oestrogen was inappropriately high for the age of the participants. This was also true for a study in over 1000 women with CHD, mean age 62 years, using oestradiol valerate 2 mg daily, which showed a non-significant reduction in cardiac mortality [29]. There was a high dropout rate. Another secondary prevention study in only 255 women, mean age 67 years, used an inappropriately high dose of transdermal oestradiol 80 μg and showed no overall benefit or harm but again had a high dropout rate [30]. Finally, in a pilot study, 100 women with CHD, mean age 68 years, were randomised to a lower dose of oral oestradiol 1 mg daily plus NETA or placebo and showed a non-significant 30% reduction in CHD events after 12 months [31]. The largest primary prevention randomised clinical trial was the Women's Health Initiative (WHI) [32]. Over 16,500 postmenopausal women, mean age 63 years, were randomised to conjugated equine oestrogens 0.625 mg plus MPA 2.5 mg daily. After 5.6 years of intervention, there was no overall benefit for CHD events. Almost 11,000 hysterectomised women, mean age 63 years, received conjugated equine oestrogens 0,625 mg alone or placebo; after just over 7 years of intervention, there was no overall CHD benefit. However, in the oestrogen-alone arm, there was a significant reduction in a composite CHD outcome in those initiating treatment below age 60 years, and with long-term follow-up post-intervention, there was a significant reduction in CHD events compared with placebo. A 10-year prospective clinical trial of over 1000 women in the early postmenopause randomised healthy women to oral oestradiol 2 mg daily plus NETA if non-hysterectomised or to no treatment [33]. There was an additional 6-year observational post-trial follow-up. Women on HRT had a significant reduction of a composite endpoint of myocardial infarction, death, or hospital admission with heart failure. There was no increase in adverse outcomes with the HRT, including stroke, VTE, and breast cancer, during the 16 years. A meta-analysis of 23 randomised clinical trials of HRT versus placebo or no treatment included over 39,000 women [34]. Those initiating HRT below age 60 years or within 10 years of menopause had a one-third reduction in the endpoint of myocardial infarction or death. Those initiating HRT above age 60 years or beyond 10 years of menopause had an increase in events during the first year but then showed a 20% reduction after 2 years. A more recent meta-analysis of 19 randomised clinical trials of HRT versus placebo or no treatment included over 49,000 women [35]. Those initiating HRT within 10 years of menopause had a 50% reduction in the endpoint of myocardial infarction or death, whilst there was no significant effect in those initiating HRT beyond 10 years postmenopause.

Conclusion

Both menopause and HRT have profound effects on metabolic risk factors for CHD. Loss of ovarian function leads to adverse changes in lipids and lipoproteins, glucose and insulin metabolism, and body fat distribution. There are also adverse changes in arterial function. These changes result in an increased incidence of CHD. HRT will reverse many of these changes and may result in decreases in CHD. However, this benefit is dependent on a number of factors. The age at initiation of HRT is clearly very important, with the greatest benefits of CHD event reduction being seen in those initiating treatment close to the onset of menopause, although it should be emphasised that initiating HRT at later ages does not necessarily result in overall CHD harm. But lack of benefit in terms of CHD events in older women, including those with established CHD, may well be due to inappropriate dosing of oestrogen. Many of the beneficial arterial effects of oestrogen are dose dependent, and it is likely that using appropriately lower starting doses in older women would avoid any cardiovascular harm and may prove of benefit. Not only the dose at initiation but also the route of administration of HRT could be important, certainly in terms of athero-thrombotic events. There are haemostatic advantages for non-oral oestrogen administration compared with oral administration, although this could in part be related to dosage. There appear to be differences according to the type of progestogen used in HRT, with some adverse metabolic and vascular effects seen with androgenic, compared with non-androgenic, progestogens. The totality of current data suggests that HRT is beneficial for the primary prevention of CHD in postmenopausal women. Age at initiation requires individualisation of doses and types of hormones, and their route of administration also needs to be considered. The optimal duration of HRT use for CHD prevention remains unknown. For women wishing to come off HRT, it would seem prudent at present to reduce the dose gradually rather than stop abruptly.

References

1. Yusuf S, Hawken S, Ounpuu S et al (2004) Effect of potentially modifiable risk factors associated with myocardial infarction in 52 countries (the INTERHEART study): case-control study. Lancet 364:937–952
2. Lokkegaard E, Jovanovic Z, Heitmann BE et al (2006) The association between early menopause and risk of ischaemic heart disease: influence of hormone therapy. Maturitas 53:226–233
3. Stevenson JC, Crook D, Godsland IF (1993) Influence of age and menopause on serum lipids and lipoproteins in healthy women. Atherosclerosis 98:83–90
4. Walton C, Godsland IF, Proudler AJ, Wynn V, Stevenson JC (1993) The effects of the menopause on insulin sensitivity, secretion and elimination in non-obese, healthy women. Eur J Clin Investig 23:466–473
5. Ley CJ, Lees B, Stevenson JC (1992) Sex- and menopause-associated changes in body-fat distribution. Am J Clin Nutr 55:950–954
6. Coylewright M, Reckelhoff JF, Ouyang P (2008) Menopause and hypertension. Hypertension 51:952–959
7. Taddei S, Verdis A, Ghiadoni L et al (1996) Menopause is associated with endothelial dysfunction in women. Hypertension 28:576–582
8. Levine ME, Lu AT, Chen BH et al (2016) Menopause accelerates biological aging. PNAS 113:9327–9332
9. Godsland IF (2001) Effects of postmenopausal hormone replacement therapy on lipid, lipoprotein, and apolipoprotein (a) concentrations: analysis of studies published from 1974–2000. Fertil Steril 75:898–915
10. Stevenson JC, Rioux JE, Komer L, Gelfand M (2005) 1 and 2 mg 17β-estradiol combined with sequential dydrogesterone have similar effects on the serum lipid profile of postmenopausal women. Climacteric 8:352–359
11. Spencer CP, Godsland IF, Cooper AJ, Ross D, Whitehead MI, Stevenson JC (2000) Effects of oral and transdermal 17 β-estradiol with cyclical oral norethindrone acetate on insulin sensitivity, secretion, and elimination in postmenopausal women. Metabolism 49:742–747
12. Manassiev NA, Godsland IF, Crook D et al (2002) Effect of postmenopausal oestradiol and dydrogesterone therapy on lipoproteins and insulin sensitivity, secretion and elimination in hysterectomised women. Maturitas 42:233–242
13. Gambacciani M, Ciaponi M, Cappagli B et al (1997) Body weight, body fat distribution, and hormonal replacement therapy in early postmenopausal women. J Clin Endocrinol Metab 82:414–417
14. Scarabin P-Y, Oger E, Plu-Bureau G (2003) Differential association of oral and transdermal oestrogen-replacement therapy with venous thromboembolism risk. Lancet 362:428–432
15. Stevenson JC, Gerval MO (2014) The influence of sex steroids on affairs of the heart. In: Genazzani AR, Brincat M (eds) Frontiers in gynecological endocrinology. Volume 1. From symptoms to therapies. Springer, Heidelberg, pp 225–231
16. Archer DF, Thorneycroft IH, Foegh M et al (2005) Long term safety of drospirenone-estradiol for hormone therapy: a randomized, double-blind, multicenter trial. Menopause 12:716–727
17. Wingrove CS, Garr E, Godsland IF, Stevenson JC (1998) 17 β-Oestradiol enhances release of matrix metalloproteinase-2 from human vascular smooth muscle cells. Biochim Biophys Acta 1406:169–174
18. Tuomikoski P, Lyytinen H, Korhonen P et al (2014) Coronary heart disease mortality and hormone therapy before and after the Women's Health Initiative. Obstet Gynecol 124:947–953
19. Mikkola TS, Tuomikoski P, Lyytinen H et al (2015) Increased cardiovascular mortality risk in women discontinuing postmenopausal hormone therapy. J Clin Endocrinol Metab 100:4588–4594
20. Clarkson TB, Anthony MS, Jerome CP (1998) Lack of effect of raloxifene on coronary artery atherosclerosis of postmenopausal monkeys. J Clin Endocrinol Metab 83:721–726

21. Clarkson TB, Morgan TM (2001) Inhibition of postmenopausal atherosclerosis progression: a comparison of the effects of conjugated equine estrogens and soy phytoestrogens. J Clin Endocrinol Metab 86:41–47
22. Williams JK, Anthony MS, Honore EK et al (1995) Regression of atherosclerosis in female monkeys. Arterioscler Thromb Vasc Biol 15:827–836
23. Hodis HN, Mack WJ, Lobo RA et al (2001) Estrogen in the prevention of atherosclerosis. A randomized, double-blind, placebo-controlled trial. Ann Intern Med 135:939–953
24. Herrington DM, Reboussin DM, Brosnihan BK et al (2000) Effects of estrogen replacement on the progression of coronary-artery atherosclerosis. N Engl J Med 343:522–529
25. Hodis HN, Mack WJ, Henderson VW et al (2016) Vascular effects of early versus late postmenopausal treatment with estradiol. N Engl J Med 374:1221–1231
26. Harman SM (2012) Effects of oral conjugated estrogen or transdermal estradiol plus oral progesterone treatment on common carotid artery intima media thickness (CIMT) and coronary artery calcium (CAC) in menopausal women: initial results from the Kronos Early Estrogen Prevention Study (KEEPS). In: North American Menopause Society Annual Meeting
27. Stevenson JC (2009) HRT and cardiovascular disease. In: Lumsden MA (ed) Best practice and research clinical obstetrics and gynaecology, vol 23. Elsevier, Amsterdam, pp 109–120
28. Hulley S, Grady D, Bush T et al (1998) Randomized trial of estrogen plus progestin for secondary prevention of coronary heart disease in postmenopausal women. JAMA 280:605–613
29. Cherry N, Gilmour K, Hannaford P, Heagerty A et al (2002) Oestrogen therapy for prevention of reinfarction in postmenopausal women: a randomized placebo controlled trial. Lancet 360:2001–2008
30. Clarke SC, Kelleher J, Lloyd-Jones H, Slack M, Schofield PM (2002) A study of hormone replacement therapy in postmenopausal women with ischaemic heart disease: the Papworth HRT Atherosclerosis Study. BJOG 109:1056–1062
31. Collins P, Flather M, Lees B, Mister R, Proudler AJ, Stevenson JC (2006) Randomized trial of effects of continuous combined HRT on markers of lipids and coagulation in women with acute coronary syndromes: WHISP pilot study. Eur Heart J 27:2046–2053
32. Manson JE, Chlebowski RT, Stefanick ML et al (2013) Menopausal hormonal therapy and health outcomes during the intervention and poststopping phases of the Women's Health Initiative randomized trials. JAMA 310:1353–1368
33. Schierbeck LL, Rejnmark L, Tofteng CL et al (2012) Effect of hormone replacement therapy on cardiovascular events in recently postmenopausal women: randomized trial. Br Med J 345:e6409
34. Salpeter SR, Walsh JME, Greyber E, Salpeter EE (2006) Coronary heart disease events associated with hormone therapy in younger and older women. J Gen Intern Med 21:363–366
35. Boardman HMP, Hartley L, Eisinga A et al (2015) Hormone therapy for preventing cardiovascular disease in postmenopausal women. Cochrane Database Syst Rev 4:CD002229

How to Prevent Cardiovascular Disorders: Influence of Gonadal Steroids on the Heart

16

Svetlana Vujovic, Milina Tancic-Gajic, Ljiljana Marina, Zorana Arizanovic, Zorana Stojanovic, Branko Barac, Aleksandar Djogo, and Miomira Ivovic

In the ancient Rome, average life duration was 23 years; in Sweden at the end of the eighteenth century, 36.6 years for women and 33.7 for men; and in many European countries at the beginning of the twenty-first century, life expectancy was 72 and 76 years, respectively. The menopause (period in women's life 1 year after the last menstruation until the end of life) and involutive hypoandrogenism in males (testosterone below 12 nmol/L and typical symptoms) are characterized by decrease of gonadal steroids and initiating of cardiovascular diseases (CVD). Rahman [1] found that women who entered early menopause (40–45 years) had 40% increase of heart disease. Meta-analysis confirmed these data (Table 16.1).

Table 16.1 Cardiovascular risks and mortality in postmenopausal women—meta-analysis

Authors	Study	Location	Follow-up (years)	Number	Nos.
Li (2013)	BWHS	USA	13	11,052	6
Amagal (2009)	Jichi medical school cohort study	Japan	9.2	3824	6
Gallagher (2011)	Textile worker study	China	9.11	267,400	5
Jacobsen (2003)	Norwegian women cohort study	Norway	20.6	19,731	7

P.S. NOS—Newcastle-Ottawa scale for cohort study; 6–8—higher quality study

S. Vujovic (✉) • M. Tancic-Gajic • L. Marina • Z. Arizanovic
Z. Stojanovic • B. Barac • A. Djogo • M. Ivovic
Faculty of medicine, University of Belgrade, Clinic of endocrinology, diabetes and diseases of metabolism, Clinical center of Serbia, Belgrade, Serbia
e-mail: prof.svetlana.vujovic@gmail.com

M. Birkhaeuser, A.R. Genazzani (eds.), *Pre-Menopause, Menopause and Beyond*, ISGE Series, https://doi.org/10.1007/978-3-319-63540-8_16

Decrease of estradiol in women and testosterone in men represents independent risk factor for dyslipidemia, inflammation, obesity, insulin resistance, hypertension, endothelial dysfunction, and autonomous nervous system disturbances leading to CVD. Menopausal replacement therapy with estradiol regulates eating behavior, increases lipolytic adrenaline effects, decreases orexigenic peptides, protects from hepatic steatosis, improves insulin sensitivity, and decreases mortality rate of ischemic heart disease (IHD) 10 years after stopping therapy in a case that therapy was initiated before 60 years of age [2].

Estradiol increases hepatic excretion of apolipoprotein A and low-density lipoproteins, decreases apolipoprotein B, lipoprotein lipase transcription, adipose proliferation, plasminogen activator inhibitor (PAI), C-reactive protein and interleukin 6, and regulates PPAR γ [3]. In men testosterone decreases cholesterol, LDL, and proinflammatory cytokines and increases insulin sensitivity. Rossano [4] found that cholesterol and HDL are more important for male cardiovascular system and triglycerides and LDL for women's.

Low estradiol induces hyperaldosteronism, endothelial dysfunction, autonomous nervous system dysfunction, ventricular arrhythmias, natrium retention and potassium loss, prothrombotic activity, myocardial fibrosis, and necrosis. Hormone replacement therapy with estradiol corrects all these disturbances. Total testosterone is inversely correlated with blood pressure in men (BP) [5].

Markers of autonomous dysfunction, heart rate variability, and baroreceptor sensitivity (short-term regulation of BP) are changed in hypoestrogenic milieu. Estradiol therapy increases antioxidant enzymes (catalase, superoxide dismutase) [6].

Estradiol exerts direct vascular effects:

- Acute: Ca antagonism, antioxidant, dilatation, decreased endothelin and angiotensinogen II, and anti-inflammation.
- Chronic: Ca antagonist and decrease of oxidative stress, ACE activity, protection from vascular hypertrophy, and myocyte hypertrophy.
- Women have less obstructive coronary artery disease and preserved systolic function.

Coronary arteries are twice more normal in coronary disease (compared to men), but intramural plaques are more frequent, and they have subintimal atherosclerosis and vasospastic disease. In a case of discontinuation of estradiol therapy before age of 60 years, increase mortality rate in the first year due to plaque rupture, arrhythmia, and myocardial infarction was observed [7]. Enzyme aromatase converts testosterone and androstenedione to estradiol in cardiac myocytes. Testosterone regulates cardiac action potential and calcium homeostasis in women's heart cells and has positive effects on endothelial cells.

Testosterone therapy in male dilatates blood vessels. In the acute myocardial infarction, high estradiol and low testosterone were found. Intracoronary infusion of testosterone induced coronary dilatation and increased coronary blood flow in men with coronary disease [8]. Fourts Tromso Study (1994–1995) analyzed on 1568 subjects the impact of endogenous testosterone on risk for myocardial infarction

Table 16.2 Myocardial response to acute ischemia

Characteristics	Female	Male
Apoptotic rate in periinfarction region	Lower	Tenfold higher
Bax expression in periinfarction region	Lower	Greater
Duration of cardiomyopathy	Longer	Shorter
Myocardial healing	Earlier	Delayed
Infarction expansion index	Lower	Higher
Mortality rate	Three times lower	Greater
Cardiac decompensation	Later onset	Earlier onset
Cardiac function	Better	Worse
Remodelling	Better	Maladaptive

and all-cause mortality [9]. Men with free testosterone in a lowest quartile had a 24% greater risk for all-cause mortality due to ischemic heart disease [10]. Gender differences in myocardial response to ischemia are found (Table 16.2).

Polymorphic variants in genes including estrogen receptor, MDR1, APOZ, ACE, preproendothelin-1, and microsomal triglyceride transfer protein (MTP) have been identified that have gender-specific effects on the action of specific common drugs to treat age-associated CVD.

16.1 The Role of Mitochondria in Aging

Mitochondria play essential role during the initial steps of sex steroid hormone biosynthesis. Import of cholesterol from the outer to the inner mitochondrial membrane is a rate-limiting step involving interaction between the steroid acute regulatory protein (StAR) and molecular complex. Cholesterol is converted by cytochrome P450 side-chain cleavage to pregnenolone. In male, pregnenolone is converted to 17 αOH pregnenolone, dehydroepiandrosterone (DHEA), androstenedione, and testosterone. In female it is converted to estradiol.

Decline of sex steroids and accumulation of mitochondrial damage may create a positive feedback loop that contributes to the progressive degeneration in tissue function. Mitochondrial reactive oxygen species (ROS) promotes mitochondrial damage in ovarian follicles, too. Estradiol can inhibit mitochondrial ROS generating in cardiomyocytes. While estradiol protects normal cells from oxidative stress, it exacerbates oxidative stress in damaged cells. So, the most important fact is to initiate therapy on time.

Low testosterone in male reduces expression of mitochondrial respiratory genes. Androgen receptor overexpression in myocytes increases mitochondrial enzyme activity and oxygen consumption. Testosterone therapy increases mitochondrial biogenesis, improves mitochondrial quality, and increases physical activity [11].

Experiments on *Macaca fascicularis* monkeys showed decrease in the expression of key enzymes in glycolysis (pyruvate kinase, alpha enolase, triosephosphate isomerase), glucose oxidation (pyruvate dehydrogenase E1 beta subunit), and the tricarboxylic acid cycle in left ventricular samples from old male monkeys.

Table 16.3 Gender-dependent factors influencing cardiovascular prognosis

Characteristics	Female	Male
Cardiac weight	Preserved	Reduction (1 g/year
Myocyte number	Preserved	Reduction 64 million/year
Myocyte volume	Preserved	Increased
Mononucleate/binucleate myocytes	Constant	Decreased
Apoptotic index	Low	3 times higher
Apoptotic rate	Increased	Decreased

These glycolytic glucose oxidation and TCA enzymes were not observed in young males and old females. The changes in glycolytic and mitochondrial metabolic pathway in old monkeys' hearts were similar to changes observed in hearts affected by diabetes mellitus or left ventricle dysfunction and could be involved in cardiomyopathy of aging.

Heart muscles of males grow bigger and thicker with age, while in females it retains its size or gets smaller. So, aging does not lead to myocyte loss and myocyte cellular reactive hypertrophy in women indicating that gender difference may play detrimental effects on the aging process (Table 16.3).

In study group of subjects aged 54–94 years during 10 years, weight of the left ventricle increased in men 8 g and decreased 1.6 g in women. The difference in size, volume, and pumping ability occurred independently of other risk factors (weight, blood pressure, cholesterol levels, exercise). Myocardial apoptosis is increased in aging males compared to females. Changes in myocardial ERα expression, localization, and association with structural proteins have been found in end-stage failing hearts of patients with dilating cardiomyopathy.

16.2 Gonadal Hormones and Arrhythmias

Steroid hormones are regulators of calcium channel expression. Membrane density of the cardiac L-type Ca channel is regulated by estradiol in women and suggests that estradiol decrease leads to an increase in the number of cardiac L-type Ca channels, abnormality in excitability, and increase risk of arrhythmias. Therapy with 17 beta-estradiol has antagonistic effects on Ca channels when acutely administered through smooth muscles and cardiac myocytes decreases [12] .

Estrogen, via estrogen receptor-dependent mechanism, differentially alters the response of male and female cells to hypoxia. Intrinsic electrical difference resulting from variable ion channel expression and diverse sex hormone regulation via long-term genomic and acute non-genomic pathway was found [13].

Receptors for estradiol alpha and beta are found on cardiomyocytes, fibroblasts, and endothelial cells. In women, lower expression levels of K+ channel α and β subunits were found. QT interval is a period of ventricle activation and repolarization. Women show higher basic heart rate than men as well as LONGER QT interval, shorter QRS duration, and lower QRS voltage.

While estrogen may exacerbate arrhythmia susceptibility, during reproductive period, progesterone is protective and decreases QT interval [14]. Progesterone receptors are located at vascular smooth muscle cells and cardiac myocytes. The ratio between estradiol and progesterone is very important in sudden, unexpected, transient arrhythmias in the luteal phase, especially in women with premenstrual syndrome. QT interval is longer in the follicular phase than in luteal phase. Progesterone inhibits L-type Ca channels currents, and action potentials are shorter in the luteal phase protecting from arrhythmias [15]. Testosterone increases repolarizing K+ current density and protects against arrhythmias in women. Women with long QT tend to have a higher prevalence of sick sinus node syndrome, atrioventricular tachycardia, idiopathic right ventricle tachycardia, and dysrhythmic events.

In heart failure, prolonged action potential duration, decreased cell excitability, increased Na/Ca exchange, preserved β adrenergic responsiveness, and decreased outward K currents were observed. Therapy with estradiol may regulate Ca influx through reverse Na/Ca exchange by lessening the magnitude of the rise in Na during myocardial infarction in ischemic heart. Biomarkers of cardiovascular disease including troponin, C-reactive protein, phosphorylase, A2, E-selectin, adiponectin, lipid peroxides, and resistin have gender-specific distribution and expression.

The greatest density of androgen receptors is in the heart! Cardiac fibroblasts derived from male rats were more susceptible to hypoxia compared to females.

In males with heart failure, the hearts are prone to arrhythmias and contractile dysfunction. Testosterone therapy induces rapid vasodilatation. Acute application of testosterone increases intracellular calcium in osteoblasts, platelets, skeletal muscles, and cardiac myocytes. Testosterone rapidly elicits voltage-dependent calcium oscillations and IP3 receptor-mediated calcium release from cardiomyocytes. Cardiac excitation triggers a rise in intracellular calcium and contraction known as excitation contraction coupling (EC). ECE is initiated when calcium enters the cell via L-type calcium channels during phase 2 of the action potential (AP). The small influx of calcium triggers the release of much larger amount of calcium through Ca release channels in the sarcoplasmic reticulum (SR) in the process known as Ca-induced Ca release. Calcium is released from SR in the form of discrete subcellular units called Ca sparks that fuse to form Ca transient. Calcium then binds to contractile proteins (myofilaments) which results in sarcomere shortening and cardiac contraction. One of the important regulators of cardiac contractility functions is phospholamban (PLB). During systole, PLB binds to Ca pump and prevents Ca from being pumped back into the sarcoplasmic reticulum (SR). During muscle relaxation PLB is in its phosphorylated state which removes its inhibitory effects out of SR Ca ATPase (SERCA) and restores low Ca levels in the cytoplasm. PLB is highly expressed in the failing heart and may be a mechanism of systolic contractile dysfunction. In men the expression of PLB is increased. PLB has also been shown to be phosphorylated by cAMP-dependent protein kinase and Ca/calmodulin-dependent protein kinase. Calmodulin 3 has a low expression in men. In failing hearts induced expression of Na/K–ATPase-α1 induces decrease of Ca efflux, increasing cytoplasmatic Ca, and Ca-depending arrhythmia occurs.

Chronic testosterone withdrawal influences cardiac calcium-handling mechanism in ventricular myocytes, and AP is prolonged. The decrease of SR calcium release is a consequence of:

- Decreased density of L-type Ca channels, so less calcium is available to trigger SR calcium release.
- The magnitude of calcium sparks may decline. The decline in SR Ca uptake arises through a reduction in PLB. Contractions are attenuated in myocytes and relaxation is slowed. Prolonged AP can increase probability of early depolarization which can trigger arrhythmias [15].

Brugada syndrome is present in males eight times more compared to females. Ventricular tachycardia is characterized by ST-segment elevation in the right precordial leads (V1–3) and right bundle branch block. Lower expression of repolarizing ion channel subunits was found.

Conclusion

Gonadal hormones show sex-specific characteristics on cardiovascular system. Follow-up and treating of all disturbances of estradiol, progesterone, and testosterone, predominantly, are necessary in order to avoid diseases and improve quality of life.

References

1. Rahman I (2015) Relationship between age at natural menopause and risk of heart failure. Menopause 1:12–16
2. Rossouw JE, Prentice RL, Manson JE et al (2007) Postmenopausal hormone therapy and risk of cardiovascular disease by age and years since menopause. JAMA 297:1465–1477
3. Genevieve A (2011) Lipids, menopause and early atherosclerosis in SWAN heart women. Menopause 18:376–384
4. Rossano (2012) Lancet 673:60367–60365
5. Laughlin GA, Barret-Connor E (2008) Low serum testosterone and mortality in older men. J Clin Endocr Metab 93:68–75
6. Goldmeyer S (2014) Cardiovascular autonomic dysfunction in primary ovarian insufficiency:clinical and experimental evidence. Am J Trans Res 6:91–101
7. Mendelsohn ME (2005) Molecular and cellular basis of cardiovascular gender differences. Science 10:1583–1587
8. Webb CM, Mc Neil JG et al (1999) Effects of testosterone on coronary vasomotor regulation in men with coronary heart disease. J Am College Cardiol 83:437–439
9. Maranon R, Reckelhoff J (2013) Sex and gender differences in control of blood pressure. Clin Sci (Lond) 125:311–318
10. Vikam T, Schirmer H, Hjolstad I (2009) Endogenous sex hormones and the prospective association with cardiovascular disease and mortality in men: the Tromso study. Eur J Endo 161:435–442
11. Velarde M (2014) Mitochondrial and sex steroid hormone cross talk during aging. Longevity Health Span 3:2–10
12. Johnson B, Zheng W, Korach K et al (1997) Increased expression of the cardiac L-type Ca channel in ER-deficient mice. J Gen Psychiolo 110:135–140

13. Yang P, Clausy CE (2011) Gender-based differences in cardiac diseases. J Biomed Res 25:81–83
14. Dogan M, Akpak Y, Yiginer O (2016) The effects of menstrual cycle on cardiac conduction system. Crescent J Med Biol Sci 3:37–39
15. Ayaz O, Howlett SE (2015) Testosterone modulates cardiac contraction and calcium homeostasis: cellular and molecular mechanism. Biol Sex Differ 6:9

Part V

Benign Breast Diseases, BRCA Mutation and Breast Cancer

Risk-Reducing Surgery and Treatment of Menopausal Symptoms in BRCA Mutation Carriers (and Other Risk Women)

17

Piero Sismondi, Marta D'Alonzo, Paola Modaffari, Viola Liberale, Valentina Elisabetta Bounous, Andrea Villasco, and Nicoletta Biglia

17.1 Introduction and Risk Assessment

In developed countries breast cancer (BC) occurs in one out of eight women during her lifetime, estimating the life expectancy of 85 years. About 10% of BC is associated with genetic risk factors, essentially mutations of BRCA1 and BRCA2, however, but the majority of BC are sporadic. Risk factors for BC are primarily related to age and to estrogen exposure (early menarche, late menopause, nulliparity, use of exogenous hormones); in addition high-risk population also includes women with atypical hyperplasia and patients with ductal or lobular carcinoma in situ.

The lifetime cumulative risk of breast cancer for women with *BRCA1 or BRCA2 mutations* is very high ranging from 45 to 65%; this population has an elevated ovarian cancer risk as well [1]. The Ovarian cancer estimated lifetime risks is 36–46% and 10–27% in *BRCA1* and *BRCA2* mutation carriers, respectively. Therefore for these women, a close surveillance is suggested as well as medical and surgical options, including chemoprevention, bilateral salpingo-oophorectomy, and mastectomy.

Outside of genetic risk factors, for *the general population*, it is important to identify women at *high risk of breast cancer*: patients with previous thoracic RT < 30 y of age, women diagnosed with lobular carcinoma in situ, and women with an estimated 5-year breast cancer risk ≥1.7% [2]. Several mathematical models to estimate this risk have been proposed; currently the most used is the National Cancer

P. Sismondi (✉) • M. D'Alonzo • P. Modaffari • V. Liberale • V.E. Bounous
A. Villasco • N. Biglia
Department of Obstetrics and Gynaecology, University of Turin,
"Umberto I Hospital", Turin, Italy
e-mail: piero.sismondi@unito.it; p.sismondi@tin.it

M. Birkhaeuser, A.R. Genazzani (eds.), *Pre-Menopause, Menopause and Beyond*, ISGE Series, https://doi.org/10.1007/978-3-319-63540-8_17

Institute (NCI) Breast Cancer Risk Assessment Tool which is a modified version of the Gail model that consider age, race, age at first pregnancy, family history, and history of atypical hyperplasia; individuals with a 5-year risk of 1.66% or greater are considered at risk [3]. All the models have a limited reliability, and, as a matter of fact, up to 60% of BC occurs in women with no known risk factors; the available models do not include some risk factors such as obesity, diet, mammographic density, and use of HRT. A higher accuracy could be obtained by incorporating information on genotypes as well.

A recent report published in the *New England Journal of Medicine* [4] underlines the importance of *atypical hyperplasia* as an independent factor for the inclusion of patients in chemoprevention programs. Atypical hyperplasia is a high-risk benign lesion that is found in approximately 10% of biopsies with benign findings. In studies with long-term follow-up, atypical hyperplasia has been shown to confer a relative risk for future breast cancer of 4. Another large cohort study at the Mayo Clinic [5] published on 2014 confirms the cumulative high risk of breast cancer among women with atypical hyperplasia. Indeed, 25 years after a biopsy showing atypical hyperplasia, breast cancer (either in situ or invasive) developed in 30% of the women, with greater numbers of foci associated with a higher risk. Hartman and co. conclude suggesting that absolute risk data about women diagnosed with atypical hyperplasia should be used instead of models to describe breast cancer risk in this population. Guidelines for high-risk women should be updated to include women with atypical hyperplasia. Analyses of data from the subgroup of women with atypical hyperplasia were performed in four of the placebo-controlled trials (NSABP P-1, MAP.3, IBIS-I, and IBIS-II). A total of 2009 women with atypical hyperplasia were randomly assigned to receive an active agent or placebo in these trials. Relative-risk reductions in the atypical hyperplasia subgroup ranged from 41 to 79%, which suggested an even greater benefit than in the total population treated with the active agent in these trials.

Women with a life expectancy of ≥10 years and no diagnosis or history of breast cancer who are considered to be at increased risk for breast cancer based on any of the above-mentioned assessments, should receive individualized counseling to decrease breast cancer risk. *Strategies for prevention of breast cancer include* lifestyle factors (avoidance of obesity, maintaining physical activity, moderation in alcohol intake), chemoprevention therapy with risk reduction agents, and risk reduction surgery [2].

17.2 Risk Reduction Mastectomy (RRM)

Retrospective analyses with median follow-up periods of 13–14 years have indicated that bilateral risk-reducing mastectomy decreased the risk of developing breast cancer by approximately 90% in moderate- and high-risk women and in known *BRCA1/2* mutation carriers [6]. Further results from smaller prospective studies with shorter follow-up support the conclusion that RRM provides a high degree of protection against breast cancer in women with a *BRCA1/2* mutation. A recent meta-analysis including 2635 patients demonstrated a significant risk reduction in breast cancer incidence in BRCA1 and BRCA2 mutation carriers receiving RRM (HR 0.07; 95% CI 0.01–0.44; $p = 0.004$).

In the 2007 guidelines issued by the Society of Surgical Oncology, *indications for bilateral prophylactic mastectomies* in patients without a cancer diagnosis included BRCA mutations or other genetic susceptibility genes, strong family history with no demonstrable mutation, histological risk factors (including atypical ductal or lobular hyperplasia, or lobular carcinoma in situ confirmed on biopsy); a further indication was a difficult surveillance [7]. The position statement states that rarely, bilateral prophylactic mastectomies may be warranted for an exceptional patient with no family history or high-risk histology such as patient with extremely dense fibronodular tissue that is difficult to evaluate with standard breast imaging, several prior breast biopsies for clinical and/or mammographic abnormalities, and strong concern about breast cancer risk. In the same guidelines, potential indications for prophylactic contralateral mastectomy in patients with a current or previous diagnosis of breast cancer were risk reduction (see indications as listed above), difficult surveillance (patients with clinically and mammographically dense breast tissue or diffuse indeterminate microcalcifications in the contralateral breast), or reconstructive issues (symmetry/balance).

The 2017 NCCN Breast Cancer Risk Reduction Panel supports the use of RRM for carefully selected women at high risk for breast cancer who desire this intervention, exclusively considering BRCA1/2 or other genetic mutations and previous history of LCIS [2]. There are no data regarding RRM in women with prior mantle radiation exposure. As regards atypical hyperplasia, the Society of Surgical Oncology recognizes it as a possible but not routine indication for bilateral prophylactic mastectomy [7]. The recent report published in the *New England Journal of Medicine* on atypical hyperplasia and possible surgical risk reduction interventions concludes that, in current practice, with minimal data available on this topic and with chemopreventive agents for risk reduction available, atypical hyperplasia is generally not an indication for prophylactic mastectomy [8].

Women considering RRM should first have *appropriate multidisciplinary consultations*, a clinical breast examination and bilateral mammogram if not performed within the past 6 months. If results are normal, women who choose RRM may undergo the procedure with or without immediate breast reconstruction. *Axillary node* assessment has limited utility at the time of RRM. Women undergoing RRM do not require an axillary lymph node biopsy unless breast cancer is identified on the pathologic evaluation of the mastectomy specimen. *Following RRM*, for monitoring breast health, women should continue with annual exams of the chest and the reconstructed breast because there is still a small residual risk of developing breast cancer. Mammograms are not recommended in this situation [2].

17.3 Bilateral Risk-Reducing Salpingo-Oophorectomy (RRSO)

The absence of reliable methods of early detection and the poor prognosis associated with advanced ovarian cancer have lent support for the performance of bilateral risk-reducing salpingo-oophorectomy (RRSO) that *decreases the risk* of developing ovarian and fallopian cancer by 85–95% in BRCA1/2 mutation carriers when performed before age 50 [9]. RRSO is also reported to reduce by approximately 50% the risk for breast cancer in BRCA mutation carriers when performed in premenopausal age. The results of several studies suggest that RRSO may be associated with a greater reduction in breast cancer risk for BRCA1 mutation carriers compared with BRCA2 mutation carriers [10, 11].

The decreased hormonal exposure following surgical removal of the ovaries is the basis for the reductions in breast cancer risk after RRSO; results from Eisen et al. suggest the reductions in breast cancer risk is greater when the surgery is performed in younger women (OR 0.41 (95% CI, 0.25–0.68) for RRSO performed at age 40 years or younger versus odds ratio 0.47 (95% CI, 0.28–0.80) for RRSP performed in carriers aged 41–50 years). Nonsignificant risk reduction of breast cancer was found for women aged 51 years or older [11]. Data are limited about the *optimal age for RRSO*. Considering that the mean age at diagnosis of ovarian cancer is 50.8 years for BRCA1/2 mutation carriers [12], current guidelines for ovarian cancer risk management recommended bilateral salpingo-oophorectomy at the completion of childbearing or by age 35 to 40 [2]. Considering the slight advance of the diagnosis in BRCA 1 carriers than in BRCA 2, in the first group of patients, the RRSO could be proposed as soon as possible after the completion of childbearing, delaying the surgery after 40 years only after careful consideration of risks and benefits. In BRCA2-mutated patients, instead, the action may be brought between 40 and 50 years considering the progressive reduction of the protective effect against breast cancer [13].

Following prophylactic salpingo-oophorectomy, a 1–4.3% *residual risk for a primary peritoneal carcinoma* in BRCA1 and BRCA2 mutation carriers still exists [14]. It cannot be excluded that in some cases peritoneal carcinoma foci are actually metastases of subclinical disease that was present at the time of surgery (occult carcinomas), so that undiagnosed cancers at the time of surgery will be considered primary peritoneal cancer when they become clinically apparent. Possibly fewer peritoneal cancers will be diagnosed after salpingo-oophorectomy if the comprehensive pathology review of the specimens is performed on all patients [15]. Fisch et al. in paper based on a series of 159 female BRCA1 or BRCA2 carriers who underwent prophylactic oophorectomy showed that 2–10% of BRCA1/2 carriers who undergo prophylactic salpingo-oophorectomy will be found to have occult carcinomas if the ovaries and the tubes are rigorously examined. No cancers were detected among women who had the operation at age 39 or younger [16]. The conclusion is that a rigorous operative and pathologic protocol for RRSO increases the detection rate of occult ovarian malignancy in BRCA mutation carriers, influencing the postoperative management with additional staging, chemotherapy, and follow-up in affected women. Also, the *peritoneal lavage cytology* can detect occult carcinoma at the time of RRSO [17] and should always be performed [2]. The additional benefit of *concurrent hysterectomy* is not clear. Even if careful ligation of the fallopian tube at the uterine origin is performed, a small portion of interstitial fallopian tube in the cornua of the uterus is left in situ if hysterectomy is not performed, however, in the largest study on fallopian tube cancer to date, 92% of cancers originated in the distal or midportion of the tube. The concurrent hysterectomy can simplify HRT allowing estrogen-only supplementation and can reduce the endometrial cancer risk associated with tamoxifen treatment for a previous breast cancer [13]. However, the risk and benefits of concomitant hysterectomy should be discussed with each individual woman. As the majority of BRCA-associated ovarian cancers appear to originate in the fallopian tube, some authors propose *prophylactic salpingectomy*; data on short- and long-term outcomes of this prophylactic surgery is limited, and there are no studies directly comparing prophylactic salpingectomy with bilateral salpingo-oophorectomy for BRCA-mutated women. A clinical trial led by Leblanc et al. is currently recruiting young BRCA mutation carriers for radical fimbriectomy (NCT016808074), but it is not expected to be complete until 2019 (http://clinicaltrials.gov). *A two-stage procedure* has been proposed: bilateral salpingectomy with delayed oophorectomy to prevent the adverse consequences of premature menopause. Know et al. developed a Markov Monte Carlo simulation model to compare three strategies for risk reduction in women with BRCA mutations: bilateral salpingo-oophorectomy, bilateral salpingectomy, and bilateral salpingectomy with delayed oophorectomy. The model estimates the number of future breast and ovarian cancers and cardiovascular deaths attributed to premature menopause with each strategy: bilateral salpingo-oophorectomy offers the greatest risk reduction for breast and ovarian cancer, but when considering quality-adjusted life expectancy, bilateral salpingectomy with delayed oophorectomy is a cost-effective strategy and may be an acceptable alternative for those unwilling to undergo immediate bilateral salpingo-oophorectomy [18]. Finally, some authors proposed the *tubal ligation* as a feasible option to reduce the risk of ovarian cancer in women with BRCA mutations who have completed childbearing. Four main mechanisms are invoked: a screening effect, the alteration of ovarian function, a mechanical barrier to the ascent of endometrial or proximal fallopian tube cells into the peritoneal cavity, and the prevention of retrograde transport of carcinogenic substances from the vagina. A meta-analysis of 13 studies shows a reduced risk of epithelial ovarian cancer by 34%. The protective effect of tubal ligation was confirmed even in a subgroup of women 10–14 years after the procedure. The risk reduction was confirmed for the endometrioid and serous cancers but not for mucinous [19].

17.4 Treatment of Menopausal Symptoms in BRCA Mutation Carriers

The absence of reliable methods of early detection and the poor prognosis associated with advanced ovarian cancer have lent support for the performance of bilateral risk reduction RRSO; however, there are many concerns and worries about the resulting premature menopause.

The most *common symptoms* are vasomotor symptoms (hot flashes, night sweats, palpitations), vaginal dryness, sexual dysfunction, cognitive dysfunction, poor sleep, and tiredness. Women who were premenopausal at the time of surgery experienced a worsening of hot flashes, night sweats and sweating, and a decline in sexual function 1 year after surgery. Menopausal disorders are more severe if RRSO is performed in premenopausal women than in postmenopausal women [20].

Premenopausal oophorectomy is also associated with an increased risk of *osteopenia, osteoporosis, and fracture*. Following oophorectomy, there is an increased prevalence of osteoporosis within 3 to 6 years of surgery; the loss of trabecular bone has been reported to be as high as 20% during the first 18 months following surgery. Several recent cross-sectional studies have examined bone health after salpingo-oophorectomy in women with a BRCA mutation. Cohen et al. published a study of 226 BRCA carriers after salpingo-oophorectomy [21]: among women who underwent surgery before the age of 50 years, high rates of osteopenia (62%) and osteoporosis (9%) were reported. The 2010 Canadian guidelines for diagnosis and management of osteoporosis propose bone density measurement with DXA at the time of salpingo-oophorectomy and again 1–2 years after surgery; the timing of further bone density measurements should be individualized based on the results of these two measurements; to prevent osteoporosis, a recommended daily intake of 1500 mg calcium from dietary and supplemental sources and supplementation with 800 IU/day of vitamin D daily is suggested. In women with premature menopause, hormone replacement therapy (HRT), if not contraindicated, is advised to preserve bone mineral density; however, the duration of use is not clear [2].

Bilateral oophorectomy has also been shown to be a risk factor *for coronary heart disease*. A positive association between bilateral oophorectomy and increased risk of cardiovascular disease has been observed in a number of observational studies, including the Nurses' Health Study (rate ratio 2.2) and the Mayo Clinic Cohort of Oophorectomy and Aging (HR 1.4). A recent study [22] links BRCA1 gene function with cardiovascular function, (RCA1 gene products work to prevent DNA damage). The loss of BRCA1 in cardiomyocytes may result in adverse cardiac remodeling, poor ventricular function, and increased mortality in response to ischemic or genotoxic stress. Therefore BRCA1-mutated women may be at an increased risk for cardiovascular disease, even if there are no clinical studies to date to evaluate this issue. Also in this context, HRT may mitigate the increase in cardiovascular risk associated with surgical menopause.

Several studies show that *short-term HRT use* does not negate the protective effect of RRSO on subsequent breast cancer risk in BRCA1/2 mutation carriers [23]. In a matched case-control study of 472 postmenopausal women with a BRCA1 mutation, Eisen et al. examined whether or not the use of HRT was associated with subsequent risk of breast cancer [24]. The adjusted OR for breast cancer associated with ever use of HRT compared with never use was 0.58 (95% CI 0.35–0.96; $P = 0.03$); they concluded that HRT use was not associated with increased risk of breast cancer; indeed, in BRCA1-mutated women, it was associated with a decreased risk. In a recent review, Marchetti et al. [25] conclude that HRT generally reduces symptoms related to surgical menopause; short-term HRT seems to improve the quality of life and does not seem to have an adverse effect on oncologic outcomes in BRCA1 and BRCA2 mutation carriers without a personal history of breast cancer. The 2013 NICE guidelines recommend HRT for women with no personal history of breast cancer, including BRCA1 or BRCA2 mutation carriers, having had bilateral salpingo-oophorectomy before their natural menopause. They should take combined HRT or estrogens only depending on having the uterus or not, until the time they would have expected natural menopause.

Estrogen therapy, however, is *contraindicated for breast cancer survivors* [26]. The Stockholm trial [27] was prematurely stopped in 2003 when the parallel HABITS trial [28] reported a higher recurrence rate in breast cancer patients who received systemic estrogens compared to women treated with placebo. At 4 years of follow-up, the HABITS study still found an increased risk of recurrence [29], whereas a recently updated analysis of the data from the Stockholm trial at 10.8 years of follow-up did not show any excess of recurrence risk [30]. An alternative compound to conventional estrogen/progestogen treatment, tibolone, was tested versus placebo in the LIBERATE trial, showing a significant superiority to placebo in reducing vasomotor symptoms and improving sleep quality, sexual behavior, mood, and attraction but unfortunately also a significant increase in the recurrence rate [31].

Because of this concern, research efforts have focused on *nonhormonal drugs* to alleviate climacteric symptoms. Several substances have been tested: some of them give similar results to placebo that in itself provides a response in around 20–30% of women, while others have shown promising results.

Conclusion

Women with a life expectancy ≥10 years and no diagnosis/history of breast cancer who are considered to be at increased risk for breast cancer should receive counseling to decrease breast cancer risk, considering lifestyle factors, therapy with risk reduction agents, and risk reduction surgery (in BRCA1/2 mutation carriers).

Bilateral risk-reducing mastectomy decreases the risk of developing breast cancer by at least 90%; it should be proposed to carefully selected women at high risk for breast cancer considering BRCA1/2 or other genetic mutations and previous history of LCIS. In current practice, atypical hyperplasia is not an indication for prophylactic mastectomy.

Bilateral risk-reducing salpingo-oophorectomy decreases the risk of developing ovarian and fallopian cancer by 85–95% and breast cancer by 50% in BRCA1/2 mutation carriers when performed in premenopausal age. Peritoneal washing should be performed at surgery, and pathologic assessment should include fine sectioning of the ovaries and fallopian tubes. The additional benefit of concurrent hysterectomy is not clear at the time. In women with no personal history of breast cancer, short-term HRT use does not negate the protective effect of RRSO on subsequent breast cancer risk, and it should be offered until the time of expected natural menopause.

References

1. Antoniou A, Pharoah P, Narod S, Risch HA et al (2003) Average risks of breast and ovarian cancer associated with BRCA1 or BRCA2 mutations detected in case series unselected for family history: a combined analysis of 22 studies. Am J Hum Genet 72(5):1117–1130
2. NCCN Guidelines 1 (16 Dec 2016) Breast cancer risk reduction
3. Gail MH, Costantino JP (2001) Validating and improving models for projecting the absolute risk of breast cancer. J Natl Cancer Inst 93(5):334–335
4. Hartmann LC et al (2015) Atypical hyperplasia of the breast, risk assessment and management options. N Engl J Med 372:78–89
5. Hartmann LC, Radisky DC, Frost MH et al (2014) Understanding the premalignant potential of atypical hyperplasia through its natural history: a longitudinal cohort study. Cancer Prev Res (Phila) 7:211–217
6. Hartmann LC et al (1999) Efficacy of bilateral prophylactic mastectomy in women with a family history of breast cancer. N Engl J Med 340:77–84
7. Giuliano AE, Boolbol S, Degnim A et al (2007) Society of Surgical Oncology: position statement on prophylactic mastectomy. Approved by the Society of Surgical Oncology Executive Council, March 2007. Ann Surg Oncol 14(9):2425–2427
8. Giuliano AE, Boolbol S, Degnim A, Henry K, Marilyn Leitch A, Morrow M (2007) Annals of. Surg Oncol 14(9):2425–2427. doi:10.1245/s10434-007-9447-z
9. Rebbeck TR, Kauff ND, Domchek SM (2009) Meta-analysis of risk reduction estimates associated with risk-reducing salpingo oophorectomy in BRCA1 or BRCA2 mutation carriers. J Natl Cancer Inst 101:80–87
10. Kauff ND, Domchek SM, Friebel ME et al (2008) Risk-reducing salpingooophorectomy for the prevention of BRCA1- and BRCA2-associated breast and gynecologic cancer: a multicenter, prospective study. J Clin Oncol 26:1331–1337
11. Eisen A, Lubinski J, Klijn J et al (2005) Breast cancer risk following bilateral oophorectomy in BRCA1 and BRCA2 mutation carriers: an international case-control study. J Clin Oncol 23:7491–7496
12. Rebbeck TR, Lynch HT, Neuhausen SL et al (2002) Prophylactic oophorectomy in carriers of BRCA1 or BRCA2 mutations. N Engl J Med 346(21):1616–1622
13. RIGENIO Guidelines (2007) Regione Piemonte
14. Finch A, Beiner M, Lubinski J et al (2006) Salpingo-oophorectomy and the risk of ovarian, fallopian tube, and peritoneal cancers in women with a BRCA1 or BRCA2 mutation. JAMA 296:185–192
15. Lavie O, Hornreich G, Ben-Arie A, Rennert G, Cohen Y et al (2004) BRCA germline mutations in Jewish women with uterine serous papillary carcinoma. Gynecol Oncol 92:521–524
16. Finch A, Shaw P, Rosen B et al (2006) Clinical and pathologic findings of prophylactic salpingo-oophorectomies in 159 BRCA1 and BRCA2 carriers. Gynecol Oncol 100:58–64
17. Colgan TJ, Boerner SL, Murphy J, Cole DE, Narod S, Rosen B (2002) Peritoneal lavage cytology: an assessment of its value during prophylactic oophorectomy. Gynecol Oncol 85(3):397–403
18. Kwon JS, Tinker A, Pansegrau G et al (2013) Prophylactic salpingectomy and delayed oophorectomy as an alternative for BRCA. Obstet Gynecol 121:14–24
19. Cibula D, Widschwendter M, Májek O, Dusek L (2011) Tubal ligation and the risk of ovarian cancer: review and meta-analysis. Hum Reprod Update 17(1):55–67
20. Finch A, Metcalfe KA, Chiang JK, Elit L, McLaughlin J, Springate C et al (2011) The impact of prophylactic salpingo-oophorectomy on menopausal symptoms and sexual function in women who carry a BRCA mutation. Gynecol Oncol 121(1):163–168
21. Cohen JV, Chiel L, Boghossian L, Jones M, Domchek SM et al (2012) Non-cancer endpoints in BRCA1/2 carriers after risk-reducing salpingo-oophorectomy. Familial Cancer 11(1):69–75
22. Shukla PC, Singh KK, Quan A et al (2011) BRCA1 is an essential regulator of heart function and survival following myocardial infarction. Nat Commun 2:593

23. Rebbeck TR, Friebel T, Wagner T et al (2005) Effect of short-term hormone replacement therapy on breast cancer risk reduction after bilateral prophylactic oophorectomy in BRCA1 and BRCA2 mutation carriers: the PROSE Study Group. J Clin Oncol 23:7804–7810
24. Eisen A, Lubinski J, Gronwald J, Moller P, Lynch HT et al (2008) Hormone therapy and the risk of breast cancer in BRCA1 mutation carriers. J Natl Cancer Inst 100(19):1361–1367
25. Marchetti C, Iadarola R, Palaia I, di Donato V, Perniola G, Muzii L, Panici PB (2014) Hormone therapy in oophorectomized BRCA1/2 mutation carriers. Menopause 21(7):763–768
26. International Menopause Society (IMS) (2013) Updated 2013 International Menopause Society recommendations on menopausal hormone therapy and preventive strategies for midlife health. Climacteric 16:316–337
27. Von Schoultz E, Rutqvist LE, Stockholm Breast Cancer Study Group (2005) Menopausal hormone replacement therapy after breast cancer: the Stockholm randomised trial. J Natl Cancer Inst 97:533–535
28. Holmberg L, Anderson H (2004) For the HABITS steering and data monitoring committees. HABITS (hormonal replacement therapy after breast cancer – is it safe?), a randomised comparison: trial stopped. Lancet 363:453–455
29. Holmberg L, Iversen OE, Rudenstam CM et al (2008) Increased risk of recurrence after hormone replacement therapy in breast cancer survivors. J Natl Cancer Inst 100:475–482
30. Fahlén M, Fornander T, Johansson H et al (2013) Hormone replacement therapy after breast cancer: 10 year follow up of the Stockholm randomised trial. Eur J Cancer 49(1):52–59
31. Kenemans P, Bundred NJ, Foidart JM et al (2009) Safety and efficacy of tibolone in breast-cancer patients with vasomotor symptoms: a doubleblind, randomised, non-inferiority trial. Lancet Oncol 10:135–146

Benign Breast Disease During Women's Life

18

Svetlana Vujovic

The breasts are fountain of life, intimacy, and love. Gonadal hormones, predominantly, life style, and eating habits create changes in breast tissue.

18.1 Puberty

Breast buds, in which networks of tubules are formed, are generated from ectoderm. Until puberty male and female breast do not show any differences. The master regulators of breast growth are estradiol, progesterone, growth hormone (GH), insulin-like growth factor (IGF-1), and prolactin [1]. Estradiol and GH/IGF-1, through activating estrogen receptor α (ERα), specifically induce growth and transformation of the tubules into the maturated ductal system (Table 18.1).

The development of the female breast (thelarche) begins 3 years before menarche and fully developed by age 18.

18.2 Reproductive Period

In contrast to progesterone receptor (PR), ER expression in the breast is stable and differs relatively little in correlation with reproductive status, menstrual cycle phase, or exogenous hormone therapy [3]. Estradiol, progesterone, prolactin, and GH/IHG-1 modulate growth factors (Table 18.2).

They regulate cellular growth, proliferation, and differentiation via activation of intracellular signaling cascades that control cell functions such as Erk, Akt, JNK, and Ark/Stat [4]. The liver is the source of approximately 80% of circulating IGF-1.

S. Vujovic
Clinic of Endocrinology, Diabetes and Diseases of Metabolism, Clinical Center of Serbia, Faculty of Medicine, University of Belgrade, Belgrade, Serbia
e-mail: prof.svetlana.vujovic@gmail.com

M. Birkhaeuser, A.R. Genazzani (eds.), *Pre-Menopause, Menopause and Beyond*, ISGE Series, https://doi.org/10.1007/978-3-319-63540-8_18

Table 18.1 Estradiol and progesterone effects

Estradiol effects	Progesterone effects
Induction of duct sprout	Induction of ductal development and growth [2] via amphiregulin
Elongation of terminal duct buds	Lobular development
Induction of bulbous structures penetration into the fat pad and branches	Complete maturation of ductal alveolar system
Stromal tissue growth	
Adipose tissue growth	
Nipple-areola complex increase	
Prolactin increase	

Table 18.2 Growth factors in breasts

Insulin-like growth factor 1	Tissue necrosis factor β
Insulin-like growth factor 2	Transforming growth factor α
Amphiregulin	Transforming growth factor β
Epidermal growth factor	Heregulin
Fibroblast growth factor	Wnt
Hepatocyte growth factor	RANKL
Tissue necrosis factor α	Leukemia inhibiting factor

Although IGF-1 is responsible for most of the role of GH in mediating breast development, GH itself has been found to play a direct augmentation role as well as it increases ER expression in the breast stromal (connective) tissue, while IGF-1 has been found not to do this. EGF receptor is molecular target of EGF, TGFα, amphiregulin, and heregulin. Estradiol and progesterone mediate ductal development through induction of amphiregulin expression and this downstream EGFR activation.

Insulin, glucocorticoids (cortisol), and thyroxin play permissive poorly understood role. Leptin induces mammary gland epithelial cell proliferation. Androgens suppress the action of estradiol by decreasing the expression of ER [5]. Calcitriol, via vitamin D receptor, may be a negative regulator of ductal development but a positive regulator of lobuloalveolar development [6]. Vitamin D supplementation suppresses cyclooxygenase-2 expression and reduces and increases, respectively, the levels of prostaglandin E2 and TGF β2, known as inhibitory factors [7]. Overexpression of COX 2 induces hyperplasia of breast volume.

Adiponectin acts as insulin sensitizer and has anti-inflammatory actions. It can inhibit proliferation of endothelial cells and has been shown to exert antiproliferative effects on breast tissue [8]. In obese women adiponectin is low. Obesity is considered to be a chronic pro-inflammatory status. Adipose tissue contributes up to 30% of circulating interleukin 6, an inflammatory cytokine which induces hepatic synthesis of C-reactive protein.

About 69% of women experience cyclical breast pain during luteal phase. [illegible] in breast tissue relating to stromal, ductal, and glandular tissue [illegible] age. In early reproductive period, glandular component may respond to cyclic hormonal stimuli and exaggerated development of fibroadenoma. In late reproductive period, glandular tissue may become hyperplastic with sclerosing adenosis or lobular hyperplasia. During menopause atrophic changes of glandular tissue and stromal and fatty tissue occur, and with estradiol and progesterone replacement therapy, lobular tissue changes persist.

18.3 Benign Breast Disease

Benign breast diseases (BBD) represent all benign breast changes in women between 30 and 50 years of age. Eponyms are fibrocystic breast disease, Schimmelbusch's disease, Recklus disease, Cooper's disease, and Tillaux-Phocas diseases. Microscopic examinations can show fibrosis, adenosis, cysts, epitheliosis, and papillomatosis. Fibrocystic breast disease is not associated with increased risk of breast carcinoma.

18.3.1 Fibroadenoma

Fibroadenoma is a benign tumor in which epithelial cells are arranged in a fibrous stroma. They represent a hyperplasia or proliferative process in a single terminal duct unit. The peak of incidence is between 20 and 24 years. About 10% of fibroadenoma disappear each year. They stop growing after reaching 3–4 cm. Types of fibroadenoma are:

- Pericanalicular
- Intracanalicular
- Giant intracanalicular

They are presented as painless firm, discrete, round, rubbery tumors, with well distinct Borders, and are freely mobile lumps. Fibroadenoma need not to be removed because they tend to remain unchanged or decrease in size approaching the menopause and usually becomes nonpalpable. Phyllode tumors are often larger and reach 3–6 cm.

18.3.2 Cysts

Breast cysts result from involution of the lobules primarily during perimenopausal years in anovulatory cycles or cycles with changed estradiol/progesterone ratio and higher insulin levels. Cystic disease is characterized by the presence of fluid-filled structures greater than 3 mm which are lined by a layer of epithelial cells. In about 7–8% of women, macrocysts are present, in 50% cysts are solitary, and in 30% cysts can be detected. They are apocrine structures lined by secretory epithelial. It is possible to make a distinction between:

1. Type 1 cysts: high potassium, low natrium, and chloride (Na:K < 3). Increased melatonin, estradiol, dehydroepiandrosterone sulfate (DHEAS), EGF, and decreased levels of TGF β2
2. Type 2 cysts: low potassium, high natrium, and chloride (Na:K > 3)
3. Type 3 cysts: intermediate electrolyte to types 1 and 2 [9]

Platelet-derived growth factor PDGF0, IGF, and gastrin-related peptide are found in cyst fluid. While PDGF is several times higher in cysts than in serum, IGF1 and IGF2 are lower in cyst fluid. Melatonin was found 5–23 times higher in cyst fluid compared to daytime melatonin and three- to fourfold higher than night levels [10]. Melatonin suppressed all proliferation and counteracts effects of growth hormone.

18.3.2.1 Pathophysiology of Benign Breast Disease

Benign breast disease is characterized by increased blood perfusion, capillary permeability, and mucocutaneous substances accumulation. Hyalinization, swelling, and organization, due to albumin accumulation, are key factors developing diffuse synchronous hyperplasia of epithelial tissue and interlobar connective tissue. Vascular, neural, and epithelial factors are involved in BBD.

(a) Higher estradiol/progesterone ratio in the luteal phase

Progesterone levels begin dropping from about 35 years of age more frequently when anovulatory cycles start occurring. Progesterone insufficiency initiates benign breast disease.

Dynamic changes in estradiol and progesterone ratio become out of balance. Progesterone inhibits estrogen-induced mitosis and proliferation and causes differentiation of the cells. It, also, inhibits prolactin production. Intramammary estradiol levels are 20 times higher compared to that one in peripheral blood. Estrogen increases mitosis and secretory activity in the pituitary but particularly the proliferation of prolactin cells. High prolactin levels suppress ovulation. Progesterone has many roles: protection against breast cysts, nocturnal diuretic, carcinoma prevention agent, antianxiety agent, contributes to the formation of bones, and improves sexual drive during menopause. There is progesterone deficiency in cases of premenstrual syndrome, insomnia, early miscarriages, painful or lumpy breasts, infertility, unexplained weight gain, and anxiety.

The most important fact in the etiology of BDD is dynamic changes during the luteal phase in the ratio between estradiol and progesterone. Many women have ovulatory cycles but progesterone rapidly decreases after the midluteal phase inducing the increase of E2/P. Estradiol has an impact on breast cell proliferation of 230%; however, progesterone decreases it by 400%. When given together with estradiol, progesterone inhibited estrogen-induced breast cell proliferation [11]. Progesterone has natriuretic effect due to suppression of renal tubular reabsorption and increment of cell filtration preventing retention of liquid within the breast gland. That is the mechanism of treating painful breasts. Also, progesterone has an effect on vascular network by decreasing capillary permeability and breast tissue edema.

We examined effects of progesterone gel on the cyst volume and pain in the breast. During the sixth month of therapy with progesterone gel twice daily locally on the breast from day 16 to 26 of menstrual cycle, significant reduction of cyst number and size and decreased mastalgia were observed. There was a reduction of E2/P ratio on day 24 during therapy, compared to the ratio before therapy as well as ratio on day 21 of the cycle during therapy. The increase of progesterone on day 24 was found in comparison with progesterone before therapy on the same day [12]. In a double-blind Italian study of the effects of micronized progesterone vaginal cream on the breast, decreased pain was observed in 64.9% of women with mastalgia versus 22% in control group [13].

Synthetic progestins have different effects on breast tissue depending on the progestin form. Some of them are androgenic, and others induce water retention. In oral contraceptives, especially monophasic, the ratio between estradiol and progesterone is stable. No increase of E2/P is seen in the luteal phase and cysts decrease, as well as mastalgia. Drospirenone, as a progestin component, has the best results, concerning mastalgia.

(b) Transient hyperprolactinaemia

In the luteal phase, during higher estradiol levels, prolactin can increase. The addition of dopamine agonists can reduce prolactin levels. Such a therapeutic option treats consequences:

(c) Suboptimal thyroid hormone secretion in the luteal phase can induce BBD but in a broader complex of other etiological factors.
(d) Eating habits: methylxanthines (caffeine, chocolate, and cold drinks).

18.3.2.2 Clinical Characteristics of Benign Breast Disease

1. Cyclical mastalgia represents pain severe enough to interfere with daily life or lasting over 2 weeks per month.
2. It appears between30 and 40 years of age.
3. Premenstrual syndrome is associated with BBD.

18.3.2.3 Diagnostic Procedures

- Clinical examinations
- Breast ultrasound
- Mammography
- Cyst fluid aspiration
- Nuclear magnetic resonance

18.3.2.4 Therapy

1. Progesterone – is the drug of choice as previously described and first-line therapy for BBD.
2. Oral contraceptives – individually given which is a good choice.
3. Dopamine agonists.

4. Insulin sensitizers – not yet approved. In decreasing high insulin levels in the luteal phase and changing eating habits, they increase progesterone, change E2/P ratio, and decrease mastalgia and cysts volume (our unpublished data).
5. Danazol
   Food and Drug Administration advised danazol for mastalgia treatment. Unfortunately, many side effects (gaining weight, acne, hirsutism, etc.) make it not just unacceptable but harmful.
6. Tamoxifen
   With antiestrogen effects, it causes many side effects and is not acceptable.
7. Vitamin E (400 IU), magnesium (600 mg), and vitamin B6 (50 mg)

18.3.2.5 Benign Breast Disease and Breast Carcinoma

Fibrocystic changes are associated with no risk of breast carcinoma. Latest studies of Carrol [14] indicate the antiproliferative effects of progesterone. Progesterone receptors counteract with estrogen receptors following stimulation of both hormonal pathways. Progesterone induces RANKL, and breast carcinoma with RANKL expression has lower Ki-67, a growth marker. Loss of progesterone receptors was found in 20% of breast cancer cases. Treatment of breast carcinoma with progesterone is comparable to tamoxifen, and it lowers risk for estrogen-positive breast carcinoma. Meta-analysis provides evidence for the association between MTHFR genes; C677T in exon 4 at nucleotide C677T plays an important role in breast carcinoma [15].

References

1. Hynes NE, Watson CJ (2010) Mammary gland growth factors: roles in normal development and in cancer. Cold Spring Herb Perspect Biol 2:8
2. Aupperlee MD, Leipprandt JR, Bennet JM et al (2013) Amphiregulin mediates progesterone-induced mammary ductal development during puberty. Breast Cancewr Res 15:44
3. Haslam S, Osuch J (2006) Hormones and breast cancer in postmenopausal women. Breast Dis 42:69
4. Rawlings JS, Rosler KM, Harrison DA (2004) The JAK/STST signaling pathway. J Cell Sci 117:1281–1283
5. Zhou J, Ng S, Adesanya-Famuiya O et al (2000) Testosterone inhibits estrogen-induced mammary epithelial proliferation and suppress estrogen receptor expression. FASEB J 14:1725–1730
6. Welsh J (2011) Vitamin D metabolism in mammary gland and breast cancer. Mol Cell Endocrinol 347:55–60
7. Qin W, Smith C, Jensen M et al (2013) Vitamin D favourably alters the cancer promoting prostaglandin cascade. Anticancer Res 33:4496–4499
8. Catsburg C, Gunter M, Chen C et al (2014) Insulin, estrogen, inflammatory markers and risk of benign proliferative brest disease. Cancer Res 74:3248–3258
9. Ness J, Sedghinasab M, Moe RE et al (1993) Identification of multiple proliferative growth factors in breast cyst fluid. Am J Surgery 166:237–243
10. Burch JB, Walling M, Rush A et al (2007) Melatonin and estrogen in breast cyst fluids. Breast Cancer Res Treat 103:331–341

11. Foidart JM, Cohn C, Denoo X (1998) Estrogen and progesterone regulate the proliferation of human breast epithelial cells. Fertil Steroid 69:963–969
12. Brkic M, Vujovic S, Franic Ivanisevic M et al (2016) The influence of progesterone gel therapy in the treatment of fibrocystic breast disease. Open J Obstet Gynecol 6:334–341
13. Nappi C, Affinito P, Carlo D et al (1992) Double blind control trial of progesterone vaginal cream treatment of cyclical mastalgia in women with benign breast disease. J Endocrinol Invest 15:801–806
14. Carrol JS, Hickey TE, Tarulli GA et al (2017). Deciphering the divergent roles of progestogens in breast cancer. Nat Rev Cancer 17:54–64
15. Yan W, Zhang Y, Zhao E et al (2016) Association between the MTHFR C667T polymorphism and breast carcinoma risk: a meta analysis of 23 case control studies. The Breast J 22:593–594

Treatment of Menopausal Symptoms in Breast Cancer Survivors

19

Piero Sismondi, Valentina Elisabetta Bounous, Valentina Tuninetti, Viola Liberale, Martina Gallo, and Nicoletta Biglia

19.1 Introduction

Breast cancer is increasing worldwide and affects up to one in eight women who survive up to the age of 85 years in Western countries. Four out of five new cases of breast cancer are diagnosed in women over 50 years, with the peak in the 50–64 years age range. The survival rate of breast cancer patients has significantly increased due to earlier diagnosis and advances in adjuvant treatment: at 5 years after initial diagnosis is 89%. There are now more than 2.5 million breast cancer survivors (BCSs) in the USA [1].

Advances in the early detection and treatment of breast cancer have provided gains in patients' survival time. However, these gains are often accompanied by a variety of treatment-associated toxicities that influence the quality of life (QoL).

19.2 Menopausal Symptoms in Breast Cancer Survivors

Many of BCSs suffer from symptoms, which result directly from breast cancer adjuvant treatment with chemotherapy, tamoxifen, aromatase inhibitors, and ovarian suppression [2, 3].

The most frequent symptoms are hot flushes, but also the genitourinary syndrome of menopause (GSM), a new terminology referring to the wide range of vaginal and urinary symptoms related to menopause, has become the main problem for BCSs [4].

These women experience vasomotor symptoms such as hot flashes, night sweats and palpitations, vaginal dryness, sexual dysfunction, cognitive dysfunction, poor

P. Sismondi (✉) • V.E. Bounous • V. Tuninetti • V. Liberale • M. Gallo • N. Biglia
Department of Obstetrics and Gynaecology, University of Turin,
"Umberto I Hospital", Turin, Italy
e-mail: piero.sismondi@unito.it

M. Birkhaeuser, A.R. Genazzani (eds.), *Pre-Menopause, Menopause and Beyond*, ISGE Series, https://doi.org/10.1007/978-3-319-63540-8_19

sleep and tiredness, osteoporosis, and fertility problems. Up to 20% of BCSs consider stopping or actually cease endocrine therapy [2, 3].

Women can experience menopausal symptoms if chemotherapy results in premature cessation of ovarian function or as an adverse effect of endocrine therapies. Vasomotor symptoms are typically more severe in younger survivors because of the abrupt change in hormones and, when present, can have a significant impact on QoL. For younger women on endocrine therapies, 50–70% will likely experience hot flushes while on tamoxifen [5].

Sexual complaints are a common problem among BC survivors. They include sexual desire disorder/decreased libido (23–64% of patients), arousal or lubrication concerns (20–48% of patients), orgasmic concerns (16–36% of patients), and dyspareunia (35–38% of patients). Patients who receive chemotherapy tend to have more of these sexual concerns than those treated only with surgery and/or radiation. Treatment with aromatase inhibitors may cause vaginal dryness, dyspareunia (which can be severe), menopausal symptoms, and loss of sexual desire [5].

General psychosocial long-term and late effects are depression, worry, anxiety, fear of recurrence and fear of pain, challenges with body image and self-image, difficulties in relationship and in other social role, and end-of-life concerns such as death and dying [5].

These symptoms can be so troublesome that BCSs refer to doctors. The more frequent reasons for consulting a menopause clinic among BCSs are hot flushes (64%), vulvovaginal atrophy (44%), osteoporosis (29%), and mood changes (22%) [6].

19.3 Management of Symptoms

Management of menopause symptoms in BCSs is an unsolved problem during and after adjuvant therapy [7]. Much debate is ongoing about the safety of prescription of estrogens, even for a short period of time, and available guidelines do not help physicians and women to make a decision [8, 9]. At present, many trials have explored the safety of very low-dose vaginal estrogens that use new delivery modalities. Some hope might derive from new drugs and/or physical therapy that were not previously available.

Hormonal supplementation is the most effective strategy in reducing menopausal symptoms in healthy postmenopausal women [7, 10]. Unfortunately, the safety of hormone replacement therapy (HRT) in BCSs has been seriously criticized after the results of randomized controlled trials (RCTs). Three RCTs on HRT after breast cancer diagnosis closed prematurely due to concern about the safety of treatment [11–13]. The HABITS [11] open RCT allocated either to HRT or to best treatment without hormones, and the main endpoint was any new breast cancer event. Until September 2003, 434 women were randomized; 345 had at least one follow-up report. After a median follow-up of 2.1 years, 26 women in the HRT group and 7 in the non-HRT group had a new breast cancer event. All women with an event in the

HRT group and two of those in the non-HRT group were exposed to HRT. These findings indicated an unacceptable risk for women exposed to HRT in the HABITS trial, and the trial was terminated on December 17, 2003. The Stockholm trial [12] was started in 1997 and designed to minimize the dose of progestogen in the HRT arm. Disease-free women with a history of breast cancer were randomized to HRT (n = 188) or no HRT (n = 190). The trial was stopped in 2003 after the HABITS study reported increased recurrence. However, the Stockholm material showed no excess risk after 4 years of follow-up. Reasons for different results were the greater progestogen exposure in HABITS trial (preferential use of continuous combined HRT), less concomitant use of tamoxifen in HABITS trial (21% versus 52% in Stockholm trial), and the shorter duration since primary treatment surgery and randomization to HRT in HABITS trial (2.1 years) as compared to Stockholm trial (2.6 years).

At long-term follow-up, analysis of the data of the two RCTs confirmed the same results, with a significant increase of recurrence in patients in the HABITS trial (HR, 2.4; 95% CI, 1.3–4.2) [14] and no excess of the risk in the patients in the Stockholm trial (HR, 1.3; 95% CI, 0.9–1.9) [15].

The LIBERATE trial [13], started in 2002, was a multicenter, double-blind, placebo-controlled RCT designed to assess the safety and efficacy of tibolone (a compound that displays estrogenic, progestogenic, and androgenic properties) in women with climacteric symptoms and a history of breast cancer. After 1 year of treatment, tibolone significantly improved vasomotor symptoms and sleep quality, sexual behavior, mood, and attraction, compared to placebo [16]. The trial was stopped prematurely 6 months before the planned end because of a significant increase in the recurrence rate in women treated with tibolone as compared to the placebo group.

Current safety data do not support the use of systemic HRT in BCSs [17], however, in selected women and in conjunction with each woman's oncologist, it can be considered for compelling reasons after nonhormonal and complementary options have been unsuccessful. Because there is a lack of safety data supporting the use of estrogen therapy or estrogen-progesterone therapy in BCSs [18], treatment of menopausal symptoms without hormones should be explored and may be the sole option in women with contraindications to HRT.

19.4 Nonhormonal Treatments for Hot Flushes in Breast Cancer Survivors

Alternative nonhormonal treatments for vasomotor symptoms are pharmacological and non-pharmacological. Several substances have been tested: some of them give similar results to placebo that in itself provide a response in around 20–30% of women. Pharmacological treatments include antidepressant such as selective serotonin reuptake inhibitors (SSRIs), fluoxetine, citalopram, paroxetine, sertraline, and mirtazapine; selective noradrenaline reuptake inhibitors (SNRIs), venlafaxine and desvenlafaxine and gabapentin; and phytoestrogen, black cohosh, and vitamin E. Non-pharmacological treatments include acupuncture, yoga, paced respiration, hypnosis, and diet. It is recommended that primary care clinicians should offer SNRIs, SSRIs, gabapentin, lifestyle modifications, and/or environmental modifications to help mitigate vasomotor symptoms [5].

The Cochrane Collaboration [19] analyzed 16 RTCs: 6 studies on SSRIs and SNRIs, 2 on clonidine, 1 on gabapentin, 2 each on relaxation therapy and homeopathy, and 1each on vitamin E, magnetic devices, and acupuncture. Data on continuous outcomes were presented inconsistently among studies, which precluded the possibility of pooling the results. Three pharmacological treatments (SSRIs and SNRIs, clonidine, and gabapentin) reduced the number and severity of hot flushes. One study assessing vitamin E did not show any beneficial effect. One of two studies on relaxation therapy showed a significant benefit. None of the other non-pharmacological therapies had a significant benefit. Side effects were inconsistently reported. Clonidine, SSRIs and SNRIs, gabapentin, and relaxation therapy showed a mild to moderate effect on reducing hot flushes in BCSs.

The SSRIs and SNRIs can reduce hot flushes by 65% and begin working within the first week [20]. Patient response is variable, and if one drug does not improve hot flushes, another can be tried after 1–2 weeks drug trial. Paroxetine, citalopram, and escitalopram appear to have the fewest adverse effects.

Venlafaxine is an effective treatment for the relief of vasomotor symptoms in BCSs. The use of the low dose (37.5 mg/day) is associated with minimal side effects and produces a good improvement in hot flushes if pursued over 8 weeks [21].

Mirtazapine appears to be effective in reducing hot flushes in BCSs. The efficacy and safety of mirtazapine 30 mg/daily for 12 weeks reduce hot flushes in BCSs 55.6% ($p < 0.05$) reduction in HF frequency and 61.9% ($p < 0.05$) reduction in HF score as compared to baseline [22].

Duloxetine and escitalopram showed a significant reduction in hot flush frequency and in hot flush score with no significant differences between two groups. The beneficial effect is fast, with a reduction of more than 50% of hot flushes in the first month for both drugs [23].

Treatment with SSRIs/SNRIs may cause or complicate sexual dysfunction by reducing libido and causing anorgasmia. Most studies in depressed populations report sexual function does not vary by SSRI type. Others suggest that female orgasm disorder is most commonly associated with paroxetine and venlafaxine.

Treatment with SSRIs/SNRIs may interfere with tamoxifen by inhibiting the CYP2D6 enzyme. For women treated with tamoxifen, there may be a preference to avoid some SSRIs and SNRIs that are potent inhibitors of CYP2D6 enzyme with a consequent decrease in the efficacy of tamoxifen: among SSRIs, citalopram and escitalopram have a mild effect and can be given with tamoxifen, unlike paroxetine and fluoxetine, which both have large effect. As regards SNRIs, venlafaxine and desvenlafaxine are the safest choices for tamoxifen users, whereas duloxetine has a moderate effect. Although evidence supports SSRI and SNRI efficacy in reducing hot flushes [24], only paroxetine has been approved by the Food and Drug

Administration (FDA) for the treatment of moderate to severe vasomotor symptoms associated with menopause [25].

The use of gabapentin 900 mg/day compared to vitamin E for the control of vasomotor symptoms in 115 women with breast cancer has demonstrated the reduction of frequency by 57.05% in the gabapentin group. The effect of vitamin E was fairly small: hot flush frequency was reduced by 10.02%. Gabapentin was also particularly effective in improving the quality of sleep [26].

Phytoestrogens are a family of plant compounds with estrogenic and antiestrogenic properties depending on dose and menopausal status. They are divided into two classes: isoflavones (with soy high concentration) and lignans (with flaxseed high concentration). The estrogenic activity is much less than 17-beta estradiol, and like other weak estrogens, such as tamoxifen, they can act like selective estrogen receptor modulators (SERMs). They have been considered as chemopreventive and chemotherapeutic and have nonhormonal antioxidant properties that may contribute to their physiological effect [27]. There is no evidence of effectiveness in the alleviation of menopausal symptoms with the use of phytoestrogen treatments. A review of the Cochrane Collaboration [28] that includes 43 RCTs showed significant difference overall in the frequency of hot flushes between red clover extract and placebo. Some trials found that the frequency and severity of hot flushes and night sweats were alleviated when compared to placebo but they are of low quality and underpowered. There was no evidence of estrogenic stimulation of the endometrium when used for up to 2 years. The limit of this review was that nobody of the trial includes patients with previous breast cancer. Two studies [29, 30] on the use of phytoestrogen on BCSs suggest that soy-based supplements might affect the efficacy of breast cancer treatment with aromatase inhibitors. Considering the high number of breast cancer patients using soy supplements to treat menopausal symptoms, the increased risk for adverse interactions with breast cancer treatment is of major concern and should be considered with care.

Also for the use of black cohosh, there is currently insufficient evidence to support its application on menopausal symptoms [31].

Including in non-pharmacological treatments, yoga and relaxation had a greater improvement in hot flush frequency, sleep disturbances, and levels of joint pain and fatigue on 37 BCSs suffering from vasomotor symptoms [32]. Also, acupuncture is better than placebo in relieving the burden of hot flushes, and after 3 months of treatment, it has the same results as venlafaxine. Women refer more libido and well-being [27, 33, 34].

Another nonhormonal option to reduce hot flushes is the stellate ganglion block (SGB). The stellate ganglion is a sympathetic ganglion located at the level of C7. The mechanism of action of SGB in reducing hot flushes is unclear: it was suggested that the SGB resets the temperature-regulating mechanisms by interrupting the connections between the central and sympathetic nervous systems. In the study by Lipov, SGB decreases the frequency of hot flushes and their severity [35]. Thus SGB in BCSs seems both safe and efficacious; however, it is an invasive procedure.

19.5 Genitourinary Syndrome of Menopause and Vulvovaginal Atrophy

Management of GSM in BCSs is an unsolved problem during and after adjuvant therapy. Recently, the new terminology GSM has been proposed instead of vulvovaginal atrophy, to better describe the constellation of symptoms and signs associated with menopause [4]. The syndrome includes genital symptoms such as dryness, burning, and irritation; sexual symptoms such as lack of lubrication, discomfort, and pain; and urinary symptoms such as urgency, dysuria, and recurrent urinary tract infections.

Lubricants and moisturizers are the first-line therapies [7], but they only provide poor benefit. Much debate is ongoing about the safety of prescription of vaginal estrogens, even for a short period of time, and available guidelines do not help physicians and women to make a decision [8, 9]. At present, many trials have explored the safety of very low-dose vaginal estrogens that use new delivery modalities. Some hope might derive from new drugs and/or physical therapy that were not previously available.

In BCSs vaginal dryness has been reported by 19–23% and 42–70% of pre- and postmenopausal patients, respectively, whereas dyspareunia has been reported by 10–16% and 27–39%, respectively [36].

Up to 74% of women experience urogenital symptoms during breast cancer treatment [37, 38], and sexual intimacy and loving relationship with a partner are the spheres that are most negatively influenced by vaginal atrophy [39]. Breast cancer diagnosis and treatment may dramatically impair the quality of the couple relationship. Data indicate that the emotional intimacy and the sense of bonding, affection, and commitment may be improved in the majority of couples (60–70%), while the physical, erotic intimacy may be variably affected. The longer the time between surgery and having intercourse again, the higher the probability of sexual dysfunction. Patients and their partners should be reassured that there is no medical contraindication to sexual intimacy including touching the operated breast during breast cancer therapy and afterward [40].

Nonhormonal water-based lubricants and polycarbophil moisturizers are the first-line treatments for women with a history of hormone-dependent cancers, and they imply a moderate decrease of symptoms both for vaginal dryness and dyspareunia; they are not more effective than placebo in relieving urogenital symptoms, and they present only a transient benefit. Vaginal estrogens are more effective than systemic estrogens to treat symptoms of urogenital atrophy, and the use of them in women with a history of hormone-dependent cancer is controversial. Low-dose vaginal estrogen improves vaginal symptoms in the majority of treated women, with plasma estradiol levels remaining in the range of postmenopausal levels, and the lowest dose possible should be used to obtain improvement [41]. The first studies on the topic directly analyzed breast cancer recurrence risk in BCSs using vaginal estrogen. In the study of Dew on 1472 BCSs, 23.2% used a vaginal estrogen and about half (47%) were using tamoxifen. No increase in recurrence was observed after a mean follow-up of 5.5 years, but the design of this study does not confirm any absence of risk [42]. Kendall et al. (2006) demonstrated that the vaginal estradiol tablet 25 mcg significantly raises systemic estradiol levels, at least in the short term. This reverses the estradiol suppression achieved by aromatase inhibitors in BCSs [43]. Wills demonstrated that vaginal estrogen treatment, regardless of type, results in elevated circulating estradiol levels in the study population and suggests caution [44].

A recent committee opinion [45] assess that in women with a history of estrogen-dependent breast cancer, vaginal estrogen should be reserved for those patients who are unresponsive to nonhormonal remedies, and the decision to use vaginal estrogen may be made in coordination with a woman's oncologist. Additionally, it should be preceded by an informed decision-making and consent process in which the woman has the information and resources to consider the benefits and potential risks of low-dose vaginal estrogen.

A new nonhormonal solution for treating GSM in BCSs is the vaginal laser. It acts by inducing the production of new collagen and elastic fibers. The Laser procedure is an efficient, easy-to-use, quick, and safe procedure, without the need for long-term hormonal therapy [46, 47]. Fractional microablative CO_2 [46] and Erbium laser [47] treatment are both associated with a significant improvement of sexual function and satisfaction with sexual life in postmenopausal women with VVA symptoms.

Another alternative to hormonal treatment for VVA in postmenopausal women is the novel SERM ospemifene. Ospemifene is a new oral compound that was originally developed as a treatment for postmenopausal osteoporosis. It has been approved by the US Food and Drug Administration and recently also by the European Medicines Agency for the treatment of moderate to severe symptomatic VVA in postmenopausal women who are not candidates for vaginal estrogens. Preclinical [48], clinical [49–52], and SERM class effects [53] assess ospemifene breast safety. SERM are a class of drugs that have antiestrogenic or neutral effects on the breast: clinical trials with tamoxifene and raloxifene have shown antiestrogenic or neutral effects on the breast [53]. These observations suggest that ospemifene might be proposed as a likely safe treatment option for BCSs suffering from VVA. In women with previous breast cancer, ospemifene can be used for the treatment of VVA after the end of adjuvant treatments.

Conclusion

Menopausal symptoms are common among BCSs and can adversely affect QoL and sexual health. Because a wide range of possible treatments is now available for BCSs, menopause after breast cancer should no longer be considered an unsolved problem but an interesting area of further clinical research.

References

1. The Surveillance, Epidemiology, and End Results (SEER) Program of the National Cancer Institute, 2011
2. Hickey M (2008) Practical clinical guidelines for assessing and managing menopausal symptoms after breast cancer. Ann Oncol 19(10):1669–1680
3. Loprinzi CL et al (2008) Symptom management in premenopausal patients with breast cancer. Lancet Oncol 9(10):993–1001
4. Portman DJ, Gass ML, On Behalf of the Vulvovaginal Atrophy Terminology Consensus Conference Panel (2014) Genitourinary syndrome of menopause: new terminology for vulvovaginal atrophy from the International Society for the Study of Women's Sexual Health and The North American Menopause Society. Maturitas 79(3):349–354
5. Runowicz CD et al (2016) American Cancer Society/American Society of Clinical Oncology Breast Cancer Survivorship Guidelines. J Clin Oncol 34(6):611–635. doi:10.1200/JCO.2015.64.3809
6. Biglia N, Cozzarella M, Cacciari F, Ponzone R, Roagna R, Maggiorotto F, Sismondi P (2003) Menopause after breast cancer: a survey on breast cancer survivors. Maturitas 45:29–38
7. The North American Menopause Society (NAMS) (2012) The 2012 hormone therapy. Position statement of the North American Menopause Society Menopause. Menopause 19:257–271
8. The North American Menopause Society (NAMS) (2013) Management of symptomatic vulvovaginal atrophy: 2013 position statement of the North American Menopause Society. Menopause 20:888–902
9. Rees M, Pérez-López FR, Ceasu I et al (2012) EMAS clinical guide: low-dose vaginal estrogens for postmenopausal vaginal atrophy. Maturitas 73:171–174
10. The International Menopause Society (IMS) (2013) Updated 2013 International Menopause Society recommendations on menopausal hormone therapy and preventive strategies for midlife health. Climacteric 16:316–337
11. Holmberg L, Anderson H, HABITS Steering and Data Monitoring Committees (2004) HABITS (hormonal replacement therapy after breast cancer is it safe?), a randomised comparison: trial stopped. Lancet 363:453–455
12. Von Schoultz E (2005) Menopausal hormone therapy after breast cancer: the Stockholm randomized trial. JNCI 97(7):533–535
13. Kenemans P, Bundred NJ, Foidart JM et al (2009) Safety and efficacy of tibolone in breast-cancer patients with vasomotor symptoms: a double blind, randomised, noninferiority trial. Lancet Oncol 10:135–146
14. Holmberg L et al (2008) On behalf of the HABITS study group: increased risk of recurrence after hormone replacement therapy in breast cancer survivors. JNCI 100(7):475–482
15. Fahlen M et al (2013) Hormone replacement therapy after breast cancer: 10 years follow up of the Stockholm randomized trial. Eur J Cancer 49:52–59
16. Sismondi P et al (2011) Effects of tibolone on climacteric symptoms and quality of life in breast cancer patients—data from LIBERATE trial. Maturitas 70:365–372
17. De Villiers TJ, Hall JE, Pinkerton JV, Pérez SC, Rees M, Yang C, Pierroz DD (2016) Revised global consensus statement on menopausal hormone therapy. Maturitas 91:153–155
18. Baber RJ, Panay N, Fenton A (2016) The IMS writing group 2016. IMS recommendations on women midlife health and menopause hormone therapy. Climacteric 19(2):109–150. doi:10.3109/13697137.2015.1129166
19. Rada G, Capurro D, Pantoja T, Corbalán J, Moreno G, Letelier LM, Vera C (2010) Non-hormonal interventions for hot flushes in women with a history of breast cancer. Cochrane Database Syst Rev (9). doi:10.1002/14651858.CD004923.pub2
20. Handley A, Williams M (2015) The efficacy and tolerability of SSRI/SNRIs in the treatment of vasomotor symptoms in menopausal women: a systematic review. J Am Assoc Nurse Pract 27(1):54–61
21. Biglia N et al (2005) Evaluation of low-dose venlafaxine hydrochloride for the therapy of hot flushes in breast cancer survivors. Maturitas 52(1):78–85

22. Biglia N, Kubatzki F, Sgandurra P, Ponzone R, Marenco D, Peano E, Sismondi P (2007) Mirtazapine for the treatment of hot flushes in breast cancer survivors: a prospective pilot trial. Breast J 13(5):490–495
23. Biglia N, Bounous VE, Susini T, Pecchio S, Sgro LG, Tuninetti V, Torta R (2016) Duloxetine and escitalopram for hot flushes: efficacy and compliance in breast cancer survivors. Eur J Cancer Care. doi:10.1111/ecc.12484
24. Carroll DG, Kelley KW (2009) Use of antidepressants for Management of Hot Flashes. Pharmacotherapy 29:1357–1374
25. Orleans RJ, Li L, Kim MJ, Guo J, Sobhan M, Soule L, Joffe HV (2014) FDA approval of paroxetine for menopausal hot flushes. N Engl J Med 370:1777–1779
26. Biglia N, Sgandurra P, Peano E, Marenco D, Moggio G, Bounous V, Tomasi Cont N, Ponzone R, Sismondi P (2009) Non-hormonal treatment of hot flushes in breast cancer survivors: gabapentin vs. vitamin E. Climacteric 12(4):310–318
27. Morrow PK, Mattair DN, Hortobagyi GN (2011) Hot flashes: a review of pathophysiology and treatment modalities. Oncologist 16(11):1658–1656
28. Lethaby A, Marjoribanks J, Kronenberg F, Roberts H, Eden J, Brown J (2013) Phytoestrogens for menopausal vasomotor symptoms. Cochrane Database Syst Rev 10(12):CD001395
29. Du M, Yang X, Hartman JA, Cooke PS, Doerge DR, Ju YH, Helferich WG (2012) Low-dose dietary genistein negates the therapeutic effect of tamoxifen in athymic nude mice. Carcinogenesis 33(4):895–901
30. Van Duursen MB, Nijmeijer SM, de Morree ES, de Jong PC, van den Berg M (2011) Genistein induces breast cancer-associated aromatase and stimulates estrogen-dependent tumor cell growth in in vitro breast cancer model. Toxicology 289(2–3):67–73
31. Leach MJ, Moore V. Black cohosh (Cimicifuga spp.) for menopausal symptoms. Cochrane Database Syst Rev. 2012 Sep 12;(9):CD007244
32. Carson JW, Carson KM, Porter LS, Keefe FJ, Seewaldt VL (2009) Yoga of awareness program for menopausal symptoms in breast cancer survivors: results from a randomized trial. Support Care Cancer 17:1301–1309
33. Walker EM et al (2010) Acupuncture versus venlafaxine for the management of vasomotor symptoms in patients with hormone receptor-positive breast cancer: a randomized controlled trial. J Clin Oncol 28:634–640
34. Venzke L, Calvert JF, Gilbertson B (2010) A randomized trial of acupuncture for vasomotor symptoms in post-menopausal women. Complement Ther Med 18:59–66
35. Lipov EG, Joshi JR, Lipov S, Sanders SE, Siroko MK (2008) Cervical sympathetic blockade in a patient with post-traumatic stress disorder: a case report. Ann Clin Psychiatry 20:227–228
36. Crandall C, Petersen L, Ganz PA et al (2004) Association of breast cancer and its therapy with menopause-related symptoms. Menopause 11:519–530
37. Baumgart J, Nilsson K, Stavreus-Evers A, Kask K, Villman K, Lindman H et al (2011) Urogenital disorders in women with adjuvant endocrine therapy after early breast cancer. Am J Obstet Gynecol 204(1):26.e 1-7
38. Baumgart J, Nilsson K, Evers AS, Kallak TK, Poromaa IS (2013) Sexual dysfunction in women on adjuvant endocrine therapy after breast cancer. Menopause 20(2):162–168
39. Nappi RE, Kokot-Kierepa M (2012) Vaginal health: insights, views and amp; attitudes (VIVA) – results from an international survey. Climacteric 15:36–44
40. Újhelyi M et al (2016) A European Society of Breast Cancer Specialists (EUSOMA). Orv Hetil 157:1674–1682
41. Biglia N et al (2015) Genitourinary syndrome of menopause in breast cancer survivors: are we facing new and safe hopes? Clin Breast Cancer 15:413–420. doi:10.1016/j.clbc.2015.06.005
42. Dew JE, Wren BG, Eden JA (2003) A cohort study of topical vaginal estrogen therapy in women previously treated for breast cancer. Climacteric 6:45–52
43. Kendall A, Dowsett M, Folkerd E, Smith I (2006) Caution: vaginal estradiol appears to be contraindicated in postmenopausal women on adjuvant aromatase inhibitors. Ann Oncol Off J Eur Soc Med Oncol 17:584–587

44. Wills S et al (2012) Effects of vaginal estrogens on serum estradiol levels in postmenopausal breast cancer survivors and women at risk of breast cancer taking an aromatase inhibitor or a selective estrogen receptor modulator. J Oncol Pract 8:144–148
45. American College of Obstetricians and Gynecologists' Committee on Gynecologic Practice, Farrell R (2016) ACOG Committee opinion no. 659: the use of vaginal estrogen in women with a history of estrogen-dependent breast cancer. Obstet Gynecol 127(3):e93–e96. doi:10.1097/AOG.0000000000001351
46. Salvatore S, Nappi RE, Zerbinati N et al (2014) A 12 week treatment with fractional CO2 laser for vulvovaginal atrophy: a pilot study. Climateric 17:363–369
47. Gambacciani M, Levancini M, Cervigni M (2015) Vaginal erbium laser: the second-generation thermotherapy for the genitourinary syndrome of menopause. Climateric 18:757–763
48. Burich RA, Mehta NR, Wurz GT, McCall JL, Greenberg BE, Bell KE, Griffey SM, DeGregorio MW (2012) Ospemifene and 4-hydroxyospemifene effectively prevent and treat breast cancer in the MTag.Tg transgenic mouse model. J Am Menopause Soc 19:96–103
49. Bachmann GA, Komi JO, Ospemifene Study Group (2010) Ospemifene effectively treats vulvovaginal atrophy in postmenopausal women: results from a pivotal phase 3 study. Menopause 17:480–486
50. Simon J, Lin V, Radovich C, Bachmann GA, The Ospemifene Study Group (2012) One year long-term safety extension study of ospemifene for the treatment of vulvar and vaginal atrophy in postmenopausal women with a uterus. Menopause 20:418–427
51. Portman DJ, Bachmann GA, Simon JA, Ospemifene Study Group (2013) Ospemifene, a novel selective estrogen receptor modulator for treating dyspareunia associated with postmenopausal vulvar and vaginal atrophy. Menopause 20:623–630
52. Goldstein SR, Bachmann GA, Koninckx PR et al (2014) Ospemifene 12-month safety and efficacy in postmenopausal women with vulvar and vaginal atrophy. Climacteric 17:173–182
53. Cuzick J et al (2013) Selective oestrogen receptor modulators in prevention of breast cancer: an updated meta-analysis of individual participant data. Lancet 381:1827–1834

Myoinositol and Inositol Hexakisphosphate in the Treatment of Breast Cancer: Molecular Mechanisms

20

Mariano Bizzarri, Simona Dinicola, and Alessandra Cucina

20.1 Introduction

Myo-Ins is among the oldest components of living beings, undergoing complex evolutionary modifications ultimately leading to the current multiplicity of functions for inositol-containing molecules in eukaryotes [1]. Besides the biological role sustained in its free form, Myo-Ins and its phosphate derivatives—chiefly represented by InsP6—also serve as important components of structural lipids and secondary messengers.

Deregulation of inositol-based cellular pathways has been established in several pathological conditions [1]. Namely, both InsP6 and Myo-Ins showed to play critical roles in both carcinogenesis and breast cancer development. Conversely, InsP6 and Myo-Ins display significant chemopreventive effects in vitro and in vivo, as they modulate a number of processes, including mRNA transcription, chromatin

M. Bizzarri (✉)
Department of Experimental Medicine, Sapienza University of Rome, via A. Scarpa 14, 00161 Rome, Italy
e-mail: mariano.bizzarri@uniroma1.it

S. Dinicola
Department of Experimental Medicine, Sapienza University of Rome, via A. Scarpa 14, 00161 Rome, Italy

Department of Surgery "Pietro Valdoni", Sapienza University of Rome, via A. Scarpa 14, 00161 Rome, Italy
e-mail: simona.dinicola@uniroma1.it

A. Cucina
Department of Surgery "Pietro Valdoni", Sapienza University of Rome, via A. Scarpa 14, 00161 Rome, Italy

Azienda Policlinico Umberto I, viale del Policlinico 155, 00161 Rome, Italy
e-mail: alessandra.cucina@uniroma1.it

M. Birkhaeuser, A.R. Genazzani (eds.), *Pre-Menopause, Menopause and Beyond*, ISGE Series, https://doi.org/10.1007/978-3-319-63540-8_20

remodeling, cytoskeleton configuration, and p53 activity, just to mention a few. These new findings prompted reassessing under a new light the molecular mechanistic anticancer effect of inositols.

20.2 Molecular Mechanisms of Action

20.2.1 Cell Cycle Control and Apoptosis

Several studies have investigated the inhibitory activity of InsP6 on cancer cell growth. Results show that InsP6 induces G_1 phase arrest and shortens S phase of cancer cells, mainly by modulation of cyclins; upregulation of p53, p57, p27, and p21; and downregulation of phosphorylated pRB. InsP6, by increasing the hypophosphorylated form of pRB, increases pRB/E2F complexes formation thus blocking further progression along the cell cycle [2]. Furthermore, InsP6 downregulates several genes involved in cell cycle advancement while upregulating those activated in cycle inhibition. Downregulation of breast cancer proliferation occurs independently from the estrogen receptor (ER) status, as cell growth arrest has been achieved in both ER-negative and ER-positive cells [3]. While early studies suggested that InsP6 effect is rather cytostatic than cytotoxic [4], it has been later showed that InsP6 actively induces apoptosis. In fact, InsP6 triggers both cell growth inhibition and programmed cell death in numerous cancer cell lines including breast cancer [5]. Moreover, InsP6 synergizes with doxorubicin and tamoxifen in inducing apoptosis in drug-resistant cancer cell lines [6]. However, Myo-Ins has been shown having only a minimal pro-apoptotic activity, even if it significantly synergize with InsP6, both in vitro and in vivo, in inducing cancer inhibition [7].

According to the culture context, as an alternative of apoptosis or growth inhibition, cell differentiation occurs after InsP6 treatment. Induction of differentiation was evidenced in human erythroleukemia cells as well as in breast tumors after Insp6 addition [8, 9]. Why cancer cells respond so differently following InsP6 administration is not yet clear. Probably, other factors, namely, other inositol phosphate derivatives, may participate in such processes, thereby driving the final output into diverse fates [10].

20.2.2 The p53 Network

Selective activation of p53 activity is a critical step when cells are selectively committed toward apoptosis and/or inhibition of proliferation. It is noteworthy that InsP6 increases p53 levels several folds, at both mRNA and protein level [11], even if p53 is not mandatory for InsP6/Myo-Ins pro-apoptotic activity as both apoptosis and inhibition of cell growth have been both observed in cancer cells lacking p53 [12, 13]. Activation of p53, in turn, increases the endogenous synthesis of Myo-Ins through ISYNA1 gene modulation, thus reinforcing the apoptotic commitment through to a positive feedback [14]. Furthermore, p53-dependent increase in intracellular Myo-Ins synthesis is mandatorily required to sustain growth inhibition as well as for inhibiting chemotherapy-induced resistance in cancer cells [14]. Downstream of p53 InsP6 reduces pro-survival factors and upregulates caspases and other pro-apoptotic factors [15], while in normal cells, addiction of either InsP6 or Myo-Ins did not induce any significant apoptotic effect. It is noteworthy that breast cancer cells show significantly reduced levels of Myo-Ins, as documented by metabolomic studies [16].

20.2.3 Inhibition of the PI3K/Akt Pathway

The PI3K/Akt pathways are a pivotal hub, upstream the activation of many survival pathways. PI3K triggers the phosphorylation-dependent activation of Akt. In turn, activated Akt modulates the function of numerous substrates involved in the regulation of cell cycle progression, ultimately allowing cancer cells becoming more aggressive. Both InsP6 and Myo-Ins significantly reduce PI3K expression [17] (at both mRNA and protein level) and Akt activation by inhibiting its phosphorylation [18, 19]. InsP6 impairs directly PI3K activity and the PI3K-dependent activation of the tumor promoter-induced AP-1, as well as the phosphorylation-dependent activation of ERK and other mitogen-activated kinases (MAPK), both in vitro and in vivo [20, 21]. Given that PI3K/Akt pathway activity is mandatory required for triggering EMT, blocking PI3K would hinder the transformation of cancer cells into a more aggressive phenotype. Indeed, breast cancer cells treated in vitro with Myo-Ins showed increased E-cadherin, downregulation of metalloproteinase-9, and redistribution of β-catenin behind cell membrane, while motility and invading capacity were severely inhibited [19]. Those changes were associated with the downregulation of PI3K/Akt activity, leading to a decrease in downstream signaling effectors: NF-κB, COX-2, and SNAI1. Moreover, Myo-Ins decreases presenilin-1 (PS1) levels and inhibits its activity, thus decreasing both Notch-1 and SNAI1 levels. Furthermore, InsP6 impairs NF-κB in cancer cells, by inhibiting its activation or by preventing the nuclear translocation of NF-κB and NF-κB-luciferase transcription activity [5]. Those changes are associated with a dramatic cytoskeleton remodeling [19] thereby suggesting that Myo-Ins inhibits the principal molecular pathway supporting EMT in breast cancer cells.

20.2.4 Inhibition of Invasiveness and Motility

Myo-Ins significantly hampers both motility and invasiveness of breast cancer cells [19]. This effect is due to cytoskeleton remodeling and the concomitant inhibition of metalloproteinases (MMPs) release [19]. Similarly, InsP6 significantly reduces the number of lung metastatic colonies in a mouse metastatic tumor model [22], while in MDA-MB-231 breast cancer cells, this effect is facilitated by reduced adhesion and MMP release [23].

20.2.5 Wnt Signaling and Anti-Inflammatory Effects

Overexpression of the Wnt ligand—usually in association with deregulated γ-secretase activity—may lead to altered expression and redistribution of β-catenin and of several molecular factors belonging to the so-called inflammatory pathway, like COX-2 and PGE2. Increased expression of the aforementioned molecules has been associated with carcinogenesis in numerous tissues, chiefly in colon cancer [24]. InsP6 downregulates both in vitro and in vivo the Wnt pathway via β-catenin inhibition, hence significantly reducing COX-2 at the mRNA and protein level [25]. Similarly, in breast cancer cells, Myo-Ins has proven to downregulate both NF-κB and COX-2 while relocating β-catenin behind cell membrane and inhibiting its nuclear translocation [19]. Inhibition on inflammatory markers is not limited to epithelial cells as inositol activity also probably interferes with the pro-inflammatory activity of stroma cells. Indeed, both InsP6 and Myo-Ins have demonstrated to prevent pulmonary fibrosis, breast density, and chronic inflammatory damage, likely by influencing the cross talk among cells and their milieu [26, 27]. Additionally, Myo-Ins modulates the expression of both TGFβ and its receptors, thus mitigating its pro-inflammatory effects [28]. Furthermore, InsP6 has been shown to exert valuable effects on fibroblasts by blocking the syndecan-4-dependent focal adhesion and microfilament bound [29]. Syndecan-4, a heparan sulfate proteoglycan embedded into cellular membranes where it regulates cell-matrix interactions, binds to the fibroblast growth factor (FGF), fostering its coupling with the FGF receptor. InsP6 disrupts such interaction, thus preventing the FGF-based signaling [30]. Additionally, inositol-related effects on the cell microenvironment involve modulation of angiogenesis. Formation of new blood vessels is required for sustaining cancer growth and invasiveness. Disruption of the structural relationships among cancer cells and their microenvironment promotes neo-angiogenesis, mainly through the release of vascular endothelial growth factor (VEGF) and basic fibroblast growth factor (bFGF). InsP6 negatively modulates both VEGF and bFGF release from tumor cells and impairs endothelial cell growth [31]. Likely, VEGF-reduced synthesis may be due to InsP6-mediated inhibition on PI3K/Akt and MAPK/ERK pathways, given that both of them are deemed to modulate VEGF upregulation [22]. Furthermore, the synergistic activity of hypoxia and insulin-like growth factor II (IGF-II) increases VEGF mRNA expression and upregulates IGF-1 protein that, in turn, reinforces VEGF release. Given that InsP6 has been shown to antagonize IGF-II activity by inhibiting the IGF-II receptor binding [32], it is likely that some InsP6 anti-angiogenic effects can be ascribed to this mechanism.

Overall, these data (Fig. 20.1) suggest that inositol and its phosphate derivatives exert several anticancer effects by interfering with numerous key biochemical pathways.

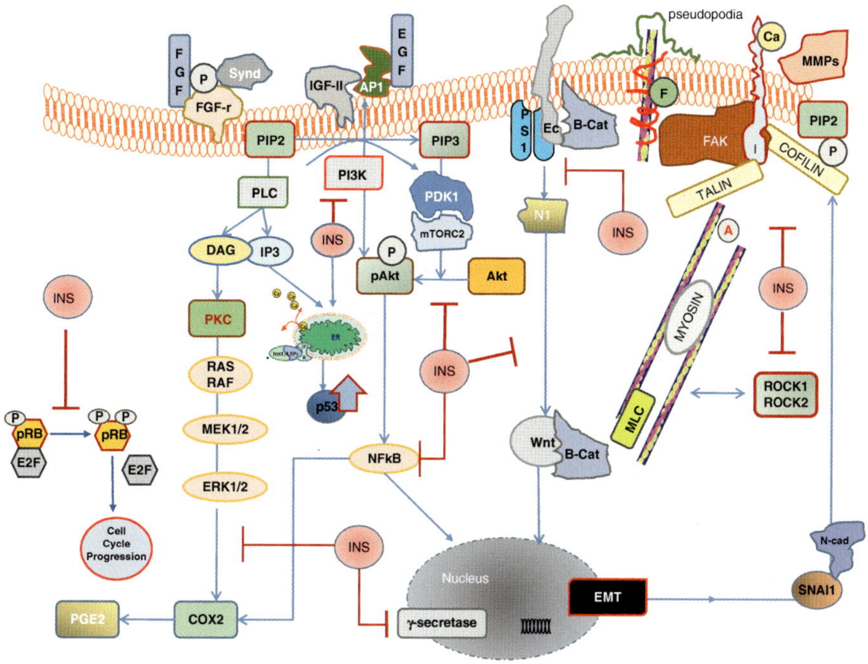

Fig. 20.1 Anticancer mechanisms of inositol in breast cancer cells. Inositols (Ins)—including both InsP6 and Myo-Ins—modulate several biochemical pathways. Inositols inhibit pRB phosphorylation (P), thus fostering the pRB/E2F complexes formation and blocking further progression along the cell cycle. Phosphatidylinositol-4,5-bisphosphonate (PIP2) is metabolized to diacylglycerol (DAG) and Ins-trisphosphate (IP3) by phospholipase-C (PLC). Increased levels of IP3 and Myo-Ins enhance p53 activity and mitochondria-dependent apoptosis through increased Ca^{2+} release. Moreover, PI3K catalyzes the synthesis of PIP3 from PIP2. PIP3 is required for enabling the activation of ERK and Akt pathways. Indeed, by reducing both PI3K levels and its activity, inositols counteract the activation of the PKC/RAS/ERK pathway. Upstream of that pathway, inositols disrupt the ligand interaction between FGF and its receptor (FGF-r) by interfering with syndecan (Synd) activity as well as with the EGF-transduction processes involving IGF-II receptor and AP-1 complexes. Downstream of PI3K inhibition, Akt activation through selective phosphorylation promoted by PDK and mTORC2 is severely impaired upon inositol addition. Downregulation of both Akt and ERK leads consequently to NF-κB inhibition and reduced expression of inflammatory markers, like COX-2 and PGE2. Inositol-induced downregulation of presenilin-1 (PS1), when associated with inhibition of the PI3K/Akt pathway, counteracts the epithelial-mesenchymal transition (EMT), thus reducing Wnt activation, *β*-catenin (*β*-cat) translocation, Notch-1, N-cadherin (N-cad), and SNAI1 release. Inositols interfere also directly with different cytoskeleton components by upregulating focal adhesion kinase (FAK) and E-cadherin (Ec) and decreasing fascin (F) and cofilin, two main components of the pseudopodia. Reduced formation of membrane ruffling and pseudopodia, as well as inhibited release of metalloproteinases (MMPs), severely impairs both motility and invasiveness of cancer cells. This effect is also supported by the inositol-induced inhibition on ROCK1/2 release and by the decreased levels of phosphorylated myosin light chain (MLC). Overall, these effects enable inositols to remodel F-actin (A) assembly and thus to reshape the cytoskeleton architecture. *Blue arrow* indicates promoting effect; *red line* with bar indicates inhibitory effect

20.3 Anticancer Activity Through Insulin Modulation

Myoinositol, as well as its isomer D-chiro-inositol (D-chiro-Ins), participates in both insulin and glucose metabolism, and deregulated Myo-Ins metabolism has been documented in several conditions associated with diabetes or insulin resistance [1]. When insulin binds to its receptor, two distinct inositol phosphoglycans (IPG), incorporating either Myo-Ins or D-Chiro-Ins, are released by insulin-stimulated hydrolysis of glycosyl-phosphatidylinositol lipids located on the outer leaflet of the cell membrane. IPGs affect intracellular metabolic processes, namely, by activating key enzymes controlling the oxidative and non-oxidative metabolism of glucose. Given that Myo-Ins may efficiently counteract insulin resistance and its metabolic complications [33], it is tempting to speculate that it may also prevent IGF-I increase associated to those conditions. In turn, insulin resistance and increased levels of IGF-I are frequently associated with cancer, and it is therefore conceivable that Myo-Ins modulation of insulin activity may efficiently contribute in reducing tumor risk. Indeed, InsP6 has been already shown to inhibit the IGF-I/IGF-II receptor pathway-mediated sustained growth in cancer cells [23, 32].

20.4 Antioxidant and Other Effects

Myo-Ins displays an appreciable antioxidant activity, while InsP6 is among the strongest antioxidants present in nature. By chelating polyvalent cations, InsP6 and Myo-Ins suppress the Fenton reaction and the consequent release of hydroxyl radicals [34]. In biological tissues, InsP6 inhibits xanthine oxidase and reactive oxygen species production, thus dramatically inhibiting the free radical-based damage occurring in cells and tissues following inflammation, hypoxia, or exposition to radiation injury [35]. Myo-Ins counteracts oxidative damage in fish exposed to environmental stresses and significantly inhibits systemic markers of oxidative stress in gynecological patients [1]. InsP6 scavenges superoxide radicals in vitro and in vivo, thus preventing formation of ADP-iron-oxygen complexes that trigger lipid peroxidation. Indeed, after InsP6 administration lipid peroxidation is significantly inhibited [36]. As an increase in both reactive oxygen species and lipid peroxidation has been associated with cancer development, it can be surmised that the antioxidant capabilities of InsP6 and Myo-Ins could account for their anticancer chemopreventive effects.

20.5 Chemopreventive and Therapeutic Efficacy in Human Clinical Trials

Only a few pilot studies have been performed in order to ascertain the usefulness of inositols in clinical setting. InsP6 plus Myo-Ins treatment of colon cancer patients is associated with appreciable reduction in tumor burden and improved quality of life [37]. Furthermore, significant longer survival and better quality of life have been obtained in breast and lung cancer patients treated with InsP6 and Myo-Ins [38]. Again, InsP6 and Myo-Ins ameliorate the responsiveness to chemotherapy in breast cancer patients and markedly reduce the burden of side effects [38]. As previously noticed in animal studies, Myo-Ins has been demonstrated to exert a significant chemopreventive activity. A study enrolling 26 smokers showed that Myo-Ins in a daily dose up to 18 g/p.o. is safe and well tolerated while inducing a significant regression of individual pulmonary dysplastic lesions (91% in the inositol-treated group versus 48% in control group) in a sample of heavy smoker individuals [39]. This effect is probably linked to the observed inhibition of PI3K activity in dysplastic lesions.

Conclusion

Myoinositol and InsP6 play major biological functions, including modulation of cell cycle progression, apoptosis, and differentiation. Evidence is mounting that inositol acts on both cytosolic and nuclear targets in enabling cells to successfully copy with many different stressors, namely, during developmental processes and cellular differentiation [1]. Cancer can be considered a kind of "development gone awry," in which the deregulation in the cross talk among cells and their microenvironment plays a relevant role. Given that inositol participates in the cell-stroma interplay, by modulating metalloproteinases, E-cadherin, focal kinase complexes, and many other cytoskeletal components, it can be hypothesized that inositol and its derivatives may counteract cancer-related processes by specifically acting at this level, i.e., by restoring a "normal" cell-stroma relationship. A recent paper, indeed, strongly supports this hypothesis. In fact, InsP6 and Myo-Ins prevent the development and metastatic progression of colon cancer in mice by modifying extracellular matrix proteins (collagen IV, fibronectin, and laminin), integrin-1, matrix metalloproteinase 9, as well as several growth factors (VEGF, bFGF, TGFβ) [40].

Studies in this field are welcome in order to deepen our understanding of inositol mechanisms.

References

1. Bizzarri M, Fuso A, Dinicola S et al (2016) Pharmacodynamics and pharmacokinetics of inositol(s) in health and disease. Expert Opin Drug Metab Toxicol 12(10):1181–1196
2. Vucenik I, Tantivejkul K, Ramakrishna G et al (2005) Inositol hexaphosphate (IP6) blocks proliferation of breast cancer cells through PKCδ-dependent increase in p27Kip1 and decrease in retinoblastoma protein (pRb) phosphorylation. Breast Cancer Res Treat 91:35–45
3. Shamsuddin AM, Yang GY, Vucenik I (1996) Novel anti-cancer functions of IP6: growth inhibition and differentiation of human mammary cancer cell lines in vitro. Anticancer Res 16:3287–3292
4. Vucenik I, Kalebic T, Tantivejkul K et al (1998b) Novel anticancer function of inositol hexaphosphate: inhibition of human rhabdomyosarcoma in vitro and in vivo. Anticancer Res 18:1377–1384

5. Ferry S, Matsuda M, Yoshida H, Hirata M (2002) Inositol hexakisphosphate blocks tumor cell growth by activating apoptotic machinery as well as by inhibiting the Akt/NFkB-mediated cell survival pathway. Carcinogenesis 23:2031–2041
6. Tantivejkul K, Vucenik I, Eiseman J et al (2003) Inositol hexaphosphate (IP6) enhances the anti-proliferative effects of adriamycin and tamoxifen in breast cancer. Breast Cancer Res Treat 79:301–312
7. Vucenik I, Shamsuddin AM (2003) Cancer inhibition by inositol hexaphosphate (IP6) and inositol: from laboratory to clinic. J Nutr 133:3778S–3784S
8. Sakamoto K, Venkatraman G, Shamsuddin AM (1993) Growth inhibition and differentiation of HT-29 cells in vitro by inositol hexaphosphate (phytic acid). Carcinogenesis 14:1815–1819
9. Yang GY, Shamsuddin AM (1995) IP6-induced growth inhibition and differentiation of HT-29 human colon cancer cells: involvement of intracellular inositol phosphates. Anticancer Res 15:2479–2487
10. Pittet D, Schlegel W, Lew DP et al (1989) Mass changes in inositol tetrakis- and pentakisphosphate isomers induced by chemotactic peptide stimulation in HL-60 cells. J Biol Chem 264:18489–18493
11. Weglarz L, Molin I, Orchel A et al (2006) Quantitative analysis of the level of p53 and p21WAF1 mRNA in human colon cancer HT-29 cells treated with inositol hexaphosphate. Acta Biochim Pol 53(2):349–356
12. Roy S, Gu M, Ramasamy K et al (2009) p21/Cip1 and p27/Kip1 are essential molecular targets of inositol hexaphosphate for its antitumor efficacy against prostate cancer. Cancer Res 69(3):1166–1173
13. Zhang Z, Liu Q, Lantry LE et al (2000) Germ-line p53 mutation accelerates pulmonary tumorigenesis: p53-independent efficacy of chemopreventive agents green tea or dexamethasone/myo -inositol and chemotherapeutic agents taxol or adriamycin. Cancer Res 60(4):901–907
14. Koguchi T, Tanikawa C, Mori J et al (2016) Regulation of myo-inositol biosynthesis by p53-ISYNA1 pathway. Int J Oncol 48(6):2415–2424
15. Diallo JS, Betton B, Parent N et al (2008) Enhanced killing of androgen independent prostate cancer cells using inositol hexakisphosphate in combination with proteasome inhibitors. Br J Cancer 99:1613–1622
16. Beckonert O, Monnerjahn J, Bonk U et al (2003) Visualizing metabolic changes in breast-cancer tissue using ^{1}H-NMR spectroscopy and self-organizing maps. NMR Biomed 16(1):1–11
17. Liu G, Song Y, Cui L et al (2015) Inositol hexakisphosphate suppresses growth and induces apoptosis in HT-29 colorectal cancer cells in culture: PI3K/Akt pathway as a potential target. Int J Clin Exp Pathol 8(2):1402–1410
18. Huang C, Ma W, Hecht SS et al (1997) Inositol hexaphosphate inhibits cell transformation and activator protein 1 activation by targeting phosphatidylinositol-3′ kinase. Cancer Res 57:2873–2878
19. Dinicola S, Fabrizi G, Masiello MG et al (2016) Inositol induces mesenchymal-epithelial reversion in breast cancer cells through cytoskeleton rearrangement. Exp Cell Res 345(1):37–50
20. Gu M, Roy S, Raina K et al (2009) Inositol hexaphosphate suppresses growth and induces apoptosis in prostate carcinoma cells in culture and nude mouse xenograft: PI3K-Akt pathway as potential target. Cancer Res 69(24):9465–9472
21. Han W, Gills JJ, Memmott RM et al (2009) The chemopreventive agent myoinositol inhibits Akt and extracellular signal-regulated kinase in bronchial lesions from heavy smokers. Cancer Prev Res 2(4):370–376
22. Vucenik I, Tomazic VJ, Fabian D et al (1992) Antitumor activity of phytic acid (inositol hexaphosphate) in murine transplanted and metastatic fibrosarcoma, a pilot study. Cancer Lett 65:9–13
23. Tantivejkul K, Vucenik I, Shamsuddin AM (2003) Inositol hexaphosphate (IP6) inhibits key events of cancer metastases: I. In vitro studies of adhesion, migration and invasion of MDA-MB 231 human breast cancer cells. Anticancer Res 23:3671–3679
24. Luu HH, Zhang R, Haydon RCC et al (2004) Wnt/β-catenin signaling pathway as novel cancer drug targets. Curr Cancer Drug Targets 4(8):653–671

25. Shafie NH, Mohd Esa N, Ithnin H et al (2013) Preventive inositol hexakisphosphate extracted from rice bran inhibits colorectal cancer through involvement of Wnt/β-catenin and COX-2 pathways. Biomed Res Int 2013:681027
26. Liao J, Seril DN, Yang AL et al (2007) Inhibition of chronic ulcerative colitis associated adenocarcinoma development in mice by inositol compounds. Carcinogenesis 28:446–454
27. Kamp DW, Israbian VA, Yeldandi AV et al (1995) Phytic acid, an iron chelator, attenuates pulmonary inflammation and fibrosis in rats after intratracheal instillation of asbestos. Toxicol Pathol 23:689–695
28. Weglarz L, Wawszczyk J, Orchel A et al (2007) Phytic acid modulates in vitro IL-8 and IL-6 release from colonic epithelial cells stimulated with LPS and IL-1beta. Dig Dis Sci 52:93–102
29. Couchman JR, Vogt S, Lim ST et al (2002) Regulation of inositol phospholipid binding and signaling through syndecan-4. J Biol Chem 277:49296–49303
30. Morrison RS, Shi E, Kan M et al (1994) Inositol hexakisphosphate (InsP6): an antagonist of fibroblast growth factor receptor binding and activity. In Vitro Cell Dev Biol Anim 30A(11):783–789
31. Vucenik I, Passaniti A, Vitolo MI et al (2004) Anti-angiogenic potential of inositol hexaphosphate (IP6). Carcinogenesis 25:2115–2123
32. Kar S, Quirion R, Parent A (1994) An interaction between inositol hexakisphosphate (IP6) and insulin-like growth factor II receptor binding sites in the rat brain. Neuroreport 5:625–628
33. D'Anna R, Di Benedetto A, Scilipoti A et al (2015) Myo-inositol supplementation for prevention of gestational diabetes in obese pregnant women: a randomized controlled trial. Obstet Gynecol 126(2):310–315
34. Graf E, Eaton JW (1990) Antioxidant functions of phytic acid. Free Radic Biol Med 8:61–69
35. Rao PS, Liu XK, Das DK et al (1991) Protection of ischemic heart from reperfusion injury by myo-inositol hexakisphosphate, a natural antioxidant. Ann Thorac Surg 52:908–912
36. Porres JM, Stahl CH, Cheng WH et al (1999) Dietary intrinsic phytate protects colon from lipid peroxidation in pigs with a moderately high dietary iron intake. Proc Soc Exp Biol Med 221:80–86
37. Druzijanic N, Juricic J, Perko Z et al (2002) IP-6 and inositol: adjuvant to chemotherapy of colon cancer. A pilot clinical trial. Rev Oncol 4:171
38. Bacić I, Druzijanić N, Karlo R et al (2010) Efficacy of IP6 + inositol in the treatment of breast cancer patients receiving chemotherapy: prospective, randomized, pilot clinical study. J Exp Clin Cancer Res 29:12
39. Lam S, McWilliams A, LeRiche J et al (2006) A phase I study of myo-inositol for lung cancer chemoprevention. Cancer Epidemiol Biomark Prev 15(8):1526–1531
40. Fu M, Song Y, Wen Z et al (2016) Inositol hexaphosphate and inositol inhibit colorectal cancer metastasis to the liver in BALB/c mice. Forum Nutr 8(5):E286

Part VI

Menopause Symptoms: The Therapies

The True Risks of HRT

21

John C. Stevenson

21.1 Introduction

Hormone replacement therapy (HRT) was widely used and considered a beneficial and relatively safe treatment for many years. But this changed with the publication in 2002 of the preliminary results of a large randomised clinical trial of HRT, the Women's Health Initiative (WHI) [1]. It purported to show that there were substantial risks of HRT that outweighed any possible benefits. In particular, it claimed that HRT use increased the risk of coronary heart disease (CHD), stroke, pulmonary embolism (PE) and breast cancer. This led to a large decrease in HRT use worldwide and resulted in suffering for many symptomatic postmenopausal women. But were these concerns about the safety of HRT actually justified? The evidence for the risks of HRT will here be examined.

21.2 Breast Cancer

An association between HRT use and increased breast cancer incidence has long been considered, with some, but not all, population studies showing such a link. WHI was the largest randomised clinical trial to look at risks and benefits in terms of clinical outcomes. Their preliminary publication [1] claimed to show an increase in breast cancer in postmenopausal women randomised to oestrogen-progestogen HRT, but this increase was not statistically significant, with the confidence interval including 1. A subsequent publication of the more complete data from the study showed a statistically significant increase in breast cancer incidence with oestrogen-progestogen HRT [2]. However, when the data were subdivided according to

J.C. Stevenson
National Heart and Lung Institute, Imperial College London, Royal Brompton Hospital, London SW3 6NP, UK
e-mail: j.stevenson@imperial.ac.uk

M. Birkhaeuser, A.R. Genazzani (eds.), *Pre-Menopause, Menopause and Beyond*, ISGE Series, https://doi.org/10.1007/978-3-319-63540-8_21

whether or not women had previously taken HRT, the survival curves for women taking HRT or placebo were identical, save for the placebo group previously exposed to HRT in whom there was an apparent decline in incidence with time [3]. Of more importance, when the data were adjusted for confounding variables, the increased breast cancer incidence in HRT users was no longer statistically significant [3]. In the oestrogen-alone arm of WHI, there was no significant increase in breast cancer incidence [4], and in a later analysis of women who were at least 80% compliant with the treatment, they had a statistically significant reduction in breast cancer incidence relative to placebo [5]. With a cumulative follow-up of 13 years after the trial had ended, the incidence of breast cancer in women who had been randomised to oestrogen became significantly lower than that in the women randomised to placebo [6]. There is therefore an apparent difference between users of combined HRT and users of oestrogen alone, presumably due to the addition of medroxyprogesterone acetate (MPA) in the former group. Observational studies have shown different incidences of breast cancer with the use of different progestogens. In particular, in both the French E3N study [7] and the Finnish Cohort study [8], no increase in breast cancer incidence was seen with the use of dydrogesterone as the progestogen. The Million Women Study (MWS) [9] was a large observational study that suggested that oestrogen-progestogen HRT doubled the incidence of breast cancer, with oestrogen-alone therapy showing a smaller but still statistically significant increase. These findings reflect the difference seen between oestrogen-progestogen users and oestrogen-alone users in the WHI, but the point estimates in the MWS are strikingly higher. MWS has been criticised because of biases which may have distorted the findings [10]. It is of note that there was no increase in breast cancer mortality in either arm of WHI [6]. Indeed, observational studies have shown a decrease in breast cancer mortality with HRT use [11]. When Shapiro et al. [12–14] applied established principles of causality to studies of HRT and breast cancer, they found that the WHI oestrogen-alone arm (suggesting a reduction in breast cancer) fulfilled five out of ten such principles, the WHI oestrogen-progestogen arm fulfilled only two out of ten and the MWS fulfilled none of them. Thus it remains unproven that HRT causes breast cancer. Certainly oestrogen can act as a growth promoter to breast cancer and it may be that any increases in diagnosis of breast cancer with HRT users simply reflect the growth of pre-existing breast cancers in these women. There are many other factors that increase the risk of breast cancer more than HRT [15], and such confounding factors may not be adjusted for in HRT studies. HRT may or may not increase the risk of breast cancer, but if it does it would appear that the magnitude of any increased risk is so small that it cannot be reliably detected by present-day studies.

21.3 Ovarian Cancer

Some observational studies have linked HRT use to an increased incidence of ovarian cancer. A meta-analysis of 42 studies included a cohort of over 12,000 cases [16]. There was a significant increase in ovarian cancer with oestrogen-progestogen therapy, but the relative risk was very small at 1.11. With oestrogen alone it was slightly higher at 1.28. The Danish Sex Hormone Study included almost 910,000 women aged over 50 years with a mean follow-up of 8 years [17]. They found a significantly increased incidence rate of 1.38 and an absolute risk increase of 1 per 8300 women per year. The type of HRT and duration of use had no effect, and rather surprisingly they found that the increased risk disappeared after 2 years of stopping HRT. The Collaborative Group looked at data from 52 epidemiological studies involving almost 21,500 women [18]. They found a significantly increased incidence, regardless of whether they had taken the HRT for less than or more than 5 years. They concluded that this increased risk may be largely or wholly causal. However, a rigorous epidemiological analysis of the study [19] found that the meta-analysis did not establish that HRT causes ovarian cancer. The findings did not satisfy the criteria of time order, bias, confounding, strength of association, dose-response, duration-response, consistency and biological plausibility. Rather than HRT causing ovarian cancer, the reverse may be true. Ovarian cancer can present symptomatically with dyspareunia, lower abdominal pain and recurrent urinary tract infections, and such symptoms may be regarded as oestrogen deficiency symptoms in postmenopausal women thereby encouraging the use of HRT. The WHI did not find any significant increase in ovarian cancer associated with oestrogen-progestogen use [6]. The EPIC cohort study [20] involving 370,000 women investigated whether any reproductive or hormonal factors influenced survival from ovarian cancer. They found that HRT use was associated with a better survival. This is probably due to improved cardiovascular health benefits from the HRT. There is thus no convincing evidence that HRT causes ovarian cancer.

21.4 Stroke

An increase in ischaemic stroke, but not haemorrhagic stroke, in users of HRT has been found in some, but not all, observational studies. One of the largest observation studies, the Nurses' Health Study, found a non-significant increase in ischaemic stroke in users of HRT [21]. No duration effect was observed. The vast majority of participants in this study used conjugated equine oestrogens in their HRT, and a dose-dependent effect was demonstrated, with a significant increase in stroke seen in those using a dose of 0.625 mg and above but not with lower doses. Observational data from the UK General Practitioners Research Database have shown that there appears to be no increased stroke risk with the use of low or standard dose (50 mcg) transdermal HRT [22], although an increased risk was seen with oral HRT and with high-dose transdermal HRT (>50 mcg). A major drawback to these findings is that age at initiation of HRT was not included in the study. In the WHI [6], an increase in stroke was seen in the intervention phase with both oestrogen-progestogen and oestrogen alone, but this was not seen in women initiating HRT below age 60 years. The overall increased risk with both therapies did not persist in the cumulative follow-up. The dose of conjugated equine oestrogens used in both arms of the WHI was 0.625 mg. The Danish Osteoporosis Prevention Study (DOPS) randomised over 1000 women in the early postmenopause to HRT with oral oestradiol 2 mg (plus cyclical norethisterone acetate in non-hysterectomised women) or to no treatment [23]. The study was stopped after 10 years, but there was a further 6-year observational period. No increase in stroke was seen with the HRT during the clinical trial or in the subsequent follow-up compared with no treatment. Overall, the risk of stroke with HRT appears to be related to age at initiation, dose of oestrogen and route of administration.

21.5 Venous Thromboembolism (VTE)

Observational studies have found an approximate doubling of VTE risk with oral HRT [24]. There is evidence of dose dependency, with a higher risk being seen with higher doses. However, an increased risk for VTE is not seen with transdermal HRT [25]. This is thought to be due to the avoidance of an hepatic first-pass effect of oestrogen affecting clotting factors. In the WHI, there was an increase in both deep vein thrombosis (DVT) and PE seen with both oestrogen-progestogen and oestrogen alone, although only DVT risk in the oestrogen-progestogen arm persisted in the cumulative follow-up [6]. No increased risk was seen in those initiating HRT below age 60 years. The original presentation of the full results of the WHI oestrogen-progestogen arm demonstrated an astonishing bias [26], with the authors demonstrating a more than sevenfold increase in VTE with HRT compared with placebo. This figure was achieved by comparing women taking HRT aged 70–79 years with those taking placebo aged 50–59 years, and age is a major risk factor for VTE. Had the authors chosen to compare VTE risk in women taking HRT aged 50–59 years with those taking placebo aged 70–79 years, they would have found a relative risk of 0.7 as opposed to 7.5! DOPS found no increased risk in VTE [23].

21.6 Coronary Heart Disease

Many observational studies have shown a reduction of CHD associated with postmenopausal HRT use, with the Nurses' Health Study demonstrating both primary and secondary prevention of CHD [21, 27]. Randomised trials of HRT for secondary prevention of CHD have not shown any overall benefit, although it should be noted that they have also not shown any overall harm [28]. The WHI oestrogen-progestogen arm initially reported a significant increase in CHD events with HRT, but this finding changed with subsequent publications of more complete data [29]. The oestrogen-alone arm showed no significant effect, but in the cumulative follow-up, women initiating oestrogen-alone HRT below aged 60 years had a significant reduction in CHD [6]. DOPS also showed a significant reduction in a composite cardiovascular endpoint [23]. In their report on guidelines for the management of menopause [30], NICE (the UK National Institute for Health and Care Excellence) concluded that HRT with oestrogen alone is associated with no, or reduced, risk of CHD, and HRT with oestrogen and progestogen is associated with little or no increase in the risk of CHD. Overall, there is no evidence of any harm for CHD from HRT, and HRT should therefore not be withheld from patients with, or at risk from, CHD providing appropriate starting doses of appropriate HRT regimens are used.

21.7 Gallbladder Disease

Findings from both observational studies and randomised clinical trials have demonstrated an increased risk of gallbladder disease with HRT use in postmenopausal women. The MWS found an overall significantly increased risk for gallbladder disease with HRT compared with no treatment, with a hazard ratio of 1.64 [31]. There was a higher risk with conjugated equine oestrogens compared with oral oestradiol, a higher risk with oestrogen alone compared with oestrogen-progestogen and a higher risk with oral compared with transdermal therapy. Greater risks for gallbladder disease were seen with higher doses of both conjugated equine oestrogens and oral oestradiol compared with lower doses. The French E3N study also found a significantly increased risk for gallbladder disease with HRT use compared with no treatment [32], although the hazard ratio of 1.10 was considerably lower than that from the MWS. They confirmed a great risk with oral versus transdermal therapy, and with oestrogen-alone versus oestrogen-progestogen therapy, but did not find any difference between conjugated equine oestrogens and oral oestradiol. The WHI found a significantly increased risk of self-reported gallbladder disease equally with both oestrogen-progestogen and oestrogen alone during the intervention phase, with the magnitude of the risk being similar to that seen in the MWS [6]. There is therefore an increased risk for gallbladder disease with HRT use, although the absolute risk is very low. The risk is influenced by dose and type of HRT regimen, with lower risks associated with oestrogen-progestogen therapy, with lower hormone doses and with nonoral administration.

21.8 All-Cause Mortality

Pooled results from 19 randomised clinical trials of HRT including 16,000 postmenopausal women initiating HRT below age 60 years showed a significant reduction in all-cause mortality [33]. These findings were confirmed in a Cochrane review of randomised clinical trials including almost 37,000 postmenopausal women where those women initiating HRT within 10 years of the onset of menopause had a significantly reduced all-cause mortality [34]. Those initiating HRT above age 60 years had no difference from those taking placebo or no treatment. The WHI showed no effect of either oestrogen-progestogen or oestrogen-alone HRT on all-cause mortality [6].

Conclusion

HRT is clearly a very safe treatment, particularly in those women initiating HRT in the age group below 60 years who are the vast majority in clinical practice. There may or may not be an increased risk of breast cancer diagnosis in women on combined oestrogen-progestogen HRT, but the magnitude of any risk is very low and less than the risk for breast cancer associated with many common lifestyle factors. Conjugated equine oestrogens alone seem to result in a reduced risk of breast cancer, and there may be differences in breast cancer risk with different types of progestogens in HRT. There may or may not be an increased risk of ovarian cancer associated with HRT, but the risk is small and may simply reflect an increase in HRT use in women with undiagnosed ovarian cancer. The risk of stroke is not increased in women initiating HRT below age 60 years and is dependent on starting dose and route of administration. VTE risk is also dependent on starting dose and route of administration. CHD is not adversely affected by HRT and may well be benefited. There is a small increased risk of gallbladder disease, again modified by starting dose and route of administration. The fact that all studies do not show any increase in all-cause mortality, and indeed show a decrease, confirms the absolute safety of HRT. Risks have been grossly overstated and are hugely outweighed by the many benefits of HRT.

References

1. Writing group for the Women's Health Initiative investigators (2002) Risks and benefits of estrogen plus progestin in healthy postmenopausal women. JAMA 288:221–232
2. Chlebowski RT, Hendrix SL, Langer RD et al (2003) Influence of estrogen plus progestin on breast cancer and mammography in healthy postmenopausal women. JAMA 289:3243–3253
3. Anderson GL, Chlebowski RT, Rossouw JE et al (2006) Prior hormone therapy and breast cancer risk in the Women's health Initiative randomized trial of estrogen plus progestin. Maturitas 55:103–115
4. The Women's Health Initiative Steering Committee (2004) Effects of conjugated equine estrogen in postmenopausal women with hysterectomy. JAMA 291:1701–1712
5. Stefanick ML, Anderson GL, Margolis KL et al (2006) Effects of conjugated equine estrogens on breast cancer and mammography screening in postmenopausal women with hysterectomy. JAMA 295:1647–1657
6. Manson JE, Chlebowski RT, Stefanick ML et al (2013) Menopausal hormone therapy and health outcomes during the intervention and extended poststopping phases of the Women's health Initiative randomised trials. JAMA 310:1353–1368
7. Fournier A, Berrino F, Clavel-Chapelon F (2008) Unequal risks for breast cancer associated with different hormone replacement therapies: results from the E3N cohort study. Breast Cancer Res Treat 107:103–111
8. Lyytinen H, Pukkula E, Ylikorkala O (2009) Breast cancer risk in postmenopausal women using estradiol-progestogen therapy. Obstet Gynecol 113:65–73
9. Million Women Study Collaborators (2003) Breast cancer and hormone-replacement therapy in the million women study. Lancet 362:419–427
10. Whitehead M, Farmer R (2004) The million women study: a critique. Endocrine 24:187–193

11. Willis DB, Calle EE, Miracle-McMahill HL, Heath CW (1996) Estrogen replacement therapy and risk of fatal breast cancer in a prospective cohort of postmenopausal women in the United States. Cancer Causes Control 7:449. doi:10.1007/BF00052671
12. Shapiro S, Farmer RDT, Mueck AO, Seaman H, Stevenson JC (2011) Does hormone replacement therapy cause breast cancer? An application of causal principles to three studies: Part 2. The Women's health Initiative: estrogen plus progestogen. J Fam Plann Reprod Health Care 37:165–172
13. Shapiro S, Farmer RDT, Mueck AO, Seaman H, Stevenson JC (2011) Does hormone replacement therapy cause breast cancer? An application of causal principles to three studies: Part 3. The Women's Health Initiative: unopposed estrogen. J Fam Plann Reprod Health Care 37:225–250
14. Shapiro S, Farmer RDT, Stevenson JC, Burger HG, Mueck AO (2012) Does hormone replacement therapy cause breast cancer? An application of causal principles to three studies: Part 4. The million women study. J Fam Plann Reprod Health Care 38:102–109
15. Bluming AZ, Tavris C (2009) Informing women about hormone replacement therapy. Cancer J 15:93–104
16. Greiser CM, Greiser EM, Doren M (2007) Menopausal hormone therapy and risk of ovarian cancer: systematic review and meta-analysis. Hum Reprod Update 13:453–463
17. Mørch LS, Løkkegaard E, Andreasen AH et al (2009) Hormone therapy and ovarian cancer. JAMA 302:298–305
18. Collaborative Group on Epidemiological Studies (2015) Menopausal hormone use and ovarian cancer risk: individual participant meta-analysis of 52 epidemiological studies. Lancet 385:1835–1842
19. Shapiro S, Stevenson JC, Mueck AO, Baber R (2015) Misrepresentation of the risk of ovarian cancer among women using menopausal hormones. Spurious findings in a meta-analysis. Maturitas 81:323–326
20. Beševic J, Gunter MJ, Fortner RT et al (2015) Reproductive factors and epithelial ovarian cancer survival in the EPIC cohort study. Br J Cancer 113:1622–1631
21. Grodstein F, Manson JE, Colditz GA, Willett WC, Spelzer FE, Stampfer MJ (2000) A prospective, observational study of postmenopausal hormone therapy and primary prevention of cardiovascular disease. Ann Intern Med 133:933–941
22. Renoux C, Dell'Aniello S, Garbe E, Suissa S (2010) Transdermal and oral hormone replacement therapy and the risk of stroke: a nested case-control study. Br Med J 340:c2519
23. Schierbeck LL, Rejnmark L, Tofteng CL et al (2012) Effect of hormone replacement therapy on cardiovascular events in recently postmenopausal women: randomised trial. Br Med J 345:e6409
24. Oger E, Scarabin P-Y (1999) Assessment of the risk of venous thromboembolism among users of hormone replacement therapy. Drugs Aging 14:55–61
25. Scarabin P-Y, Oger E, Plu-Bureau G (2003) Differential association of oral and transdermal oestrogen-replacement therapy with venous thromboembolism risk. Lancet 362:428–432
26. Cushman M, Kuller LH, Prentice R et al (2004) Estrogen plus progestin and risk of venous thrombosis. JAMA 292:1573–1580
27. Grodstein F, Manson JE, Stampfer MJ (2001) Postmenopausal hormone use and secondary prevention of coronary events in the Nurses' health study. Ann Intern Med 135:1–8
28. Hulley S, Grady D, Bush T et al (1998) Randomized trial of estrogen plus progestin for secondary prevention of coronary heart disease in postmenopausal women. JAMA 280:605–613
29. Stevenson JC, Hodis HN, Pickar JH, Lobo RA (2009) Coronary heart disease and menopause management: the swinging pendulum of HRT. Atherosclerosis 207(2):336–340
30. National Institute for Health and Care Excellence (2015). Menopause: clinical guideline – methods, evidence and recommendations (NG23), Version 1.5. https://www.nice.org.uk/guidance/ng23/evidence/fullguideline-559549261. Accessed 23 Apr 2016

31. Liu B, Beral V, Balkwill A, Green J, Sweetland S, Reeves G (2008) Gallbladder disease and use of transdermal versus oral hormone replacement therapy in postmenopausal women: prospective cohort study. Br Med J 337:a386
32. Racine A, Bijon A, Fournier A et al (2013) Menopausal hormone therapy and risk of cholecystectomy: a prospective study based on the French E3N cohort. CAMJ 185(7):555–561. doi:10.1503/cmaj.121490
33. Salpeter SR, Cheng J, Thabane L, Buckley NS, Salpeter EE (2009) Bayesian meta-analysis of hormone therapy and mortality in younger postmenopausal women. Am J Med 122:1016–1022
34. Boardman HMP, Hartley L, Eisinga E et al (2015) Hormone therapy for preventing cardiovascular disease in post-menopausal women. Cochrane Database Syst Rev 4:CD002229. doi:10.1002/14651858.CD002229.pub4

Menopause Hormone Therapy Customization

22

Irene Lambrinoudaki and Eleni Armeni

22.1 Introduction

Menopause is defined as the permanent cessation of menses which is attributed to the exhaustion of ovarian follicles [1]. The average age of menopause is usually 51–52 years. The ovarian hormone senescence is associated with the occurrence of menopausal symptoms, including hot flushes and night sweats, sleep difficulties, depressive symptoms, headaches, musculoskeletal pain, and sexual dysfunction. A further morbidity is the genitourinary syndrome of menopause, manifesting as vaginal dryness, burning, pain at intercourse, or recurrent genitourinary infections. Postmenopausal estrogen decline leads to accelerated bone loss and to unfavorable metabolic alterations, establishing the pathogenesis of postmenopausal osteoporosis and cardiovascular disease [2].

Menopausal hormone therapy (MHT) has long been used to treat menopausal symptoms and to prevent chronic disease. Evidence, however, has shown that universal uncontrolled administration of MHT may be associated with increased risks. Therefore, treatment today is based on solid indications and careful tailoring, so that efficacy is maximized with the lowest possible risk. In this context, women eligible for MHT can be classified into two treatment groups [1, 2]:

- Perimenopausal and postmenopausal women over 40 years
- Women with premature ovarian failure (POF) in whom ovarian senescence starts before the age of 40 years

Age at the final menstrual period is a significant predictor of morbidity. Women experiencing menopause before the age of 45 years have a higher risk of stroke and

I. Lambrinoudaki (✉) • E. Armeni
Department of Obstetrics and Gynecology, University of Athens, Aretaieio Hospital, 76 Vas. Sofias Ave, 11528 Athens, Greece
e-mail: ilambrinoudaki@med.uoa.gr

M. Birkhaeuser, A.R. Genazzani (eds.), *Pre-Menopause, Menopause and Beyond*, ISGE Series, https://doi.org/10.1007/978-3-319-63540-8_22

ischemic heart disease (IHD), as well as all-cause mortality [3]. Compared to women experiencing a natural menopause, women with POF have a higher risk of osteoporosis, mood disturbances, and even premature death [4, 5]. Therefore, all women with POF require hormone replacement therapy until the age of natural menopause, irrespectively of the presence of menopausal symptoms [4]. This review will address the customization of MHT in the first treatment group, namely, women experiencing natural or iatrogenic menopause at a normal age.

22.2 Indications of MHT

The indications of MHT are the following [2]:

- Management of menopausal symptoms, which include hot flushes and night sweats, mood disturbances, fatigue, sleep disturbances, headaches, muscle and join pain, and sexual dysfunction
- Management of the genitourinary syndrome of menopause (GSM)
- Prevention of osteoporosis in symptomatic women at high risk of fracture

22.3 MHT Regimens and Follow-Up

Hysterectomized women are treated with estrogen-only regimens, while women with an intact uterus require the addition of a progestogen or a SERM to prevent endometrial hyperplasia. Tibolone is a synthetic steroid with estrogenic, androgenic, and progestogenic activity which can be administered to both hysterectomized and non-hysterectomized postmenopausal women [2]. Available regimens can be classified according to the following characteristics [2]:

- Dose of estrogen (standard, low, ultra-low dose)
- Type of progestogen
- Mode of delivery (continuous combined vs sequential administration)
- Route of delivery (transdermal, oral, vaginal, subcutaneous preparations)

Doses are individualized according to the treatment goals and the woman's age, years since menopause, and risk profile. The initial follow-up of women starting MHT should be in 2–3 months, to review the efficacy of treatment and to discuss possible side effects. Persistence of menopausal symptoms usually requires an increase in the estrogen dose. Frequent complaints of MHT users include unscheduled spotting or bleeding, breast tenderness, bloating, fluid retention, headaches, and mood swings. Symptoms may be more frequent in women devoid of estrogens for a long time; however, they tend to subside with time. Management includes decrease in estrogen dose, change of the type of the progestogen, or change in the route of administration. Once the woman is satisfied with her treatment, follow-up should ensue in an annual basis, where cost-benefit evaluation is performed and estrogen dose redefined. The duration of treatment depends on patient preference, cost-benefit analysis, and estrogen dose [2].

22.4 MHT and Coronary Heart Disease

Aging is associated with reduced physical activity, sarcopenia, and increased adiposity, which promote the development of atherosclerosis [6]. Beyond aging, postmenopausal estrogen decline has both direct (i.e., activation of the renin-angiotensin system, increased endothelin 1 and angiotensin II, decreased nitric oxide synthase) and indirect adverse effects (i.e., visceral adiposity, insulin resistance, elevated blood pressure, dyslipidemia) on the cardiovascular system, further exacerbating the atherosclerotic process [6]. The formation of atherosclerotic plaques increases the odds of cardiovascular events, including ischemic heart disease (IHD) and stroke [6]. Hot flushes have been identified as an independent risk factor of cardiovascular disease in middle-aged women [7]. The results of the SWAN (Study of Women's Health Across the Nation) have shown that women experiencing bothersome vasomotor symptomatology early after the menopause have increased subclinical atherosclerosis compared to women with lower intensity of vasomotor symptoms, independently of demographic and cardiovascular risk factors [8].

The time of MHT initiation following the last menstrual period is the main determinant of the cardiovascular effect of MHT. Administration of MHT in young, recently postmenopausal women is associated with a favorable effect on cardiovascular risk factors, including an improvement of the lipid profile, body composition, insulin sensitivity, arterial stiffness, and chronic inflammation [9]. Older postmenopausal women, on the other hand, may have developed subclinical atherosclerosis with mature atherosclerotic plaques [9]. Administration of MHT in these women can promote plaque destabilization and increase the risk of an acute thrombotic event.

Customized administration of MHT has been related to favorable cardiovascular outcomes. A nationwide study from Finland, evaluating a total of 489,000 women during a follow-up period of 15 years, concluded that MHT users had 18–54% lower incidence of CHD as well as increased life expectancy by 12–38% [10]. The magnitude of the observed cardiovascular benefit was linearly associated with the duration of MHT use [10]. According to the findings of a recent Cochrane review, although MHT had no effect on cardiovascular outcomes in general, it was associated with up to 48% lower incidence of CHD and up to 30% lower mortality in the subgroups of women starting MHT within 10 years after their final menstrual period [11, 12]. The ELITE (Early vs Late Intervention Trial with Estradiol) randomized controlled trial reported a slower progression of subclinical atherosclerosis in postmenopausal women receiving low-dose MHT as compared to placebo. The effect was evident only in women starting MHT within 6 years after menopause, whereas women starting MHT 10 years or more after menopause had no benefit [13]. Recommendations with respect to the customization of MHT in the context of cardiovascular risk are presented in Table 22.1.

Table 22.1 Individualization of menopausal hormone therapy (MHT) according to cardiovascular risk

High cardiovascular risk: NO MHT	Intermediate risk: transdermal MHT	Low risk: any type of MHT
Age >60 years Menopausal age >10 years Long standing poorly controled diabetes mellitus Clinically overt cardiovascular disease	Menopausal age 5 - 10 years Dyslipidemia Obesity Smoking Hypertension Diabetes	

Table 22.2 Individualization of menopausal hormone therapy (MHT) in the context of breast cancer

Lowest effective estrogen dose	Lowest breast exposure to progestogen (vaginal route)	Natural progesterone / dydrogesterone or SERM for endometrial protection	Sequential mode of administration	Annual cost-benefit analysis and estrogen dose re-setting

22.5 MHT and Breast Cancer

MHT is associated with a small but significant risk of breast cancer, with a relative risk ranging between 1.25 and 1.35 [14–17]. The Million Women Study, a non-randomized survey, reported a higher risk of breast cancer (RR = 1.66) [18]. This effect is mainly evident with combined estrogen-progestogen preparations. On the contrary, the estrogen-only (ET) arm of the WHI (Women's Health Initiative) study identified a lower risk of breast cancer in women receiving unopposed estrogen therapy for a period of 7 years (RR = 0.77) [19]. According to the results of a large British cohort study on 39,183 postmenopausal women, estrogen-only MHT use was not associated with an increase in the risk of breast cancer [20]. Further parameters that may affect breast cancer risk are treatment duration, type of the progestogen, and mode of delivery [20–22] (Table 22.2).

A careful evaluation of the patient risk profile is mandatory to minimize the MHT-associated risk of breast cancer in the clinical setting. Conditions that may interact with MHT include a low body weight, daily alcohol consumption, and a

Table 22.3 Customization of menopausal hormone therapy in the context of thrombotic risk

Screening for risk factors	Selecting the appropriate MHT regimen
• Personal or family history of VTE • Increasing age and menopausal age • Immmobilization and Obesity • Smoking • Diabetes mellitus	• **Women with no risk factors**→Any type of MHT • **Women with risk factors for VTE**→Low dose transdermal estradiol (≤50μg) in combination with micronized progesterone, preferably through the vaginal route

high mammographic density. Risk factors of breast cancer which do not interact with MHT include low parity, family history of breast cancer, and a previous breast surgery for benign condition [23, 24].

22.6 MHT and Thrombosis

Treatment with oral MHT is associated with a slightly elevated risk of stroke (RR range, 1.3–1.5) [25, 26] and a two- to threefold elevated risk of venous thromboembolic events (VTE) [26, 27]. Pathophysiological mechanisms include atherosclerotic plaque destabilization, in the case of stroke, as well as clotting factor induction through the first pass effect in the liver [25]. The absolute risk is small in young, recently postmenopausal women; however, the risk increases progressively with age and the presence of risk factors like obesity, immobilization, hypertension, diabetes, dyslipidemia, left ventricular hypertrophy, or atrial fibrillation, as well as in the presence of genetic thrombophilia [25]. According to large epidemiological studies, low-dose (E2 < =50 μg) transdermal MHT does not increase the thrombotic risk [27, 28]. In addition, the type of progestogen in the MHT regimen might also alter the magnitude of the thrombotic risk [27, 29, 30]. Table 22.3 presents recommendations that should be considered when prescribing MHT in the context of VTE.

Conclusion

MHT is the treatment of choice for the management of menopausal symptoms and the genitourinary syndrome of menopause, as well as for the prevention of osteoporotic fractures in symptomatic women. When administered timely after menopause, MHT probably exerts cardiovascular benefit. Careful patient evaluation and individualization of the MHT regimen minimize possible risks. The duration of MHT administration is defined by cost-benefit analysis and the needs of the individual woman [31, 32].

References

1. Harlow SD et al (2012) Executive summary of the stages of reproductive aging workshop + 10: addressing the unfinished agenda of staging reproductive aging. Menopause 19(4):387–395
2. Armeni E et al (2016) Maintaining postreproductive health: a care pathway from the European menopause and andropause society (EMAS). Maturitas 89:63–72
3. Muka T et al (2016) Association of age at onset of menopause and time since onset of menopause with cardiovascular outcomes, intermediate vascular traits, and all-cause mortality: a systematic review and meta-analysis. JAMA Cardiol 1(7):767–776
4. Vujovic S et al (2010) EMAS position statement: managing women with premature ovarian failure. Maturitas 67(1):91–93
5. Faubion SS et al (2015) Long-term health consequences of premature or early menopause and considerations for management. Climacteric 18(4):483–491
6. Davis SR et al (2015) Menopause. Nat Rev Dis Primers 1(15004):4
7. Franco OH et al (2015) Vasomotor symptoms in women and cardiovascular risk markers: systematic review and meta-analysis. Maturitas 81(3):353–361
8. Thurston RC et al (2016) Trajectories of vasomotor symptoms and carotid intima media thickness in the study of women's health across the nation. Stroke 47(1):12–17
9. Schenck-Gustafsson K et al (2011) EMAS position statement: managing the menopause in the context of coronary heart disease. Maturitas 68(1):94–97
10. Mikkola TS et al (2015) Estradiol-based postmenopausal hormone therapy and risk of cardiovascular and all-cause mortality. Menopause 22(9):976–983
11. Boardman HM et al (2015) Hormone therapy for preventing cardiovascular disease in postmenopausal women. Cochrane Database Syst Rev 10(3):CD002229
12. Goulis DG, Lambrinoudaki I (2015 Aug) Menopausal hormone therapy for the prevention of cardiovascular disease: evidence-based customization. Maturitas 81(4):421–422. doi:10.1016/j.maturitas.2015.05.001
13. Hodis HN et al (2016) Vascular effects of early versus late postmenopausal treatment with estradiol. N Engl J Med 374(13):1221–1231
14. Chen WY et al (2002) Use of postmenopausal hormones, alcohol, and risk for invasive breast cancer. Ann Intern Med 137(10):798–804
15. Rossouw JE et al (2002) Risks and benefits of estrogen plus progestin in healthy postmenopausal women: principal results from the Women's health Initiative randomized controlled trial. JAMA 288(3):321–333
16. Chlebowski RT et al (2003) Influence of estrogen plus progestin on breast cancer and mammography in healthy postmenopausal women: the Women's health Initiative randomized trial. JAMA 289(24):3243–3253
17. (1997) Breast cancer and hormone replacement therapy: collaborative reanalysis of data from 51 epidemiological studies of 52,705 women with breast cancer and 108,411 women without breast cancer. Collaborative group on hormonal factors in breast cancer. Lancet 350(9084):1047–1059
18. Beral V (2003) Breast cancer and hormone-replacement therapy in the million women study. Lancet 362(9382):419–427
19. Anderson GL et al (2004) Effects of conjugated equine estrogen in postmenopausal women with hysterectomy: the Women's health Initiative randomized controlled trial. JAMA 291(14):1701–1712
20. Jones ME et al (2016) Menopausal hormone therapy and breast cancer: what is the true size of the increased risk? Br J Cancer 115(5):607–615
21. Cordina-Duverger E et al (2013) Risk of breast cancer by type of menopausal hormone therapy: a case-control study among post-menopausal women in France. PLoS One 8(11):e78016
22. Asi N et al (2016) Progesterone vs. synthetic progestins and the risk of breast cancer: a systematic review and meta-analysis. Syst Rev 5(1):016–0294

23. Hvidtfeldt UA et al (2015) Risk of breast cancer in relation to combined effects of hormone therapy, body mass index, and alcohol use, by hormone-receptor status. Epidemiology 26(3):353–361
24. Yaghjyan L et al (2015) Mammographic breast density and breast cancer risk: interactions of percent density, absolute dense, and non-dense areas with breast cancer risk factors. Breast Cancer Res Treat 150(1):181–189
25. NAMS (2012) The 2012 hormone therapy position statement of: the north American menopause society. Menopause 19(3):257–271
26. Mohammed K et al (2015) Oral vs transdermal estrogen therapy and vascular events: a systematic review and meta-analysis. J Clin Endocrinol Metab 100(11):4012–4020
27. Canonico M (2015) Hormone therapy and risk of venous thromboembolism among postmenopausal women. Maturitas 26(15):30006–30002
28. Simon JA et al (2016) Venous thromboembolism and cardiovascular disease complications in menopausal women using transdermal versus oral estrogen therapy. Menopause 23(6):600–610
29. Canonico M et al (2010) Postmenopausal hormone therapy and risk of idiopathic venous thromboembolism: results from the E3N cohort study. Arterioscler Thromb Vasc Biol 30(2):340–345
30. Sweetland S et al (2012) Venous thromboembolism risk in relation to use of different types of postmenopausal hormone therapy in a large prospective study. J Thromb Haemost 10(11):2277–2286
31. Bolton JL (2016) Menopausal hormone therapy, age, and chronic diseases: perspectives on statistical trends. Chem Res Toxicol 29(10):1583–1590
32. Stute P et al (2015) Ultra-low dose - new approaches in menopausal hormone therapy. Climacteric 18(2):182–186

23 GSM/VVA: Advances in Understanding and Management

Nick Panay

23.1 Introduction

There has been considerable debate whether the terms vulvovaginal atrophy (VVA), vaginal atrophy (VA) and atrophic vaginitis (AV) are entirely appropriate. The terms are not entirely accurate from a medical perspective and have limitations from a public perspective. From the medical point of view, (vulvo)vaginal atrophy does not necessarily lead to symptoms and does not include the urinary tract. From the public point of view, there is a reluctance to use the terms "vulva" and "vagina", and atrophy is associated with negative connotations. A working group was convened by the International Society for the Study of Women's Sexual Health (ISSWH) and North American Menopause Society (NAMS) in order to discuss the nomenclature with a view to developing new terminology [1]. The term genitourinary syndrome of menopause (GSM) was agreed as it encompasses both genital and urinary tracts, which are often both affected, the symptoms are multiple (hence syndrome) and there is avoidance of use of the term vagina which many women find embarrassing.

23.2 Impact of VVA/GSM on Quality of Life (QOL)

The impact of VVA/GSM on the quality of life of many women continues to be underestimated. Although the reasons for this are multiple and complex, it is clear that many women are reluctant to complain about the problem for risk of personal

N. Panay, B.Sc., FRCOG, MFSRH
Consultant Gynaecologist, Specialist in Reproductive Medicine,
Imperial College Healthcare, London, UK

Consultant Gynaecologist, Specialist in Reproductive Medicine,
Chelsea and Westminster Hospital, London, UK

Honorary Senior Lecturer, Imperial College, London, UK
e-mail: nickpanay@msn.com

M. Birkhaeuser, A.R. Genazzani (eds.), *Pre-Menopause, Menopause and Beyond*, ISGE Series, https://doi.org/10.1007/978-3-319-63540-8_23

embarrassment and cultural reasons. Healthcare providers do not proactively raise the issue in consultations because they are uncomfortable discussing sexual issues and for fear of opening a "can of worms", with limited time to deal with the consequences. There is lack knowledge as to the available effective treatment options, both hormonal and alternative [2, 3].

Even though we have an ageing population where more than 50% of postmenopausal women suffer with VVA, the subject is avoided both in social conversation and in the media. In a recent European survey, 54% of respondents said they discussed their sexual health concerns only when the healthcare professional asks. Thirty-three percent said they were too shy to discuss their sexual health concerns [4]. Women and their sexual partners are in effect, suffering in silence. The issue is particularly frustrating because treatment is often simple and safe and can transform a woman's quality of life.

23.3 Pathophysiology

With declining oestrogen, the mucosa of the cervix and the epithelium of the vagina and vulva thin and become susceptible to injury. The vaginal rugae diminish, leading to a smoother-appearing vaginal wall accompanied by diminished blood flow and a rise in pH (6–8). Together, these changes result in a pale appearance which may contain small petechiae and/or other signs of inflammation. The proportion of superficial to parabasal cells decreases with loss of glycogen and loss of lactobacilli. The loss of secretions leads to vaginal dryness and irritation.

23.4 Symptoms

Symptoms most commonly complained about include vaginal dryness (75%), pain during intercourse (40%) and vulval and vaginal pruritus and discharge. However, the urinary tract is also commonly affected leading to urinary frequency and urgency, nocturia, dysuria and incontinence in 15–35% of women greater than 60 years of age. Recurrent urinary tract infections occur in up to 20% of postmenopausal women due to atrophy of the urothelium in response to oestrogen deficiency. Women with lower urinary tract infections have a sevenfold greater risk for sexual pain disorders and a fourfold increased risk for sexual arousal disorders [5]. In a recent European survey, 66% of women stated that vulval and vaginal symptoms interfered with their ability to enjoy sexual intercourse [4].

23.5 Diagnosis

Women experiencing sexual and urinary symptoms due to vaginal atrophy should be diagnosed and treated without delay in order to avoid a cascade of events which do not resolve spontaneously. The diagnosis of VVA/GSM is often made on symptoms alone—many healthcare professionals avoid examination of the patient, which is a mistake. There are other vulval and vaginal conditions which can lead to similar symptoms such as vulval dermatoses, e.g. lichen sclerosis and vulval/vaginal malignancy. The diagnosis has been largely subjective with few objective measures used to confirm the diagnosis and monitor progression and response to treatment. The measurement of vaginal pH and the vaginal maturation index from vaginal smears provides some objective evidence. Although these measurements are commonly used in VVA/GSM studies, they are rarely used in day-to-day clinical practice.

23.6 Global Assessment Scales

Assessment tools have been developed to facilitate the formal diagnosis and classification of the severity of GSM. One of the most commonly used tools for assessing vaginal health has been the vaginal health index. The user is asked to rate both the appearance of the vaginal mucosa and production of secretions on a scale from 1 to 5 (Fig. 23.1) [6]. The drawback of this scale is that it does not take into account the impact on the vulva or the urinary tract. The absence of a vulval assessment tool was recently addressed by development of the vulval health index (Palacios S, 2015, The vulval health index (personal communication)) which assesses the appearance of the labia majora and minora, clitoris and introitus, colour of the tissues and the presence of other pathological features. There has also been an attempt to introduce a quality-of-life impact modality (pain on intercourse) in this tool although the value of assessing only one modality is limited (Fig. 23.2). A more comprehensive tool has recently been developed following the consensus group development of the term GSM [1]. The GSM assessment tool consists of three general categories of elasticity, lubrication and tissue integrity, an anatomical section which includes vulval, vaginal and urethral anatomy and two objective measures, vaginal pH and vaginal maturation. Each one of these seven components is scored from 0 to 3 according to severity (Fig. 23.3) to provide a semi-objective measure of vulval and vaginal atrophy. A numeric score is calculated by adding each one of the scores to give a total out of

Score	1	2	3	4	5
Elasticity	None	Poor	Fair	Good	Excellent
Fluid Volume (Pooling of Selection)	None	Scant amount, vault not entirely covered	Superficial amount, vault entirely covered	Moderate amount of dryness (small areas of dryness on cotton tip applicator)	Normal amount (fully saturates on cotton tip applicator)
pH	≥ 6.1	5.6 - 6.0	5.1 - 5.5	4.7 - 5.0	≤ 4.6
Epithelial Integrity	Petechiae noted before contact	Bleeds with light contact	Bleeds with scraping	Not friable - thin epithelium	Normal
Moisture (Coating)	None, surface inflamed	None, surface not inflamed	Minimal	Moderate	Normal

Table 1: Gloria Bachmann Vaginal Health Index (VHI).

Fig. 23.1 Vaginal health index [6]

Vulva health index

	Normal (0)	Mild (1)	Moderate (2)	Severe (3)
Labia Majora	Normal	Mild loss	Moderate loss	Severe loss or disappeared
Labia Minora	Normal	Mild loss	Moderate loss	Severe loss or disappeared
Clitoris	Normal size	Mild decrease in size	Moderate decrease in size	Severe decrease or undetected
Introitus & elasticity	Normal	Mild decrease or stenosis	Moderate decrease or stensis	Severe decrease or stenosis
Color	Normal	Mild pallor	Moderate pallor	Severe pallor
Discomfort & pain	None	Mild during intercourse	Moderate during intercourse	Severe during intercourse and any discomfort intensity beyond intercourse
Other findings (petechiae, excoriation, ulceration, etc)	None	Mild	Moderate	Severe

* This physical and clinical examination assessment tool assists in the classification of vulva health and atrophy.

** A numeric score can also be calculate by multiplying each catagory total by 1-3 depending on the category and totalling up the scores. From 0 to 21. 0-7 mild vulva atrophy 7-14, Moderate vulva atrophy. >14 severe vulva atrophy.

Fig. 23.2 Vulva health index (Palacios S, 2015, The vulval health index (personal communication))

21 (0–7 = mild atrophy, 7–14 = moderate atrophy and >14 = severe atrophy). There is some inaccuracy in that there is overlap between the categories, and even though the tool assesses GSM, the score refers to degree of "atrophy" rather than the "syndrome" itself. It should be noted that both the vulva health index and the GSM tool still require validation and publication of outcomes from clinical trial usage.

23.7 Impact of VVA/GSM on Quality of Life

Despite the development of these assessment tools, the formal evaluation of impact of VVA/GSM on quality of life (QOL) remains a poorly addressed issue both in research and clinical practice. In the absence of specific VVA/GSM QOL rating scales, sexual QOL scales have been used as "surrogate rating scales" to assess the impact of GSM symptoms; but what about the impact in women who are not sexually active? There has been some recent progress in this area through adaptation of a dermatology quality-of-life scale [7]. By the admission of the authors of this paper, there was considerable work still to be done. However, a recently developed multidimensional vaginal ageing questionnaire (the day-to-day impact of vaginal ageing questionnaire DIVA) [8] could be a major step forward in the development of a practical, validated questionnaire which accurately assesses the impact of VVA/GSM on personal, social and professional aspects of QOL. Data from a recent European survey showed positive correlation between vulval, vaginal and urinary

Points	Normal = 0	Mild = 1	Moderate = 2	Severe = 3
Elasticity	Stretchable, elastic tissue	Slightly diminished elasticity	Moderately diminished	Absent, fibrotic
Lubrication	Normal secretions, moisture	Slightly decreased moisture	Mostly dry, some moisture	Very dry
Tissue integrity	Intact epithelium, no friability or petechiae	Some friability with vigorous contact, no petechiae	Moderate friability or petechiae with some contact	Significant friability, bleeding, petechiae with minimal contact
Anatomy				
Introitus	3-Dimensional	Mostly 3-dimensional	Some contraction, stenosis, rather flat	Mostly contracted, stenotic, flat
Labia majora, minora	Normal for parity, coital activity, and anatomic variation	Most definition present	Some resorption, especially inferior aspect of labia minora	Significantly decreased size; minora mostly resorbed
Urethra	Normal size and position	Normal to slightly prominent	Moderately prominent urethral meatus	Eversion present; inner aspect protruding
Rugae	Normal	Present to slightly diminished	Moderately diminished but visible	Significantly diminished to absent
Color	Normal	Some faint pallor	Moderate pallor	Complete pallor
Supportive				
pH	<5		5-6.5	
Maturation index	No parabasal cells	Decrease in number of superficial cells, increase in number of parabasal cells	Fewer superficial cells, more parabasal cells	Few to no superficial cells, many parabasal cells

Fig. 23.3 Genitourinary syndrome of the menopause assessment tool [1]

symptom severity and DIVA scores, i.e. the more severe the symptoms the higher the DIVA scores indicating impairment of QOL [9].

In order to derive meaningful information from quality-of-life scales, we need to be clear about which questions we ask women and why we ask them. Women are often confused by the meaning of terms such as "vaginal dryness"; to them, this could mean "lack of normal discharge", "absence of lubrication during intercourse" or both. The "most bothersome symptom" question, now mandatory in FDA-approved studies, attempts to individualise the assessment of the magnitude and severity of GSM but runs the risk of devaluing the other less bothersome symptoms which still impact on overall wellbeing and quality of life [10].

23.8 Improving Information to Women and Healthcare Providers

Whilst social and cultural taboos are difficult to deal with, we believe there are a number of action points which the wider medical profession (doctors, pharma companies, health departments and regulators) should urgently address to improve the situation. Firstly, formal research into VVA/GSM should be expanded to confirm the scale of the problem and the impact it has on quality of life. Although highly informative, all VVA/GSM surveys such as VIVA [3] are unavoidably biased by the type and size of study population selected, and information is limited by the choice of questions asked. Is the scale of the VVA/GSM problem even larger than we think because women are reluctant to admit to having symptoms? Guidelines issued by the International Menopause Society and other societies [11, 12] are vitally important to improve awareness of VVA/GSM and in promoting the evidence-based management. Finally, it is imperative that menopause societies and pharma companies work with the regulators to change the labelling of vaginal oestrogen preparations, which currently carry precisely the same contraindications as systemic hormone therapy even though local oestrogen is not absorbed systemically.

23.9 The Need for New Products

The development of novel efficacious and safe interventions is essential to expand our armamentarium for managing VVA symptoms to provide approaches which suit all needs and desires. For instance, there will be some women who do not wish to use oestrogen or in whom oestrogen is genuinely contraindicated. Other women may find it uncomfortable or may not want, due to personal or cultural reasons, to use vaginal products. Emerging interventions include safe new laser treatments which avoid pharmacologically active agents [13], vaginally active oral selective oestrogen receptor modulators [10] and vaginal androgens such as DHEA [14]. Technological advances in nonhormonal physiological vaginal moisturisers should banish the use of vaginal lubricant gel to the examination couch [15]. It is vital that a wide armamentarium of treatment options exists to facilitate individualised management [16].

Conclusion

VVA/GSM has been neglected for too long by sufferers, their partners, society, the medical profession and the regulators. With an ageing population, it is likely that the problem will only grow as women live nearly half of their lives in a post-menopausal state. The development of the new GSM nomenclature, new tools for assessing the severity and impact of the condition and the new intervention modalities such as laser, SERMS and androgens will facilitate the understanding and management of this distressing condition.

References

1. Portman DJ, Gass ML (2014) Vulvovaginal atrophy terminology consensus conference panel. Genitourinary syndrome of menopause: new terminology for vulvovaginal atrophy from the International Society for the Study of Women's sexual health and the North American Menopause Society. Menopause 21(10):1063–1068
2. Nappi RE, Palacios S (2014) Impact of vulvovaginal atrophy on sexual health and quality of life at postmenopause. Climacteric 17(1):3–9
3. Nappi RE, Kokot-Kierepa M (2012) Vaginal health: insights, views & attitudes (VIVA)–results from an international survey. Climacteric 15:36–44
4. Nappi RE, Palacios S, Particco M, Panay N (2016) The REVIVE (REal Women's VIews of treatment options for menopausal vaginal ChangEs) survey in Europe: country-specific comparisons of postmenopausal women's perceptions, experiences and needs. Maturitas 91:81–90
5. Laumann EO, Paik A, Rosen RC (1999) Sexual dysfunction in the United States: prevalence and predictors. JAMA 281(6):537–544
6. Bachmann GA, Notelovitz M, Kelly SJ et al (1992) Long-term non-hormonal treatment of vaginal dryness. Clin Pract Sex 8:12
7. Erekson EA, Yip SO, Wedderburn TS, Martin DK, Li FY, Choi JN, Kenton KS, Fried TR (2013) The vulvovaginal symptoms questionnaire: a questionnaire for measuring vulvovaginal symptoms in postmenopausal women. Menopause 20(9):973–979
8. Huang AJ, Gregorich SE, Kuppermann M, Nakagawa S, Van Den Eeden SK, Brown JS, Richter HE, Walter LC, Thom D, Stewart AL (2015) Day-to-day impact of vaginal aging questionnaire: a multidimensional measure of the impact of vaginal symptoms on functioning and well-being in postmenopausal women. Menopause 22(2):144–154
9. Panay N. (2016). VVA from neglect to new treatment paradigm. IMS World Congress Prague. (Symposium)
10. Nappi RE, Panay N, Bruyniks N, Castelo-Branco C, De Villiers TJ, Simon JA (2015) The clinical relevance of the effect of ospemifene on symptoms of vulvar and vaginal atrophy. Climacteric 18(2):233–240
11. Sturdee DW, Panay N, International Menopause Society Writing Group (2010) Recommendations for the management of postmenopausal vaginal atrophy. Climacteric 13:509–522
12. Management of symptomatic vulvovaginal atrophy: 2013 position statement of the North American Menopause Society. Menopause 20(9):888–902
13. Gambacciani M, Levancini M, Cervigni M (2015) Vaginal erbium laser: the second-generation thermotherapy for the genitourinary syndrome of menopause. Climacteric 18(5):1–19

14. Labrie F, Archer DF, Bouchard C, Girard G, Ayotte N, Gallagher JC, Cusan L, Baron M, Blouin F, Waldbaum AS, Koltun W, Portman DJ, Côté I, Lavoie L, Beauregard A, Labrie C, Martel C, Balser J, Moyneur É, Members of the VVA Prasterone Group (2015) Prasterone has parallel beneficial effects on the main symptoms of vulvovaginal atrophy: 52-week open-label study. Maturitas 81(1):46–56
15. Edwards D, Panay N (2016) Treating vulvovaginal atrophy/genitourinary syndrome of menopause: how important is vaginal lubricant and moisturizer composition? Climacteric 19(2):151–161
16. Palacios S, Mejía A, Neyro JL (2015) Treatment of the genitourinary syndrome of menopause. Climacteric 18(Suppl 1):23–29

24 Intravaginal DHEA for the Treatment of Vulvovaginal Atrophy, Intracrinology at Work

Fernand Labrie

24.1 Introduction

Women now spend at least one third of their lifetime after menopause with the high probability of suffering from one or more of the menopausal problems secondary to sex steroid deficiency. These pertain to vulvovaginal atrophy (VVA) or genitourinary syndrome of menopause (GSM) [1], hot flushes, osteoporosis, muscle loss, skin atrophy, fat accumulation, type 2 diabetes, cardiovascular problems, memory loss, and cognition loss [2–4].

After menopause, any sex steroid activity becomes exclusively dependent upon the ability of each tissue to transform DHEA into estrogens and androgens for local and intracellular use [5, 6]. This mechanism provides the hormones needed in each tissue without biologically significant changes in the concentration of serum E_2 and testosterone which both remain at very low and biologically inactive concentrations in the blood during all the postmenopausal years in order to protect the uterus and probably other tissues from estrogenic stimulation in the absence of luteal progesterone [3, 7]. A critical requirement of postmenopause is thus to maintain serum E_2 at a concentration of 9.3 pg/ml or below [3, 8–13].

F. Labrie
Emeritus Professor, Laval University, Quebec, QC G1V 0A6, Canada

Endoceutics Inc., Quebec, QC G1V 4M7, Canada
e-mail: fernand.labrie@endoceutics.com

M. Birkhaeuser, A.R. Genazzani (eds.), *Pre-Menopause, Menopause and Beyond*, ISGE Series, https://doi.org/10.1007/978-3-319-63540-8_24

As mentioned above, DHEA, after menopause, becomes the exclusive source of all intracellular estrogens and androgens needed for the normal functioning of individual tissues, including the vagina [6, 11, 14, 15]. Consequently, the decrease in DHEA availability with age is responsible for the sex steroid deficiency-related menopausal symptoms which should logically be best corrected by replacing the cause of the problems, namely by replacement of the missing DHEA [3, 5, 7]. In fact, once the mechanisms of intracrinology controlling all sex steroids after menopause are known [3, 7, 14, 16], replacement with a physiological amount of DHEA administered intravaginally for a strictly local action appears as the optimal therapeutic strategy [3, 7, 17] that provides both estrogens and androgens, the two missing sex steroids involved in the normal functioning of the vagina [11, 15].

With the cessation of estrogen secretion at menopause and the longer and longer life expectancy after menopause, it remains that both estrogens and androgens are essential for the normal functioning of most tissues during the whole life of women, including the vagina [11]. In this context, it should be mentioned that women are not only missing estrogens but have declining levels of androgens starting at the age of 30 years with an average 60% decrease at time of menopause [9, 18, 19]. It should also be mentioned that postmenopausal women synthetize from DHEA in their peripheral tissues approximately 50% as much androgens as observed in men of the same age [6, 9, 11]. As a consequence of the low estrogenic and androgenic activities, the menopausal symptoms mentioned above have a major negative impact on the quality of life of the majority of postmenopausal women [20] and a proper correction of these symptoms requires both estrogenic and androgenic activity available only from treatment with DHEA.

Based upon this new understanding of the physiology of sex steroids in women, the objective was to develop a novel tissue-specific prohormone replacement therapy using prasterone. Especially after intravaginal administration, this approach should provide the appropriate physiological amounts and ratios of androgens and estrogens only in the cells and tissues of the vagina in need of specific amounts of these two sex steroids, while avoiding exposure of the other tissues and the risk of systemic side effects.

The clinical efficacy and metabolism of intravaginal DHEA have been evaluated in six clinical studies, including three 12-week efficacy studies (ERC-210, ERC-231, and ERC-238). This review is a combination of the efficacy data obtained in the three phase III clinical trials ERC-210 (NCT 01846442) [21, 22], ERC-231 (NCT 01256684) [23] and ERC-238 (NCT 02013544) [24] IRB approval was obtained in all individual clinical trials. All studies were multicenter performed in the US and Canada, placebo-controlled, double-blind, and randomized phase III clinical trials aimed at analyzing the efficacy of 12-week daily intravaginal administration of 0.50% (6.5 mg) prasterone (DHEA) inserts, compared to placebo in postmenopausal women (Table 24.1).

Table 24.1 Characteristics of the efficacy clinical studies performed with daily intravaginal 0.50% prasterone ovules

	ERC-210	ERC-231	ERC-238
Phase/Type	III/efficacy double-blind	III/efficacy double-blind	III/efficacy double-blind
Duration	12 weeks	12 weeks	12 weeks
Nb of sites (with subjects enrolled)	8 (2 US & 6 CDN)	30 (21 US & 9 CDN)	38 (24 US & 14 CDN)
Nb of women enrolled	218 (164 on DHEA)	255 (174 on DHEA)	558 (376 on DHEA)
Nb of women completed	199 (151 on DHEA)	222 (150 on DHEA)	527 (356 on DHEA)
Dose of prasterone[a]	0%, 0.25%, 0.50% and 1.0%	0%, 0.25% and 0.50%	0% and 0.50% (1:2 ratio)
Most bothersome symptom (MBS) (moderate or severe)	Any of 3 VVA symptoms[b] Pain at sexual activity[c]	Pain at sexual activity	Pain at sexual activity

CDN Canada, *DHEA* dehydroepiandrosterone, *MBS* most bothersome symptom, *US* United States, *VVA* vulvovaginal atrophy

[a]0% = placebo; 0.25% = 3.25 mg; 0.50% = 6.5 mg; 1.0% = 13 mg of prasterone (DHEA)

[b]Pain at sexual activity, vaginal dryness or irritation/itching

[c]A post-hoc analysis was made on subset of women of the ITT population who had self-identified moderate to severe dyspareunia as MBS at baseline

24.2 Results

As illustrated in Fig. 24.1, fairly close parallel effects on efficacy are observed in the three placebo-controlled, prospective, double-blind, and randomized 12-week clinical trials ERC-210 [21, 22], ERC-231 [23], and ERC-238 [24]. Combination of the data thus gives similar values for the prasterone-induced changes between baseline and Week 12 as well as comparison with placebo using the ANCOVA test.

For parabasal cells, while decreases of 43.5%, 45.8%, and 29.5% were observed with prasterone over placebo in the three independent clinical trials, an average decrease of 35.1% ($p < 0.0001$ versus placebo) was observed in the integrated set of data (Fig. 24.1). Superficial cells, on the other hand, increased by 4.9%, 4.7%, and 8.5% in studies ERC-210, ERC-231, and ERC-238, respectively (Fig. 24.2). When combining all data, an average 7.7% increase over placebo ($p < 0.0001$ versus placebo) was observed. Vaginal pH, the most easily accessible objective parameter of VVA, decreased by 0.99, 0.83, and 0.67 unit in the three above-mentioned clinical trials with a 0.72 pH unit decrease observed with prasterone over placebo in the combined set of data ($p < 0.0001$ versus placebo) (Fig. 24.3).

When the severity score of moderate to severe (MS) dyspareunia considered by women at baseline as their most bothersome symptom (MBS) of VVA is analyzed, decreases of −1.21, −0.40 and −0.35 score unit over placebo are observed in

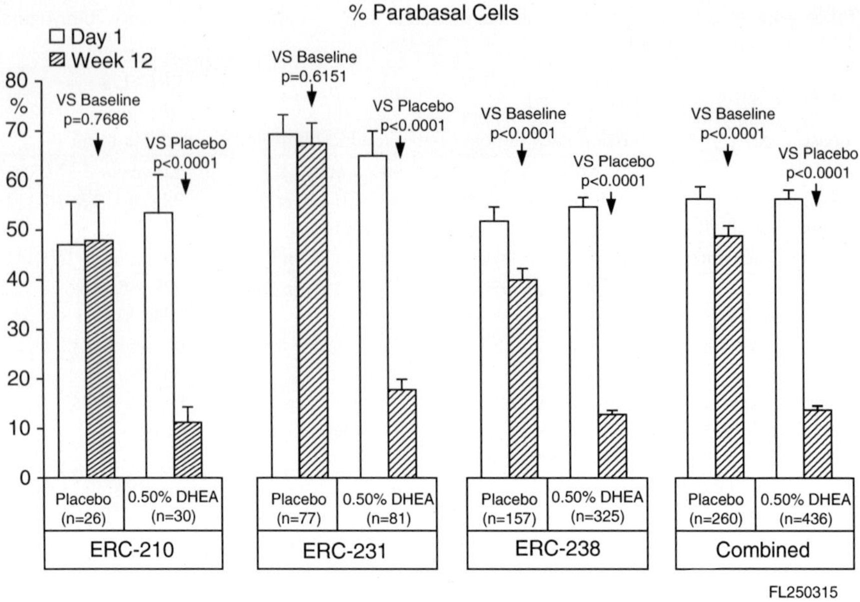

Fig. 24.1 Effect of daily intravaginal administration of 0.50% prasterone on the change in the percentage of parabasal cells from baseline to 12 weeks in clinical trials ERC-210 [22], ERC-231 [23], and ERC-238 [24] (ITT population). The combined set of data are presented at right. Data are expressed as means ± SEM. The p values are for difference from baseline for the placebo group and difference from placebo for the DHEA group

clinical trials ERC-210, ERC-231, and ERC-238, respectively, while an average decrease of −0.46 score unit (48.9% over placebo) ($p < 0.0001$) is observed in the combined set of data (Fig. 24.4).

Since a large proportion of women (about 80–85%) in studies ERC-231 and ERC-238 having MS/MBS dyspareunia also had MS vaginal dryness at baseline, it seemed important to analyze the data obtained on MS vaginal dryness, in agreement with the suggested importance of analyzing MS symptoms and not only MBS/MS symptoms in VVA studies [25].

For the 0.50% (6.5 mg) prasterone group ($n = 62$) of ERC-231, the mean severity score for vaginal dryness decreased from 2.37 ± 0.06 units at baseline to 0.92 ± 0.10 unit at 12 weeks ($p = 0.013$ versus placebo). The improvement in ERC-231 was 0.43 severity score unit (or 42%; $p = 0.013$ vs placebo) (data not shown). It is then of interest to see that of the 482 women in ERC-238 who had pain at sexual activity (dyspareunia) as their MBS VVA symptom at baseline, 283 (59%) women had moderate and 122 (25%) had severe vaginal dryness. In the ANCOVA test, the difference due to treatment shows a 0.27 severity score unit superiority in ERC-238 of prasterone compared to placebo (+23.1%, $p = 0.004$ versus placebo) (data not shown).

It should be mentioned that in addition to the efficacy data on the maturation index, vaginal pH and VVA symptoms, at each visit in all studies, the physician or gynecologist performed a visual examination of the vagina with a speculum to evaluate the severity of the four main signs of VVA, namely vaginal secretions, vaginal epithelial thickness, vaginal epithelial integrity, and vaginal color. Highly

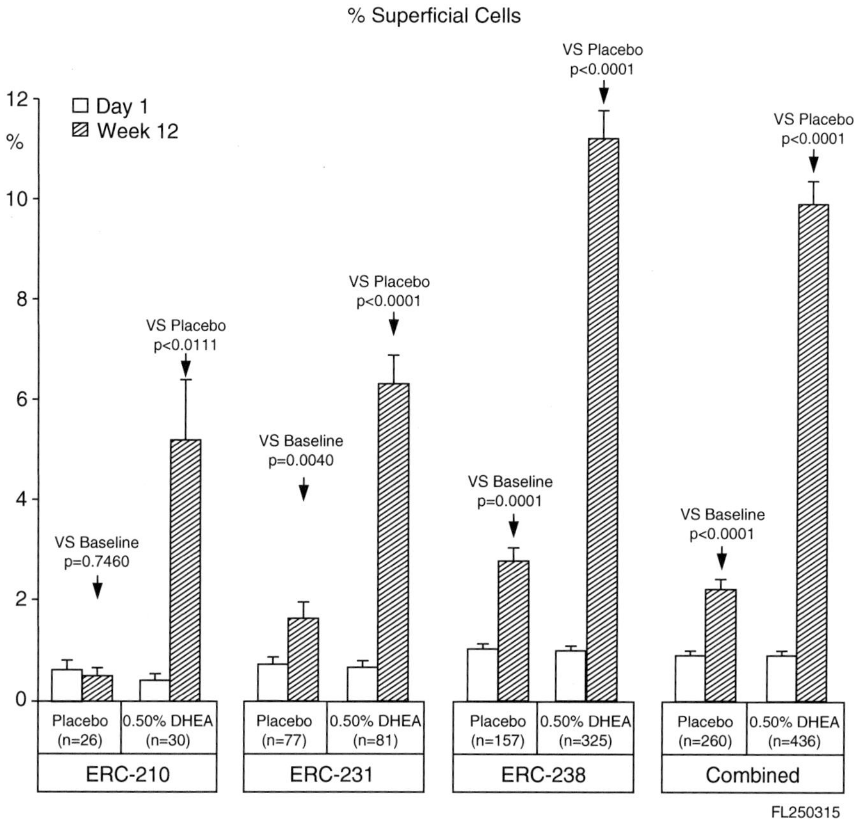

Fig. 24.2 Effect of daily intravaginal administration of 0.50% prasterone on the change in the percentage of superficial cells from baseline to 12 weeks in clinical trials ERC-210 [22], ERC-231 [23], and ERC-238 [24] (ITT population). The combined set of data are presented at right. Data are expressed as means ± SEM. The p values are for difference from baseline for the placebo group and difference from placebo for the DHEA group

statistically significant effects of daily 0.50% prasterone were observed on these four parameters over placebo in all studies performed ($p = 0.0002$ or lower).

24.2.1 Acceptability of Vaginal Administration

There was a total of 373 women in the Per-Protocol population of ERC-238 who responded at the end of the study to a questionnaire on the acceptability of the applicator in both treatment groups [26]. While it was planned that the applicator would be evaluated as suitable if at least 80% of participants have a global score ≤ 2 units, 99% and 100% of participants had a score ≤ 2 units in the placebo and prasterone groups, respectively. When asked about "like and dislike the technique of drug administration," 284 comments were positive, while 114 women gave no comment. Moreover, from 92–94% of women indicated that they were very confident to be able to use the applicator successfully in the future. The survey shows a high degree of satisfaction and of confidence to use the applicator successfully in the future [26].

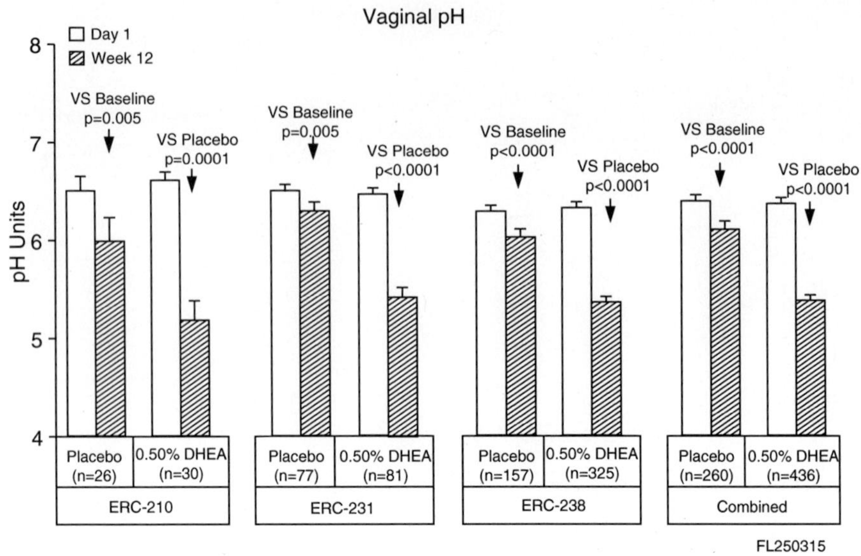

Fig. 24.3 Effect of daily intravaginal administration of 0.50% prasterone on the change in vaginal pH from baseline to 12 weeks in clinical trials ERC-210 [22], ERC-231 [23], and ERC-238 [24] (ITT population). The combined set of data are presented at right. Data are expressed as means ± SEM. The *p* values are for difference from baseline for the placebo group and difference from placebo for the DHEA group

24.2.2 Influence on the Male Partner

Sixty-six men having a partner treated with intravaginal prasterone and 34 others having a partner treated with placebo answered the questionnaires. Concerning the feeling of vaginal dryness of their female partner, the severity score following prasterone treatment improved by 81% (0.76 unit) over placebo ($p = 0.0347$). Thirty-six percent of men having a partner treated with prasterone did not feel the vaginal dryness of the partner at the end of treatment compared to 7.8% in the placebo group. When analyzing the evaluation at 12 weeks compared to baseline, an improved score of 1.09 unit was the difference found for the prasterone group compared to 0.76 for the placebo group ($p = 0.05$ versus placebo). In the prasterone group, 36% of men scored very improved compared to 18% in the placebo group. No adverse event has been reported in male partners. Moreover, the male partner had a positive evaluation of the prasterone treatment received by his female partner [27].

24.2.3 Serum Steroids Remain Within Normal Values with Intravaginal DHEA

Whereas systemic and local estrogens have been the traditional treatment of VVA [28–31] the new understanding of sex steroid physiolgoy in women, namely intracrinology [14], has led to the demonstration that DHEA exerts not only estrogenic, but both estrogenic and androgenic action in the vagina [32, 33] (Table 24.2).

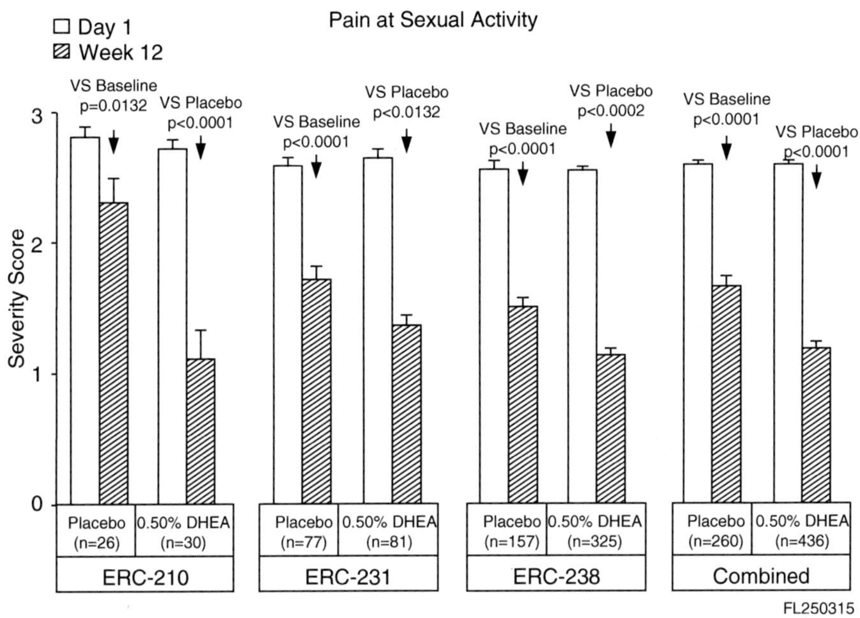

Fig. 24.4 Effect of daily intravaginal administration of 0.50% prasterone on the change from baseline to 12 weeks in the severity score of moderate to severe dyspareunia or pain at sexual activity considered as their most bothersome symptom by women at baseline in clinical trials ERC-210 [22], ERC-231 [23], and ERC-238 [24] (ITT population). The combined set of data are presented at right. Data are expressed as means ± SEM. The p values are for difference from baseline for the placebo group and difference from placebo for the DHEA group

Table 24.2 Number of subjects with treatment-emergent adverse events equal or more common than 1% by primary system organ class and preferred term in women who received daily 0.50% prasterone or placebo (MedDRA Version 16.1) (Safety Population, Preferred Terms with an Incidence ≥1% in Any Treatment Group)

Primary system organ class Preferred term[b]	Placebo $n = 474$ (percentage)	0.50% DHEA (6.5 mg)[a] $N = 1196$ (percentage)
Number (%) of subjects with at least one TEAE[c]	226 (47.7)	627 (52.4)
Gastrointestinal disorders		
Abdominal pain	14 (3.0)	21 (1.8)
Diarrhea	8 (1.7)	13 (1.1)
Nausea	14 (3.0)	19 (1.6)
General disorders and administration site complications		
Application site discharge	16 (3.4)	99 (8.3)
Fatigue	6 (1.3)	7 (0.6)
Infections and infestations		
Nasopharyngitis	22 (4.6)	40 (3.3)
Sinusitis	7 (1.5)	19 (1.6)
Urinary tract infection	21 (4.4)	57 (4.8)
Investigations		

(continued)

Table 24.2 (continued)

Primary system organ class Preferred term[b]	Placebo $n = 474$ (percentage)	0.50% DHEA (6.5 mg)[a] $N = 1196$ (percentage)
Weight increased	6 (1.3)	21 (1.8)
Musculoskeletal and connective tissue disorders		
Arthralgia	7 (1.5)	15 (1.3)
Back pain	11 (2.3)	15 (1.3)
Pain in extremity	6 (1.3)	8 (0.7)
Nervous system disorders		
Headache	14 (3.0)	35 (2.9)
Reproductive system and breast disorders		
Cervical dysplasia	6 (1.3)	21 (1.8)
Hot flush	13 (2.7)	32 (2.7)
Vaginal discharge	6 (1.3)	19 (1.6)
Vaginal hemorrhage	6 (1.3)	14 (1.2)
Vulvovaginal burning sensation	8 (1.7)	16 (1.3)
Vulvovaginal pruritus	8 (1.7)	17 (1.4)

[a]Including data of 0.50% DHEA (prasterone) doses from studies ERC-210, ERC-213, ERC-230 (up to Week 16), ERC-231, ERC-234, and ERC-238

[b]Subjects were counted only once within each preferred term

[c]TEAE (treatment-emergent adverse event): Any event that starts or worsens after the start of study treatment through 30 days after the last dose of study treatment. (AEs coded with MedDRA version 16.1)

In an analysis integrating all data obtained in women aged 40–80 years enrolled with moderate to severe symptoms of vulvovaginal atrophy (VVA) who received daily intravaginal administration of 0.50% (6.5 mg) DHEA for 12 weeks ($n = 723$; ITT-S population) as compared with placebo ($n = 266$; ITT-S population), serum steroid levels (DHEA, DHEA-sulfate (DHEA-S), androst-5-ene-3β, 17β-diol (5-diol), testosterone, dihydrotestosterone (DHT), androstenedione (4-dione), estrone (E_1), estradiol (E_2), estrone sulfate (E_1-S), androsterone glucuronide (ADT-G), and androstane-3α, 17β-diol 17-glucuronide (3α-diol-17G)) were measured at Day 1 and Week 12 by liquid chromatography-tandem mass spectrometry (LC-MS/MS) following validation performed according to the FDA guidelines [34–39].

In agreement with the mechanisms of intracrinology, all sex steroids remained well within normal postmenopausal values following administration of intravaginal DHEA. Serum estradiol, the most relevant sex steroid, was measured after 12 weeks of treatment at 3.36 pg/ml (cITT-S population) or 19% below the normal postmenopausal value of 4.17 pg/ml. On the other hand, serum E_1-S, the best recognized marker of global estrogenic activity has shown an average value of 209 pg/ml at 12 weeks compared to 220 pg/ml in normal postmenopausal women. Moreover, serum ADT-G, the main metabolite of androgens, also remained well within normal postmenopausal values. The present data shows that a low daily intravaginal dose (6.5 mg) of DHEA (prasterone) which is efficacious on the symptoms and signs of VVA permits to achieve the desired local efficacy without systemic exposure, in agreement with the stringent mechanisms of menopause established after 500 million years of evolution where each cell in each tissue is the master of its sex steroid exposure.

24.2.4 Sexual Function

Sexual dysfunction is a common problem with rates of up to 50% self-reported among women in community studies [40–42]. In the United States, it has been observed that 43% of women have sexual dysfunction of one type or another. The prevalence of sexual dysfunction increases after ovariectomy and with age [43, 44] with a higher incidence in postmenopausal women [45–48].

Our recent data have indicated the benefits of the local intravaginal action of DHEA on all domains of sexual dysfunction [49, 50], while the symptoms of VVA were also improved [21]. While it is recognized that estrogens improve the VVA symptoms by an action in the most superficial layer of the vagina, intravaginal DHEA improves both vaginal atrophy [21–23, 51] and sexual dysfunction [49, 50].

Study ERC-238 was a phase III, placebo-controlled, double-blind, prospective, and randomized study (NCT02013544, https://clinicaltrials.gov) having the primary objective to confirm the efficacy of daily intravaginal administration of 0.50% (6.5 mg) DHEA ovules (suppositories) for 12 weeks on moderate to severe (MS) pain at sexual activity as most bothersome symptom (MBS) of VVA as evaluated by a questionnaire and to evaluate, as secondary objective, the benefits on sexual dysfunction. Women were randomized in a 2:1 ratio between the 0.50% (6.5 mg) DHEA (prasterone) and placebo groups [52].

Placebo was administered daily to 157 women while 325 women received 0.50% (6.5 mg) DHEA daily for 12 weeks. All women were postmenopausal meeting the criteria of VVA, namely moderate to severe dyspareunia as their most bothersome symptom of VVA in addition to having ≤5% of vaginal superficial cells and vaginal pH > 5.0. The Female Sexual Function Index (FSFI) questionnaire was filled at baseline (screening and Day 1), 6 weeks, and 12 weeks. Comparison between DHEA and placebo of the changes from baseline to 12 weeks was made using the analysis of covariance test, with treatment group as the main factor and baseline value as the covariate.

The six domains and total score of the FSFI questionnaire were evaluated. The FSFI domain desire increased over placebo by 0.24 unit (+49.0%, $p = 0.0105$), arousal by 0.42 unit (+56.8%, $p = 0.0022$), lubrication by 0.57 unit (+36.1%, $p = 0.0005$), orgasm by 0.32 unit (+33.0%, $p = 0.047$), satisfaction by 0.44 unit (+48.3%, $p = 0.0012$) and pain at sexual activity by 0.62 unit (+39.2%, $p = 0.001$). The total FSFI score, on the other hand, has shown a superiority of 2.59 units in the DHEA group over placebo or a 41.3% greater change than placebo ($p = 0.0006$ over placebo).

The present data show that all the six domains of the FSFI are improved over placebo (from $p = 0.047$ to 0.0005), thus confirming the previously observed benefits of intravaginal DHEA on female sexual dysfunction by an action exerted exclusively at the level of the vagina, in the absence of biologically significant changes of serum steroids levels.

While psychological factors are believed to play an important role in the loss of sexual desire/interest and arousal, many studies have reported a beneficial effect of androgens on sexual function in women [53–62]. These observations have resulted in an increased use of testosterone for this indication [63, 64], although some controversy still exists concerning the efficacy of androgens on sexual dysfunction [65, 66].

There is growing evidence that low DHEA-S levels negatively correlate with sexual dysfunction in both pre- and postmenopausal women to a greater extent than testosterone levels [67–70]. Low serum DHEA has also been associated with increased sexual dysfunction over the menopausal transition [71]. In a study performed in 560 women aged 19–65 years, a correlation has been observed between sexual desire and total and free testosterone, androstenedione and DHEA-S [72]. In women aged 45–65 years, androstenedione correlated with sexual desire. Globally, a correlation was found between circulating androgens and sexual desire.

The benefits of androgens have been observed when administered alone or in association with hormone replacement therapy (HRT) [60, 73–83]. In a placebo-controlled trial performed in 60 postmenopausal women, testosterone therapy improved women's sexual desire and mood without aromatization to estrogens [84]. Moreover, an aromatase inhibitor did not prevent the beneficial effects of testosterone propionate on sexual desire in postmenopausal women [85].

Of particular relevance to the beneficial effect of intravaginal DHEA on sexual dysfunction is the observation that nerve fibers are mainly located in the muscularis, a main site of action of androgens, and that treatment with testosterone increases the number and size of the nerve terminals in the rat vagina while estrogens and progesterone have no effect [86, 87]. Recently, treatment with DHEA, through its androgenic effect, but not estrogens, has shown an increase in the number and surface area of nerve fibers in the vagina of the rat [86, 88], thus providing a potential explanation for the benefits of treatment with intravaginal DHEA on sexual function in women [49, 50]. Most importantly, these benefits are achieved by an exclusive peripheral action of DHEA limited to the vagina with no biologically significant change in the serum levels of testosterone or other steroid, which remain well within the normal postmenopausal values [12, 89, 90].

In terms of mechanism of action, it is important to indicate, as mentioned earlier, that low libido and low coital frequency was not affected in postmenopausal women who received oral or percutaneous estrogens [91] even if a significant effect was observed on vaginal dryness and pain at intercourse, thus indicating a dissociation between the effect of estrogens on vaginal atrophy and sexual dysfunction [49]. Similar findings have been reported by Lobo et al. [56] and Gonzalez et al. [92]. In patients with both vaginal atrophy and FSD who were treated for 12 weeks with Premarin (conjugated equine estrogens) cream, Premarin + testosterone cream or placebo, an improvement in the sexuality score was observed only in the Premarin + testosterone group while vaginal atrophy was improved in both the Premarin and Premarin + testosterone groups [93].

Although the role of psychological, biological, and interpersonal factors in sexual function is a matter of debate [94], the present data clearly show that local intravaginal changes induced by DHEA (prasterone) can exert beneficial effects on all aspects of sexual function, including desire/interest, a characteristic component of brain function. It thus seems possible that increased favorable outputs from a healthier vaginal mucosa could influence the brain to express increased desire/interest without the need for a direct action of hormones on the brain.

24.2.5 No Effect of DHEA on the Endometrium: Safety: No Drug-Related Effect of Intravaginal DHEA Except Application Site Discharge

As shown in Table 24.2 which indicates all treatment-emergent (which occurred from any cause during treatment) adverse events by primary system organ class and preferred term, no adverse event which could be reasonably considered drug-related was observed. This table indicates the adverse reactions of equal or more common occurrence than ≥1% in subjects who received intravaginal 0.50% prasterone (6.5 mg) or placebo. Application site discharge, the only observation with a higher incidence in the prasterone group, is likely due to melting of the hard fat used as vehicle of prasterone added to increased vaginal secretions secondary to treatment. Out of 1542 women who received intravaginal prasterone (3.25–13 mg), 0.45% ($n = 7$) discontinued due to this effect.

An atrophic or inactive endometrium was observed in all 668 non-hysterectomized women treated for 12 weeks or longer with intravaginal prasterone, including 389 treated for 1 year with a daily dose of 6.5 mg prasterone [95].

Since the menopausal symptoms and signs caused by sex steroid deficiency are such a recent phenomenon, evolution did not have the required time to build the proper feedback mechanisms able to increase DHEA secretion in response to decreased concentrations of circulating DHEA. Medicine, however, should succeed in replacing the sex steroid precursor, namely DHEA, which becomes progressively deficient during the extended years of life. The advantage of sex steroid medicine is that accurate assays of estrogens and androgens are available [37–39] and specific replacement therapy can be achieved with precision once the sex steroid deficiency has been well identified. The situation of postmenopause is somewhat facilitated by the fact that DHEA is the unique source of both estrogens and androgens after menopause [6, 90] and properly replacing DHEA can correct the deficiency in both sex steroids.

At menopause, or at the end of the reproductive years, the secretion of E_2 by the ovaries usually stops within a period of 6–12 months. Thereafter, throughout postmenopause, serum E_2 remains at biologically inactive concentrations or below the 95th centile of normal postmenopausal values, namely at or below 9.3 pg/ml [90], and not 20 pg/ml as frequently used based upon values obtained by immuno-based assays lacking specificity, thus giving approximately 100% higher values than the accurate mass spectrometry (MS)-based assays. This difference is due to unidentified compounds other than E_2, which interfere in the less specific assays. The maintenance of serum E_2 at low biologically inactive concentrations eliminates stimulation of the endometrium and avoids the risk of endometrial cancer [96].

The normal blood estrogen concentrations in women treated with physiological amounts of DHEA are not different from the situation observed in about 25% of normal postmenopausal women who have sufficiently high endogenous DHEA activity to avoid the symptoms of menopause: these women are not symptomatic and, consequently, do not need DHEA replacement. The administration of intravaginal DHEA permits to increase DHEA availability locally in the vagina where the symptoms of sex steroid deficiency are present, especially pain at sexual activity and vaginal dryness. The local addition of exogenous DHEA permits to compensate for the absence of a specific stimulator of DHEA secretion when serum DHEA decreases and becomes symptomatic.

References

1. Portman DJ, Gass ML et al (2014) Genitourinary syndrome of menopause: new terminology for vulvovaginal atrophy from the International Society for the Study of Women's sexual health and the North American Menopause Society. Menopause 21(10):1063–1068
2. Archer DF, Furst K et al (1999) A randomized comparison of continuous combined transdermal delivery of estradiol-norethindrone acetate and estradiol alone for menopause. CombiPatch study group. Obstet Gynecol 94(4):498–503
3. Labrie F, Labrie C (2013) DHEA and intracrinology at menopause, a positive choice for evolution of the human species. Climacteric 16:205–213
4. Utian WH, Shoupe D et al (2001) Relief of vasomotor symptoms and vaginal atrophy with lower doses of conjugated equine estrogens and medroxyprogesterone acetate. Fertil Steril 75(6):1065–1079
5. Labrie F (2010) DHEA after menopause–sole source of sex steroids and potential sex steroid deficiency treatment. Menopause Manag 19:14–24
6. Labrie F (2015) Androgens in postmenopausal women: their practically exclusive intracrine formation and inactivation in peripheral tissues. In: Plouffe L, Rizk B (eds) Androgens in gynecological practice. Cambridge University Press, Cambridge, pp 64–73
7. Labrie F (2015) Each tissue becomes master of its sex steroid environment at menopause. Climacteric 18:764–765
8. Labrie F, Bélanger A et al (2017) Science of intracrinology in postmenopausal women. Menopause 24:702–712
9. Labrie F, Cusan L et al (2009) Comparable amounts of sex steroids are made outside the gonads in men and women: strong lesson for hormone therapy of prostate and breast cancer. J Steroid Biochem Mol Biol 113:52–56
10. Labrie F, Martel C (2017) A low dose (6.5 mg) intravaginal DHEA permits a strictly local action while maintaining all serum estrogens or androgens as well as their metabolites within normal values. Horm Mol Biol Clin Invest 29(2):39–60
11. Labrie F, Martel C et al (2017) Androgens in women are essentially made from DHEA in each peripheral tissue according to intracrinology. J Steroid Biochem Mol Biol 168:9–18
12. Labrie F, Martel C et al (2013) Intravaginal prasterone (DHEA) provides local action without clinically significant changes in serum concentrations of estrogens or androgens. J Steroid Biochem Mol Biol 138:359–367
13. Martel C, Labrie F et al (2016) Serum steroid concentrations remain within normal postmenopausal values in women receiving daily 6.5mg intravaginal prasterone for 12 weeks. J Steroid Biochem Mol Biol 159:142–153
14. Labrie F (1991) Intracrinology. Mol Cell Endocrinol 78:C113–C118
15. Labrie F, Martel C et al (2017) Is vulvovaginal atrophy due to a lack of both estrogens and androgens? Menopause 24:1–10

16. Labrie F, Luu-The V et al (2005) Is DHEA a hormone? Starling review. J Endocrinol 187:169–196
17. Panay N, Fenton A (2015) Menopause--natural selection or modern disease? Climacteric 18(1):1–2
18. Labrie F, Bélanger A et al (2006) Androgen glucuronides, instead of testosterone, as the new markers of androgenic activity in women. J Steroid Biochem Mol Biol 99(4–5):182–188
19. Labrie F, Martel C et al (2011) Wide distribution of the serum dehydroepiandrosterone and sex steroid levels in postmenopausal women: role of the ovary? Menopause 18(1):30–43
20. Williams RE, Levine KB et al (2009) Menopause-specific questionnaire assessment in US population-based study shows negative impact on health-related quality of life. Maturitas 62(2):153–159
21. Labrie F, Archer DF et al (2009) Intravaginal dehydroepiandrosterone (Prasterone) a physiological and highly efficient treatment of vaginal atrophy. Menopause 16:907–922
22. Labrie F, Archer DF et al (2011) Intravaginal dehydroepiandrosterone (DHEA, Prasterone), a highly efficient treatment of dyspareunia. Climacteric 14:282–288
23. Archer DF, Labrie F et al (2015) Treatment of pain at sexual activity (dyspareunia) with intravaginal dehydroepaindrosterone (prasterone). Menopause 22(9):950–963
24. Labrie F, Archer DF et al (2016) Efficacy of intravaginal dehydroepiandrosterone (DHEA) on moderate to severe dyspareunia and vaginal dryness, symptoms of vulvovaginal atrophy, and of the genitourinary syndrome of menopause. Menopause 23(3):243–256
25. Chen L, Ng MJ et al (2010) Statistical considerations for the efficacy assessment of clinical studies of vulvar and vaginal atrophy. Drug Info J 44:581–588
26. Montesino M, Labrie F et al (2016) Evaluation of the acceptability of intravaginal prasterone ovule administration using an applicator. Gynecol Endocrinol 32:240–245
27. Labrie F, Montesino M et al (2015) Influence of treatment of vulvovaginal atrophy with intravaginal prasterone on the male partner. Climacteric 18:817–825
28. Archer DF (2010) Efficacy and tolerability of local estrogen therapy for urogenital atrophy. Menopause 17(1):194–203
29. Mac Bride MB, Rhodes DJ et al (2010) Vulvovaginal atrophy. Mayo Clin Proc 85(1):87–94
30. NAMS: The North American Menopause Society (2013) Management of symptomatic vulvovaginal atrophy: 2013 position statement of the North American Menopause Society. Menopause 20(9):888–902. quiz 903-884
31. Utian WH, Archer DF et al (2008) Estrogen and progestogen use in postmenopausal women: July 2008 position statement of the North American Menopause Society. Menopause 15(4 Pt 1):584–602
32. Berger L, El-Alfy M et al (2005) Effects of dehydroepiandrosterone, premarin and acolbifene on histomorphology and sex steroid receptors in the rat vagina. J Steroid Biochem Mol Biol 96(2):201–215
33. Sourla A, Flamand M et al (1998) Effect of dehydroepiandrosterone on vaginal and uterine histomorphology in the rat. J Steroid Biochem Mol Biol 66(3):137–149
34. Dury AY, Ke Y et al (2015) Validated LC-MS/MS simultaneous assay of five sex steroid/neurosteroid-related sulfates in human serum. J Steroid Biochem Mol Biol 149:1–10
35. Guidance for Industry (2001). Bioanalytical method validation. U.S. Department of Health and Human Services Food and Drug Administration Center for Drug Evaluation and Research (CDER) Center for Veterinary Medicine (CVM) May 2001 BP
36. Guidance for Industry (2013). Bioanalytical Method Validation–Revision 1. U.S. Department of Health and Human Services, Food and Drug Administration. Center for Drug Evaluation and Research (CDER), Center for Veterinary Medicine (CVM). Division of Drug Information, September 2013 (Draft Guidance). http://www.fda.gov/Drugs/GuidanceComplianceRegulatoryInformation/Guidances/default.htm
37. Ke Y, Bertin J et al (2014) A sensitive, simple and robust LC-MS/MS method for the simultaneous quantification of seven androgen- and estrogen-related steroids in postmenopausal serum. J Steroid Biochem Mol Biol 144:523–534

38. Ke Y, Gonthier R et al (2015) A rapid and sensitive UPLC-MS/MS method for the simultaneous quantification of serum androsterone glucuronide, etiocholanolone glucuronide, and androstan-3alpha, 17beta diol 17-glucuronide in postmenopausal women. J Steroid Biochem Mol Biol 149:146–152
39. Labrie F, Ke Y et al (2015) Why both LC-MS/MS and FDA-compliant validation are essential for accurate estrogen assays? J Steroid Biochem Mol Biol 149:89–91
40. Béjin A (1994) Sexual pleasures, dysfunctions, fantaisies, and satisfaction. In: Spira A, Bajos N (eds) Sexual behaviour and AIDS. Avebury, Aldershot, England, pp 163–171
41. Burwell SR, Case LD et al (2006) Sexual problems in younger women after breast cancer surgery. J Clin Oncol 24(18):2815–2821
42. Kontula O, Haavio-Mannila E (1995) Sexual pleasures. Enhancement of sex life in Finland, 1971–1992. Dartmouth, Aldershot, England
43. Laumann EO, Paik A et al (1999) Sexual dysfunction in the United States: prevalence and predictors. JAMA 281(6):537–544
44. Nathorst-Boos J, von Schoultz B (1992) Psychological reactions and sexual life after hysterectomy with and without oophorectomy. Gynecol Obstet Investig 34(2):97–101
45. Avis NE, Stellato R et al (2000) Is there an association between menopause status and sexual functioning? Menopause 7(5):297–309
46. Dennerstein L, Dudley E et al (2001) Are changes in sexual functioning during midlife due to aging or menopause? Fertil Steril 76(3):456–460
47. Hallstrom T, Samuelsson S (1990) Changes in women's sexual desire in middle life: the longitudinal study of women in Gothenburg. Arch Sex Behav 19(3):259–268
48. Osborn M, Hawton K et al (1988) Sexual dysfunction among middle aged women in the community. Br Med J (Clin Res Ed) 296(6627):959–962
49. Labrie F, Archer D et al (2014) Lack of influence of dyspareunia on the beneficial effect of intravaginal prasterone (dehydroepiandrosterone, DHEA) on sexual dysfunction in postmenopausal women. J Sex Med 11(7):1766–1785
50. Labrie F, Archer DF et al (2009) Effect of intravaginal dehydroepiandrosterone (Prasterone) on libido and sexual dysfunction in postmenopausal women. Menopause 16:923–931
51. Labrie F, Archer DF et al (2015) Prasterone has parallel beneficial effects on the main symptoms of vulvovaginal atrophy: 52-week open-label study. Maturitas 81:46–56
52. Labrie F, Archer DF et al (2015) Efficacy of intravaginal dehydroepiandrosterone (DHEA) on moderate to severe dyspareunia and vaginal dryness, symptoms of vulvovaginal atrophy and of the genitourinary syndrome of menopause. Menopause 23(3):243–256
53. Davis SR, McCloud P et al (1995) Testosterone enhances estradiol's effects on postmenopausal bone density and sexuality. Maturitas 21(3):227–236
54. Goldstat R, Briganti E et al (2003) Transdermal testosterone therapy improves well-being, mood, and sexual function in premenopausal women. Menopause 10(5):390–398
55. Hubayter Z, Simon JA (2008) Testosterone therapy for sexual dysfunction in postmenopausal women. Climacteric 11(3):181–191
56. Lobo RA, Rosen RC et al (2003) Comparative effects of oral esterified estrogens with and without methyltestosterone on endocrine profiles and dimensions of sexual function in postmenopausal women with hypoactive sexual desire. Fertil Steril 79(6):1341–1352
57. Sarrel P, Dobay B et al (1998) Estrogen and estrogen-androgen replacement in postmenopausal women dissatisfied with estrogen-only therapy. Sexual behavior and neuroendocrine responses. J Reprod Med 43(10):847–856
58. Sherwin BB, Gelfand MM (1985) Differential symptom response to parenteral estrogen and/or androgen administration in the surgical menopause. Am J Obstet Gynecol 151:153–160
59. Sherwin BB, Gelfand MM (1987) The role of androgen in the maintenance of sexual functioning in oophorectomized women. Psychosom Med 49:397–409
60. Shifren JL, Davis SR et al (2006) Testosterone patch for the treatment of hypoactive sexual desire disorder in naturally menopausal women: results from the INTIMATE NM1 study. Menopause 13(5):770–779
61. Tuiten A, Van Honk J et al (2000) Time course of effects of testosterone administration on sexual arousal in women. Arch Gen Psychiatry 57(2):149–153. discussion 155-146

62. Tuiten A, van Honk J et al (2002) Can sublingual testosterone increase subjective and physiological measures of laboratory-induced sexual arousal? Arch Gen Psychiatry 59(5):465–466
63. Davis SR, Tran J (2001) Testosterone influences libido and well being in women. Trends Endocrinol Metab 12(1):33–37
64. Hulter B, Lundberg PO (1994) Sexual function in women with hypothalamo-pituitary disorders. Arch Sex Behav 23(2):171–183
65. Basson R (2007) Hormones and sexuality: current complexities and future directions. Maturitas 57(1):66–70
66. Myers LS, Dixen J et al (1990) Effects of estrogen, androgen, and progestin on sexual psychophysiology and behavior in postmenopausal women. J Clin Endocrinol Metab 70(4):1124–1131
67. Basson R, Brotto LA et al (2010) Role of androgens in women's sexual dysfunction. Menopause 17(5):962–971
68. Davis SR, Davison SL et al (2005) Circulating androgen levels and self-reported sexual function in women. JAMA 294(1):91–96
69. Davis SR, Shah SM et al (2008) Dehydroepiandrosterone sulfate levels are associated with more favorable cognitive function in women. J Clin Endocrinol Metab 93(3):801–808
70. Genazzani AR, Pluchino N (2010) DHEA therapy in postmenopausal women: the need to move forward beyond the lack of evidence. Climacteric 13(4):314–316
71. Gracia CR, Freeman EW et al (2007) Hormones and sexuality during transition to menopause. Obstet Gynecol 109(4):831–840
72. Wahlin-Jacobsen S, Pedersen AT et al (2015) Is there a correlation between androgens and sexual desire in women? J Sex Med 12(2):358–373
73. Bachmann G, Bancroft J et al (2002) Female androgen insufficiency: the Princeton consensus statement on definition, classification, and assessment. Fertil Steril 77(4):660–665
74. Braunstein GD, Sundwall DA et al (2005) Safety and efficacy of a testosterone patch for the treatment of hypoactive sexual desire disorder in surgically menopausal women: a randomized, placebo-controlled trial. Arch Intern Med 165(14):1582–1589
75. Buster JE, Kingsberg SA et al (2005) Testosterone patch for low sexual desire in surgically menopausal women: a randomized trial. Obstet Gynecol 105(5 Pt 1):944–952
76. Davis SR, Moreau M et al (2008) Testosterone for low libido in postmenopausal women not taking estrogen. N Engl J Med 359(19):2005–2017
77. Davis SR, van der Mooren MJ et al (2006) Efficacy and safety of a testosterone patch for the treatment of hypoactive sexual desire disorder in surgically menopausal women: a randomized, placebo-controlled trial. Menopause 13(3):387–396
78. Miller KK, Biller BM et al (2006) Effects of testosterone replacement in androgen-deficient women with hypopituitarism: a randomized, double-blind, placebo-controlled study. J Clin Endocrinol Metab 91(5):1683–1690
79. Nathorst-Boos J, Floter A et al (2006) Treatment with percutanous testosterone gel in postmenopausal women with decreased libido--effects on sexuality and psychological general well-being. Maturitas 53(1):11–18
80. Panay N, Al-Azzawi F et al (2010) Testosterone treatment of HSDD in naturally menopausal women: the ADORE study. Climacteric 13(2):121–131
81. Shifren JL, Braunstein GD et al (2000) Transdermal testosterone treatment in women with impaired sexual function after oophorectomy. N Engl J Med 343(10):682–688
82. Simon J, Braunstein G et al (2005) Testosterone patch increases sexual activity and desire in surgically menopausal women with hypoactive sexual desire disorder. J Clin Endocrinol Metab 90(9):5226–5233
83. Somboonporn W, Davis S et al (2005) Testosterone for peri- and postmenopausal women. Cochrane Database Syst Rev 4:CD004509
84. Davis SR, Goldstat R et al (2006) Effects of aromatase inhibition on sexual function and well-being in postmenopausal women treated with testosterone: a randomized, placebo-controlled trial. Menopause 13(1):37–45
85. Wierman ME, Arlt W et al (2014) Androgen therapy in women: a reappraisal: an Endocrine Society clinical practice guideline. J Clin Endocrinol Metab 99(10):3489–3510
86. Pelletier G, Ouellet J et al (2013) Androgenic action of dehydroepiandrosterone (DHEA) on nerve density in the ovariectomized rat vagina. J Sex Med 10(8):1908–1914

87. Pessina MA, Hoyt RF Jr et al (2006) Differential effects of estradiol, progesterone, and testosterone on vaginal structural integrity. Endocrinology 147(1):61–69
88. Pelletier G, Ouellet J et al (2012) Effects of ovariectomy and dehydroepiandrosterone (DHEA) on vaginal wall thickness and innervation. J Sex Med 9(10):2525–2533
89. Ke Y, Labrie F et al (2015) Serum levels of sex steroids and metabolites following 12 weeks of intravaginal 0.50% DHEA administration. J Steroid Biochem Mol Biol 154:186–196
90. Labrie F (2015) All sex steroids are made intracellularly in peripheral tissues by the mechanisms of intracrinology after menopause. J Steroid Biochem Mol Biol 145:133–138
91. Long CY, Liu CM et al (2006) A randomized comparative study of the effects of oral and topical estrogen therapy on the vaginal vascularization and sexual function in hysterectomized postmenopausal women. Menopause 13(5):737–743
92. Gonzalez M, Viafara G et al (2004) Sexual function, menopause and hormone replacement therapy (HRT). Maturitas 48(4):411–420
93. Raghunandan C, Agrawal S et al (2010) A comparative study of the effects of local estrogen with or without local testosterone on vulvovaginal and sexual dysfunction in postmenopausal women. J Sex Med 7(3):1284–1290
94. Basson R, Althof S et al (2004) Summary of the recommendations on sexual dysfunctions in women. Berl Munch Tierarztl Wochenschr 1(1):24–34
95. Portman DJ, Labrie F et al (2015) Lack of effect of intravaginal dehydroepiandrosterone (DHEA, prasterone) on the endometrium in postmenopausal women. Menopause 22(12):1289–1295
96. Hammond CB, Jelovsek FR et al (1979) Effects of long-term estrogen replacement therapy. II. Neoplasia. Am J Obstet Gynecol 133(5):537–547

Part VII

Surgical Challenges After Menopause: Problems and Solutions

25 Bladder Dysfunction and Urinary Incontinence After the Menopause: Hormones, Drugs, or Surgery?

Eleonora Russo, Andrea Giannini, Marta Caretto, Paolo Mannella, and Tommaso Simoncini

25.1 Introduction

The female pelvic floor undergoes a large number of adaptive changes, related to life and endocrine events. The injuries and functional modifications of female pelvic floor due to pregnancy, life events, and aging are associated with several changes that may predispose to pelvic floor dysfunctions (PFD). Pelvic floor dysfunction globally affects micturition, defecation, and sexual activity and their incidence increases dramatically with age and menopause. Lower urinary tract dysfunctions, such as urinary incontinence (UI), detrusor overactivity (DO), overactive bladder syndrome (OAB), recurrent urinary tract infections (UTI), are prevalent in elderly women. These conditions can interfere with daily life and can lead to negative effects on health-related quality of life. Lower urinary tract symptoms and urinary incontinence have been associated with both systemic aging and menopause.

25.2 Bladder Aging: Functional and Structural Changes

Recent data suggest that several physiological and pathological bladder changes that frequently occur with aging are closely related to OAB. The International Continence Society defines overactive bladder syndrome (OAB) as urinary urgency, with or without urgency incontinence, usually with frequency and nocturia, in the absence of infection or other pathology [1]. With aging, the adaptive mechanisms that are able to adjust the functional bladder capacity to urine production become less evident. The bladder sensation and ability to empty the bladder seem to decrease with advancing age as a possible consequence of neuronal loss and remodeling of

E. Russo • A. Giannini • M. Caretto • P. Mannella • T. Simoncini (✉)
Division of Obstetrics and Gynecology, Department of Experimental and Clinical Medicine, University of Pisa, Pisa, PI, Italy
e-mail: tommaso.simoncini@med.unipi.it

M. Birkhaeuser, A.R. Genazzani (eds.), *Pre-Menopause, Menopause and Beyond*, ISGE Series, https://doi.org/10.1007/978-3-319-63540-8_25

the bladder and urethra [2]. In women suffering from lower urinary tract symptoms (LUTS), there is a persistent correlation between age and terminal detrusor overactivity and a reduction of the functional bladder capacity. These age related changes have also been detected at urodynamic testing [3]. From bladder structure point of view it seems that aging is associated with several changes in bladder properties. In bladders from OAB patients, an atypical pattern consisting of widened spaces between cells, reduction of intermediate cell junctions, increase of protrusion junctions and ultra close cell abutments was observed [4]. Some studies have showed the relationship between aging, oxidative stress, inflammation, and bladder dysfunctions [5, 6]. There is evidence that chronic bladder age related ischemia and oxidative stress in the elderly may be important factors contributing to the development of LUTS but the association between cardiovascular risk factors (such as diabetes mellitus, hypertension, nicotine use, and hyperlipidemia) and OAB has been studied only recently [2]. From this point of view therapeutic strategies such as improvement of LUT perfusion and control of oxidative stress may have beneficial effect.

25.3 Menopause, Estrogens, and Lower Urinary Tract

Most of the clinical manifestations of the bladder age-related changes become evident after menopause. The female genital and lower urinary tracts share a common embryological origin, arising from the urogenital sinus and both are sensitive to the effects of the female sex steroid hormones. Estrogen and progesterone receptors are present in the vagina, urethra, bladder, and pelvic floor musculature [7]. The genitourinary syndrome of menopause (GSM) is a new term that describes various menopausal symptoms and signs associated with physical changes of the vulva, vagina, and lower urinary tract. The GSM includes not only genital symptoms (dryness, burning, and irritation) and sexual symptoms (lack of lubrication, discomfort or pain, and impaired function), but also urinary symptoms (urgency, dysuria, and recurrent urinary tract infections [UTI]) [8]. Low levels of circulating estrogen after menopause result in physiologic, biologic, and clinical changes in the urogenital tissues. Urinary frequency and urgency are common midlife complaints; incontinence occurs in 15–35% of women over 60 years of age [9]. Recurrent UTI can affect postmenopausal women. This condition is attributable to impairment of bladder emptying with an increase in residual volume, to the presence of fecal and urinary incontinence and to the changes in vaginal flora, increased pH and change in the microbiome. These microbiological changes may be reversed with estrogen replacement following the menopause, offering a rationale for treatment and prophylaxis [10–12]. There is considerable evidence to support the use of systemic and local estrogen therapy in the management of lower urinary tract dysfunction. Particularly estrogen therapy is effective for the treatment of urge urinary incontinence, overactive bladder, and it can reduce the recurrence of urinary tract infections [13, 14]. There is evidence to show that estrogen deficiency may increase the risk of developing OAB following the menopause and estrogen replacement may lead to an improvement in physiological voiding function whilst reducing the risk of developing symptoms of overactive bladder [14]. The role of estrogens remains controversial as a beneficial effect on stress urinary incontinence. Estrogen therapy has been shown to lead to a reduction in total collagen concentration; this reduction in both quantity and strength of collagen may weaken bladder neck support and hence increase the risk of developing stress incontinence [15]. There is currently no role for systemic estrogen therapy in women with pure stress urinary incontinence [16].

25.4 Urinary Incontinence and Aging

According to the definition of the International Continence Society (ICS), UI "is the complaint of any involuntary leakage of urine." Urgency urinary incontinence is defined as involuntary leakage of urine, accompanied or immediately preceded by urgency. Stress urinary incontinence is the complaint of involuntary leakage on effort or exertion or sneezing or coughing. Mixed urinary incontinence encompasses overactive bladder syndrome and stress urinary incontinence. The complaint is of involuntary leakage associated with urgency and with exertion, effort, sneezing, or coughing [1]. Prevalence and severity of urinary incontinence increase with age.

- *Overactive bladder syndrome*

Overactive bladder syndrome is urinary urgency, with or without urgency incontinence, usually with increased daytime frequency and nocturia, if there is no proven infection or obvious pathology [1]. There is evidence to show that estrogen deficiency may increase the risk of developing OAB following the menopause [12]. The prevalence of overactive bladder syndrome increases with age (19.1% in women between 65 and 74 years of age) [17]. A wide range of treatments for OAB exists. According to the International Consultation on Incontinence (ICI) recommendations, initial management should start with conservative treatment modalities [18]. Behavior modification, which includes education about the disorder, lifestyle changes (such as avoiding caffeinated beverages, for example), as well as pelvic floor muscle training and bladder retraining, represent the first-line therapy options for this condition. Drug should be initiated after conservative methods have been tried and antimuscarinic drugs, combined with local estrogens, constitute first-line medical treatment in postmenopausal women with symptoms suggestive of an overactive bladder [16]. Antimuscarinic agents may be associated with adverse effects. The human bladder tissue, the brain, the salivary glands, the cardiovascular system, and the eye contain muscarinic receptors. As a result, antimuscarinic agents are effective in treating OAB symptoms, but they may also be associated with adverse effects such as dry mouth, constipation, cognitive impairment, tachycardia, and blurred vision. These side effects are not uncommon and may lead to failure of treatment due to people stopping the use of the drugs. The use of these medications is contraindicated in patients with narrow-angle glaucoma, urinary retention, or gastric retention. Newer generation drugs such as solifenacin and fesoterodine have been shown to be more efficacious than tolterodine [19]. A Beta-3 adrenergic agonist (Mirabegron) has been introduced as a means of medical management of overactive bladder syndrome. It is a safe, effective, and well-tolerated new class of drug. Mirabegron has a particular affinity for β3 adrenoceptors and improves the storage capacity of the bladder with little effect on the contractile ability of the bladder [20]. Mirabegron can improve the symptom in patients who had not adequate response to antimuscarinics and its tolerability profile offers potential to improve patients' adherence with treatment for OAB.

In case conservative management and medical treatment are not successful after 8–12 weeks, specialized management should be considered [18]. According to the American Urology Association and European Urology Association guidelines recommendations, OnabotulinumtoxinA intravesical injection and neuromodulation are considered the third-line treatments for patients without response to medical treatment [21]. OnabotulinumtoxinA is a neurotoxin that inhibits acetylcholine release from presynaptic neurons with decrease in acetylcholine availability in the neuromuscular junction and detrusor paralysis. The technique involves injection of onabotulinum-A in multiple sites throughout the bladder wall, avoiding injecting the trigone. This technique is being increasingly used to treat severe overactive bladder refractory to standard management both for neurogenic and idiopathic overactive bladder. The most frequent adverse effects following the administration of the toxin are urinary retention and urinary tract infection. The duration of effect of botulinum toxin type A may range from 3 to 12 months. Intravesical botulinum toxin appears to be an effective therapy for refractory OAB symptoms, but as yet little controlled trial data exist on benefits and safety compared with other interventions, or with placebo [22]. Sacral nerve stimulation can be used as an alternative to botulinum injections in patients who are dissatisfied or in whom such treatment with botulinum toxin-A treatment fails [17]. Sacral nerve stimulation follows a test phase with temporary electrodes placed next to the S3 sacral nerve root. If sufficient symptomatic improvement is given, the definitive electrode can be placed, with a subcutaneous stimulator. Incontinence episodes and voiding frequency are both reduced while receiving sacral nerve stimulation, with a significative improvement of quality of life [23]. Percutaneous tibial nerve stimulation (PTNS) is a form of peripheral neuromodulation. PTNS uses a removable device with a fine needle, penetrating the skin at the level of the posterior tibial nerve two fingers above the malleolus medialis of the ankle. The indication of proximity to the nerve is the observation for intrinsic foot muscle contraction. The stimulus is applied for half an hour. Treatment is repeated at weekly intervals. There is strong evidence for the efficacy of PTNS on frequency and urgency urinary incontinence and limited evidence for nocturia and urgency. Efficacy is comparable to that seen with antimuscarinics, but with fewer adverse effects.

Conclusion

Recent data point that several physiological and pathological modifications that frequently occur with aging, such us chronic bladder ischemia and oxidative stress, are closely related to the development of LUTS, particularly to OAB. Additionally, it is highlighted that the low levels of circulating estrogen after menopause are an important contributor to the development of structural changes associated with bladder overactivity and aging. Estrogen therapy is effective for the treatment of urge urinary incontinence, overactive bladder, and it can reduce the recurrence of urinary tract infections. Local estrogen therapy and behavior modification is a safe and effective first-line approach to lower urinary tract dysfunction in postmenopausal women. Drugs (antimuscarinic agents or beta-3 adrenergic agonist) should be initiated after conservative methods and should be combined with local estrogens. OnabotulinumtoxinA intravesical injection and neuromodulation are considered the third-line treatments, for patients without response or with contraindication to medical treatment.

References

1. Abrams P et al (2003) The standardisation of terminology in lower urinary tract function: report from the standardisation sub-committee of the International Continence Society. Urology 61(1):37–49
2. Andersson KE, Boedtkjer DB, Forman A (2017) The link between vascular dysfunction, bladder ischemia, and aging bladder dysfunction. Ther Adv Urol 9(1):11–27
3. Camoes J et al (2015) Lower urinary tract symptoms and aging: the impact of chronic bladder ischemia on overactive bladder syndrome. Urol Int 95(4):373–379
4. Elbadawi A, Yalla SV, Resnick NM (1993) Structural basis of geriatric voiding dysfunction. III. Detrusor overactivity. J Urol 150(5 Pt 2):1668–1680
5. Tyagi P et al (2014) Association of inflammaging (inflammation + aging) with higher prevalence of OAB in elderly population. Int Urol Nephrol 46(5):871–877
6. Ghoniem G et al (2011) Differential profile analysis of urinary cytokines in patients with overactive bladder. Int Urogynecol J 22(8):953–961
7. Gebhart JB et al (2001) Expression of estrogen receptor isoforms alpha and beta messenger RNA in vaginal tissue of premenopausal and postmenopausal women. Am J Obstet Gynecol 185(6):1325–1330. discussion 1330-1
8. Portman DJ, Gass ML (2014) Genitourinary syndrome of menopause: new terminology for vulvovaginal atrophy from the International Society for the Study of Women's sexual health and the North American Menopause Society. Climacteric 17(5):557–563
9. Iosif CS, Bekassy Z (1984) Prevalence of genito-urinary symptoms in the late menopause. Acta Obstet Gynecol Scand 63(3):257–260
10. Perrotta C et al (2008) Oestrogens for preventing recurrent urinary tract infection in postmenopausal women. Obstet Gynecol 112(3):689–690
11. Mac Bride MB, Rhodes DJ, Shuster LT (2010) Vulvovaginal atrophy. Mayo Clin Proc 85(1):87–94
12. Robinson D, Toozs-Hobson P, Cardozo L (2013) The effect of hormones on the lower urinary tract. Menopause Int 19(4):155–162
13. Nappi RE, Davis SR (2012) The use of hormone therapy for the maintenance of urogynecological and sexual health post WHI. Climacteric 15(3):267–274
14. Robinson D, Giarenis I, Cardozo L (2015) The management of urinary tract infections in octogenarian women. Maturitas 81(3):343–347
15. Robinson D, Cardozo L (2011) Estrogens and the lower urinary tract. Neurourol Urodyn 30(5):754–757
16. Baber RJ, Panay N, Fenton A (2016) 2016 IMS recommendations on women's midlife health and menopause hormone therapy. Climacteric 19(2):109–150
17. Wallace KM, Drake MJ (2015) Overactive bladder. F1000 Res 4:1406
18. Abrams P et al (2010) Fourth International consultation on incontinence recommendations of the International scientific committee: evaluation and treatment of urinary incontinence, pelvic organ prolapse, and fecal incontinence. Neurourol Urodyn 29(1):213–240

19. Madhuvrata P et al (2012) Which anticholinergic drug for overactive bladder symptoms in adults. Cochrane Database Syst Rev 1:Cd005429
20. Warren K, Burden H, Abrams P (2016) Mirabegron in overactive bladder patients: efficacy review and update on drug safety. Ther Adv Drug Saf 7(5):204–216
21. Gormley EA et al (2015) Diagnosis and treatment of overactive bladder (non-neurogenic) in adults: AUA/SUFU guideline amendment. J Urol 193(5):1572–1580
22. Duthie JB et al (2011) Botulinum toxin injections for adults with overactive bladder syndrome. Cochrane Database Syst Rev 12:Cd005493
23. Noblett K et al (2016) Results of a prospective, multicenter study evaluating quality of life, safety, and efficacy of sacral neuromodulation at twelve months in subjects with symptoms of overactive bladder. Neurourol Urodyn 35(2):246–251

When is Tubectomy and When Ovarectomy/Adnexectomy Indicated at Necessary Hysterectomies Beyond the Reproductive Age?

26

Liselotte Mettler

26.1 Tubectomy

Prophylactic bilateral salpingectomy (PBS) without ovariectomy has been proposed as a new preventive approach to reduce the risk of sporadic neoplasia [1, 2] in women at average risk of ovarian cancer [3], without exposing these patients to the adverse effects of iatrogenic premature menopause.

Even if opinions vary regarding short- and long-term outcomes of PBS [4], consistent preliminary data demonstrated its safety both in terms of ovarian reserve preservation and surgical complication [5, 6]; moreover, several authors have shown a significant reduction in OC risk among women with previous bilateral salpingectomy compared to tubal preservation [7, 8] or unilateral salpingectomy [8].

A 2011 position paper by the Society of Gynecologic Oncology of Canada [3] encouraged physicians to discuss the risks and benefits of PBS at the time of hysterectomy or tubal ligation with women at average risk for OC and this recommendation has been confirmed in 2015 by the American College of Obstetricians and Gynecologists [3].

The advantage of PBS has been estimated also in terms of cost-effectiveness. A recent analysis on PBS (elective salpingectomy at hysterectomy or instead of tubal ligation) showed that salpingectomy with hysterectomy for benign conditions will reduce ovarian cancer risk at acceptable cost and is a cost-effective alternative to tubal ligation for sterilization [9].

L. Mettler
Department of Obstetrics and Gynecology, University Hospitals of Schleswig-Holstein, Arnold-Heller-Str. 3/24, 24105 Kiel, Germany
e-mail: profmettler@gmx.de

M. Birkhaeuser, A.R. Genazzani (eds.), *Pre-Menopause, Menopause and Beyond*, ISGE Series, https://doi.org/10.1007/978-3-319-63540-8_26

26.1.1 Salpingectomy/Permanent Contraception

Surgical sterilization is the most used method worldwide involving 8.1% of the 15- to 49-year-old married women in developed countries, and 22.3% of women of reproductive age in less-developed countries [10].

Surgical sterilization is often achieved by resection (i.e., during a Cesarean section) or laparoscopic coagulation of the isthmic portion of the fallopian tube (FT). The remnant segment of the transected tube, however, frequently exhibits histological modifications that led to unsuccessful micro-reanastomotic procedures [11]; the most successful contraception, moreover, is recognized to be obtained by total salpingectomy [12].

For those of women (1–2%) who regret the previous decision for sterilization for any reason, it was demonstrated that the best method to obtain a pregnancy would be IVF [13], so that bilateral salpingectomy doesn't have any disadvantages in this population of women, while tubal preservation with subsequent tubal disease, definitively impair the implantation of transferred embryos [14].

Hysteroscopic sterilization was recently introduced as an attempt to provide a less invasive but similarly effective alternative to the abdominal approach. Current methodologies, unfortunately, have limitations that make the procedure less promising than expected [15].

Considering the new theory on ovarian cancer (OC) pathogenesis, even if also tubal ligation seems to reduce the risk of epithelial ovarian cancer (EOC) of 33% both in no-BRCA1 [16] and BRCA1 carriers [17, 18], recent data demonstrated that excisional tubal sterilization confers greater risk reduction (64%) than other methods [19], thus representing the more advisable sterilization procedure to be adopted in the clinical practice.

Bilateral salpingectomy, indeed, would offer to those women requesting for permanent contraception not only the absolute prevention of intrauterine pregnancies and the almost complete elimination of tubal pregnancies, but also protection against EOCs, further providing the chance to assess, along the years, the efficacy of this risk-reducing procedure [10]. With increasing reports on adnexal malignancies after the reproductive age the question whether to leave tubes and ovaries inside at hysterectomies became more and more important.

26.2 Single Center Study on Tubectomies and Partly Ovarectomies

Out of 1.014 laparoscopic hysterectomies performed between 2008 and 2015 at the Department of Obstetrics & Gynecology at the University in Kiel, Germany, 378 Subtotal (SLH) and Total Laparoscopic Hysterectomies (TLH), partially performed by conventional laparoscopic and partially by robotic assisted laparoscopic surgery resulted to be in females beyond the age of 50 years.

26.2.1 Methods

In 212 SLH and 166 TLH performed in females after the age of 50 years who were pre-menopausal or after the menopause all fallopian tubes were resected while only in 146 patients bilateral ovarectomy was performed.

26.2.2 Patients and Results

Neither intraoperatively nor in the consecutive 6 years any tubal or ovarian malignancy was detected at a retrospective evaluation of this patient collective.

26.2.3 Conclusions on Salpingectomies

While bilateral tubectomy at hysterectomy is an accepted fact to prevent adenocarcinomas of tubes and ovaries, the question of ovarectomies before the age of 65 is discussable. As ovaries also possess other function than estrogen and progesterone production their resection has to be considered individually in cases of normally looking ovaries. In our 232 patients were the ovaries remained at hysterectomy—all patients had no family history of cancer—in the whole observation period of 6 years no genital malignancies occurred.

Recently, the origin of "epithelial ovarian cancer" has been questioned. The ovary contains no epithelial cells and metaplasia of surface Müllerian cells to epithelial cells has been hypothesized to explain the types of epithelial ovarian cancer: serous, mucinous, and endometriod. The origin of epithelial ovarian cancer in the fallopian tubes is subjected at present to many studies and supports the resection of the fallopian tubes at hysterectomy as a required medical performance beyond the reproductive age.

The new proposed theory shifts the early events of carcinogenesis to the FT instead of the ovary [20], suggesting that types II tumors derive from the epithelium of the fallopian tube, whereas clear cell and endometrioid tumors derive from endometrial tissue that migrate to the ovary by retrograde menstruation [21]. These observations have been mainly collected from women carrying BRCA1/2 mutations and undergoing prophylactic salpingo-oophorectomy, in which most of the incidentally diagnosed in situ carcinomas or intraepithelial precursors of cancers (STIC) were detected not in the ovary but in the fimbrial end of the FT [22–24] (Fig 26.1).

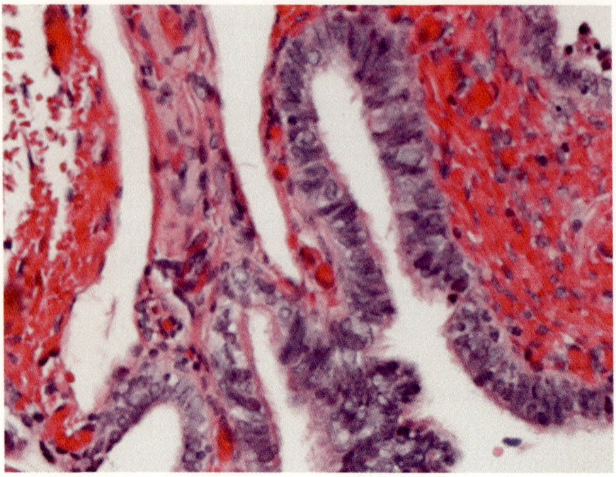

Fig. 26.1 Histologic view of a serous tubal intraepithelial cancer (STIC)

26.3 Ovariectomies/Adnexectomies

While together with ovariectomies both tubes are often also resected a tubectomy is a must with any indicated ovariectomy in nonmalignant cases.

In order to prevent the subsequent development of ovarian cancer prophylactic ovariectomy was first proposed in the 1970s. This proposal led to approximately 250,000 US females having normal ovaries removed at the time of hysterectomy for benign disease every year in the United States of America.

However, endocrine studies first performed in the 1970s and subsequently confirmed, showed that the ovaries continue to produce androgens which are converted to estrone throughout a woman's lifetime [25, 26].

In 2013, an analysis of the Nurses' Health Study cohort examined health outcomes after 28 years of follow-up for 16,873 (56.3%) women who had a hysterectomy with bilateral oophorectomy for benign disease and 13,113 (43.7%) women who had a hysterectomy with ovarian conservation [27]. Although oophorectomy was associated with a much lower mortality from ovarian cancer, less than 1% of the women with ovarian conservation died of ovarian cancer. In contrast, more women who had bilateral oophorectomy died from lung cancer (HR = 1.32), colorectal cancer (HR = 1.56), total cancers (HR = 1.18), and coronary heart disease (HR = 1.26) when compared with women who had ovarian conservation. Importantly, at no age was oophorectomy associated with an increased survival.

Studies from the Mayo Clinic had similar findings; women who had bilateral oophorectomy before age 45 had a 44% increased risk of cardiovascular mortality [28]. Rocca et al. showed higher risks of anxiety/depression, dementia/cognitive impairment, and Parkinsonism in women who had their ovaries removed [29]. In addition, after oophorectomy about 90% of premenopausal women will have vasomotor symptoms and many women will also experience mood changes, a decline in well-being, a decrease in sexual desire, sleep disturbances, and headaches [30, 31].

Additionally, vaginal dryness, painful intercourse, bladder dysfunction, and symptoms of depression may occur [32, 33].

In both the NHS and Mayo studies, these detrimental effects on health outcomes were not seen in women who took estrogen following oophorectomy. Therefore, some gynecologists have suggested that oophorectomy be performed at the time of hysterectomy for benign disease and these women be given prescriptions for menopausal hormone therapy and statins to ward off harmful cardiovascular effects. But studies show that within 5 years of a first prescription, only 17% of women continue to take estrogen and fewer than 18% are still taking statins [34].

Recently, the origin of "epithelial ovarian cancer" has been questioned. Interestingly, the ovary contains no epithelial cells and metaplasia of surface Müllerian cells to epithelial cells has been hypothesized to explain the types of epithelial ovarian cancer: serous, mucinous, and endometriod. With careful pathologic analysis of ovaries and tubes removed from BRCA positive women, precursor lesions called serous tubal intra-epithelial cancer (STIC) have been found in the fallopian tubes, but no such precursor lesions have been found in the ovary. STIC lesions have the same p53 mutations as found in high-grade serous "ovarian" cancers. The more indolent and treatable Stage I low grade cancers, found rarely inside the ovary do not have these p53 mutations. Astonishingly, the deadly form of ovarian cancer does not come from the ovary. Most aggressive "ovarian" cancers are, in fact, tubal cancers [21].

Bilateral salpingectomy has been proposed as an alternative to oophorectomy, as it removes the source of aggressive cancers but conserves functioning ovaries. Interestingly, a recent study found that women having hysterectomy and salpingectomy had similar sonographically measured antral follicle counts, mean ovarian diameters, and similar blood levels of AMH and FSH. Therefore, it appears that the ovaries function normally after salpingectomy.

26.4 Adnexal Torsion

In pre-menopausal women, detorsion of the adnexa even in apparently severely injured ovaries can be accomplished with good recovery of ovarian follicles and hormonal function. The not infrequent black–blue appearance of a torsed adnexa results from venous and lymphatic stasis, but some blood supply continues from the ovarian or uterine artery [35]. Some studies suggest that time from the onset of pain to de-torsion best predicts viability of the ovary. One study found evidence of necrosis on microscopy only after 48 hours following the onset of pelvic pain [36]. Eighteen young women, ages 23–35, undergoing in-vitro fertilization and ovarian stimulation, were studied with sonography following detorsion of the adnexa [37]. There was no difference in mean antral follicle counts when the detorsed ovary was compared with the contra-lateral ovary at 6 months following surgery.

Oophorectomy is indicated when the mass is considered suspicious for a neoplastic lesion. Criteria for suspicious lesions include a high initial morphology index, increasing size or complexity on serial sonography over a 6- to 12-week time period, or an elevated CA-125 in a postmenopausal woman.

It is well known that most ovarian tumors, even those with morphologic complexity, resolve over time. However, tumors that have an increase in MI over time should be considered for surgical exploration, oophorectomy, frozen section, and surgical staging if malignancy is found.

26.4.1 Association of Ovariectomy to Breast and Colon Cancer

Women with BRCA 1 have 40% risk of having ovarian cancer in their lifetime and BRCA 2 confers a 20% lifetime risk. Women with a BRCA 1 mutation have an increased risk of ovarian/tubal cancer as early as age 35, and 2–3% of these women will develop ovarian cancer by age 40. The risk of women with the BRCA2 mutation developing ovarian/tubal cancer occurs about one decade later [38]. Women with Lynch Syndrome, especially those with the MSH2 gene, have a lifetime risk of ovarian cancer of 33% and they also have a 40–60% risk of developing endometrial cancer.

In a BRCA positive woman, oophorectomy, or more correctly, adnexectomy, reduces the risks of ovarian/tubal cancer to less than 3%. Current recommendations suggest adnexectomy at the completion of child-bearing or: for BRCA 1, before age 35–40; for BRCA 2, before age 50; for Lynch Syndrome, adnexectomy and hysterectomy before age 40 [39].

26.4.2 Large Ovarian Masses, Endometriosis, and Oophorectomy

For women with severe, symptomatic endometriosis unresponsive to conservative management, bilateral oophorectomy concurrent with hysterectomy may decrease recurrent or persistent symptoms and the need for reoperation [40]. One study of women with symptomatic endometriosis compared outcomes between women who had a hysterectomy with ovarian conservation and women who had a hysterectomy with concurrent bilateral oophorectomy [41]. In the women who had ovarian conservation, 18/29 (62%) had recurrent pain and 9/29 (31%) required reoperation. In the group of women, who had both ovaries removed, 11/109 (10%) had recurrent pain and 4/109 (4%) required reoperation.

Another study of women with endometriosis found that of the 47 women who had a hysterectomy with ovarian conservation, 9 (19%) required further surgery over the 7 years of follow-up [42]. Of the 50 women who had a hysterectomy with bilateral oophorectomy, only 4 (8%) required reoperation. Preservation of both ovaries doubled the risk of reoperation regardless of the patient's age. Nevertheless, given the problems associated with early menopause, the authors recommended that for women younger than 40 years, hysterectomy with ovarian conservation should be considered. In patients with endometriosis and ovarian cysts (Fig. 26.2) partial ovarian resection or ovarectomy depends on symptoms as abdominal pain,

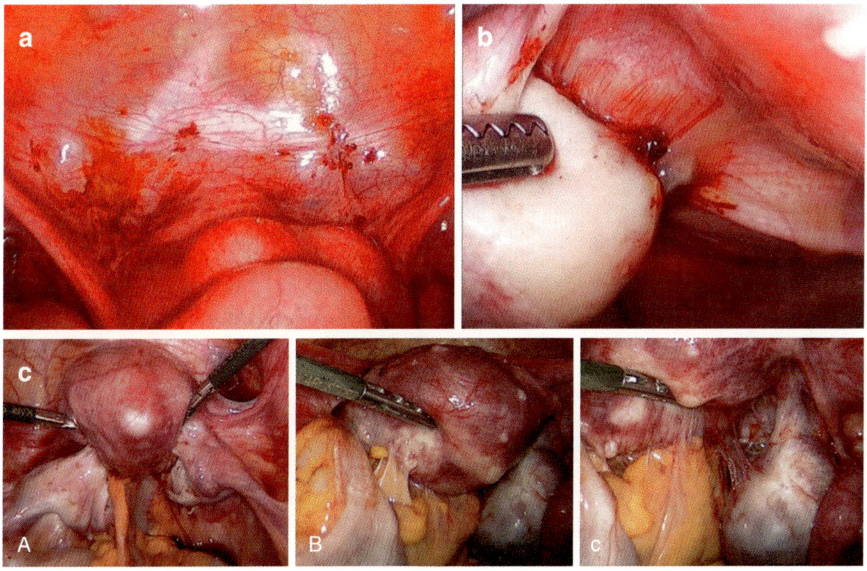

Fig. 26.2 Endoscopic image of endometriosis EEC stage I (**a**) EEC stage II (**b**) EEC stage III (**c**) *A*-frozen pelvis, *B*-right ovarian endometrioma, *C*-right ovarian endometrioma to be enucleated

dysmenorrhea, and dyspareunia as well as on the stage of endometriosis. Beyond the reproductive age an adnexectomy may be preferable.

Some women may be symptomatic from larger cysts, or they may not be comfortable with, or available for, close follow-up. For these women, surgery may be indicated. There is some evidence for removal of endometriomas, that ovarian function decreases after removal of cysts >4 cm when compared with cystectomy for cysts smaller than 4 cm [43]. However, a review of the literature found no studies showing loss of ovarian function related to the size of cyst removed. It may be prudent to conserve ovarian tissue even in large cysts clearly thought to be benign.

26.5 Summary

Tubectomy and ovarectomy at the time of hysterectomies are being reconsidered. While ovarectomy decreases definitely the long-term health outcome of females the ovarian conservation is advised till the age of 65 years. Adnexal torsion can usually treated better by detorsion than by adnexectomy. However, in cases of endometriosis ovarectomy does decrease necessary repeat surgeries.

Bilateral tubectomy should be performed in cases of hysterectomy at any age, carefully and not compromising the vascular supply of the ovaries. In addition, tubectomy definitely serves for permanent contraception. Living in the time of successful uterine transplantations even tubectomy might be reconsidered in a different way in the medical literature.

References

1. Parker WH, Broder MS, Chang E, Feskanich D, Farquhar C, Liu Z et al (2009 May) Ovarian conservation at the time of hysterectomy and long-term health outcomes in the nurses' health study. Obstet Gynecol 113(5):1027–1037
2. McAlpine JN, Hanley GE, Woo MM, Tone AA, Rozenberg N, Swenerton KD et al (2014) Opportunistic salpingectomy: uptake, risks, and complications of a regional initiative for ovarian cancer prevention. Am J Obstet Gynecol 210(5):471e1–471e11
3. Harris AL (2015) Salpingectomy and ovarian cancer prevention. Nurs Womens Health 19(6):543–549
4. Tone A, McAlpine J, Finlayson S, Gilks CB, Heywood M, Huntsman D et al (2012) It sounded like a good idea at the time. J Obstet Gynaecol Can 34(12):1127–1130
5. Morelli M, Venturella R, Mocciaro R, Di Cello A, Rania E, Lico D et al (2013) Prophylactic salpingectomy in premenopausal low-risk women for ovarian cancer: primum non nocere. Gynecol Oncol 129(3):448–451
6. Reade CJ, Finlayson S, McAlpine J, Tone AA, Fung-Kee-Fung M, Ferguson SE (2013) Risk-reducing salpingectomy in Canada: a survey of obstetrician-gynaecologists. J Obstet Gynaecol Can 35(7):627–634
7. Zhou B, Sun Q, Cong R, Gu H, Tang N, Yang L et al (2008) Hormone replacement therapy and ovarian cancer risk: a meta-analysis. Gynecol Oncol 108(3):641–651
8. Falconer H, Yin L, Gronberg H, Altman D (2015) Ovarian cancer risk after salpingectomy: a nationwide population-based study. J Natl Cancer Inst 107(2):dju410
9. Kwon JS, McAlpine JN, Hanley GE, Finlayson SJ, Cohen T, Miller DM et al (2015) Costs and benefits of opportunistic salpingectomy as an ovarian cancer prevention strategy. Obstet Gynecol 125(2):338–345
10. Dietl J, Wischhusen J, Hauslert SFM (2011) The post-reproductive fallopian tube: better removed? Hum Reprod 11:2918–2924
11. Stock RJ (1983) Histopathologic changes in fallopian tubes subsequent to sterilization procedures. Int J Gynecol Pathol 2(1):13–27
12. Bartz D, Greenberg JA (2008) Sterilization in the United States. Rev Obstet Gynecol 1(1):23–32
13. Boeckxstaens A, Devroey P, Collins J, Tournaye H (2007) Getting pregnant after tubal sterilization: surgical reversal or IVF? Hum Reprod 22(10):2660–2664
14. Cakmak H, Taylor HS (2011) Implantation failure: molecular mechanisms and clinical treatment. Hum Reprod Update 17(2):242–253
15. Creinin MD, Zite N (2014) Female tubal sterilization: the time has come to routinely consider removal. Obstet Gynecol 124(3):596–599
16. Cibula D, Widschwendter M, Majek O, Dusek L (2011) Tubal ligation and the risk of ovarian cancer: review and meta-analysis. Hum Reprod Update 17(1):55–67
17. Antoniou AC, Rookus M, Andrieu N, Brohet R, Chang-Claude J, Peock S et al (2009) Reproductive and hormonal factors, and ovarian cancer risk for BRCA1 and BRCA2 mutation carriers: results from the international BRCA1/2 carrier cohort study. Cancer Epidemiol Biomark Prev 18(2):601–610
18. Narod SA, Sun P, Ghadirian P, Lynch H, Isaacs C, Garber J et al (2001) Tubal ligation and risk of ovarian cancer in carriers of BRCA1 or BRCA2 mutations: a case-control study. Lancet 357(9267):1467–1470
19. Lessard-Anderson CR, Handlogten KS, Molitor RJ, Dowdy SC, Cliby WA, Weaver AL et al (2014) Effect of tubal sterilization technique on risk of serous epithelial ovarian and primary peritoneal carcinoma. Gynecol Oncol 135(3):423–427
20. Kurman RJ, Shih IM (2011) Molecular pathogenesis and extraovarian origin of epithelial ovarian cancer--shifting the paradigm. Hum Pathol 42(7):918–931
21. Kurman RJ, Shih IM (2010) The origin and pathogenesis of epithelial ovarian cancer: a proposed unifying theory. Am J Surg Pathol 34(3):433–443
22. Crum CP, Drapkin R, Kindelberger D, Medeiros F, Miron A, Lee Y (2007) Lessons from BRCA: the tubal fimbria emerges as an origin for pelvic serous cancer. Clin Med Res 5(1):35–44

23. Manchanda R, Abdelraheim A, Johnson M, Rosenthal AN, Benjamin E, Brunell C et al (2011) Outcome of risk-reducing salpingo-oophorectomy in BRCA carriers and women of unknown mutation status. BJOG 118(7):814–824
24. Powell CB, Chen LM, McLennan J, Crawford B, Zaloudek C, Rabban JT et al (2011) Risk-reducing salpingo-oophorectomy (RRSO) in BRCA mutation carriers: experience with a consecutive series of 111 patients using a standardized surgical-pathological protocol. Int J Gynecol Cancer 21(5):846–851
25. Judd HL, Judd GE, Lucas WE, Yen SS (1974) Endocrine function of the postmenopausal ovary: concentration of androgens and estrogens in ovarian and peripheral vein blood. J Clin Endocrinol Metab 39(6):1020–1024
26. Fogle RH, Stanczyk FZ, Zhang X, Paulson RJ (2007) Ovarian androgen production in postmenopausal women. J Clin Endocrinol Metab 92(8):3040–3043
27. Parker WH, Feskanich D, Broder MS, Chang E, Shoupe D, Farquhar CM et al (2013) Long-term mortality associated with oophorectomy compared with ovarian conservation in the nurses' health study. Obstet Gynecol 121(4):709–716
28. Rocca WA, Grossardt BR, de Andrade M, Malkasian GD, Melton LJ III (2006) Survival patterns after oophorectomy in premenopausal women: a population-based cohort study. Lancet Oncol 7(10):821–828
29. Rocca WA, Bower JH, Maraganore DM, Ahlskog JE, Grossardt BR, de Andrade M et al (2007) Increased risk of cognitive impairment or dementia in women who underwent oophorectomy before menopause. Neurology 69(11):1074–1083
30. Nathorst-Boos J, von Schoultz B, Carlstrom K (1993) Elective ovarian removal and estrogen replacement therapy--effects on sexual life, psychological well-being and androgen status. J Psychosom Obstet Gynaecol 14(4):283–293
31. Elit L, Esplen MJ, Butler K, Narod S (2001) Quality of life and psychosexual adjustment after prophylactic oophorectomy for a family history of ovarian cancer. Familial Cancer 1(3–4):149–156
32. Bachmann GA, Nevadunsky NS (2000) Diagnosis and treatment of atrophic vaginitis. Am Fam Physician 61(10):3090–3096
33. Shifren JL, Avis NE (2007) Surgical menopause: effects on psychological well-being and sexuality. Menopause 14(3 Pt 2):586–591
34. Buist DS, Newton KM, Miglioretti DL, Beverly K, Connelly MT, Andrade S et al (2004) Hormone therapy prescribing patterns in the United States. Obstet Gynecol 104(5 Pt 1):1042–1050
35. Oelsner G, Shashar D (2006) Adnexal torsion. Clin Obstet Gynecol 49(3):459–463
36. Chen M, Chen CD, Yang YS (2001) Torsion of the previously normal uterine adnexa. Evaluation of the correlation between the pathological changes and the clinical characteristics. Acta Obstet Gynecol Scand 80(1):58–61
37. Bozdag G, Demir B, Calis PT, Zengin D, Dilbaz B (2014) The impact of adnexal torsion on antral follicle count when compared with contralateral ovary. J Minim Invasive Gynecol 21(4):632–635
38. Boyd J, Sonoda Y, Federici MG, Bogomolniy F, Rhei E, Maresco DL et al (2000) Clinicopathologic features of BRCA-linked and sporadic ovarian cancer. JAMA 283(17):2260–2265
39. McCann GA, Eisenhauer EL (2015) Hereditary cancer syndromes with high risk of endometrial and ovarian cancer: surgical options for personalized care. J Surg Oncol 111(1):118–124
40. Vercellini P, Barbara G, Abbiati A, Somigliana E, Vigano P, Fedele L (2009) Repetitive surgery for recurrent symptomatic endometriosis: what to do? Eur J Obstet Gynecol Reprod Biol 146(1):15–21
41. Namnoum AB, Hickman TN, Goodman SB, Gehlbach DL, Rock JA (1995) Incidence of symptom recurrence after hysterectomy for endometriosis. Fertil Steril 64(5):898–902
42. Shakiba K, Bena JF, McGill KM, Minger J, Falcone T (2008) Surgical treatment of endometriosis: a 7-year follow-up on the requirement for further surgery. Obstet Gynecol 111(6):1285–1292
43. Tang Y, Chen SL, Chen X, He YX, Ye DS, Guo W et al (2013) Ovarian damage after laparoscopic endometrioma excision might be related to the size of cyst. Fertil Steril 100(2):464–469

Pelvic Floor Reconstructive Surgery in Ageing Women: Tailoring the Treatment to Each Woman's Needs

27

Marta Caretto, Andrea Giannini, Eleonora Russo, Paolo Mannella, and Tommaso Simoncini

27.1 Introduction

The pelvic floor is a functional unit involved in multiple functions that extend beyond the support of pelvic organs. Pelvic floor dysfunction globally affects micturition, defecation and sexual activity. Female pelvic organ prolapse (POP), sexual dysfunction, urinary incontinence (UI), chronic obstructive defecation syndrome (OFD), and constipation are just a few of the many facets of pelvic floor dysfunction, and their incidence increases dramatically with age and menopause. The pelvic floor in women is a complex and highly vulnerable structure. Injuries and functional modifications of this complex due to pregnancy, life events and aging often lead to pelvic organ prolapse. This anatomical and functional defect determines a variable association of complaints related to the urinary, genital and low intestinal tracts. Such symptoms are extremely common in aging individuals. They also often impair significantly quality of life. Pathophysiology of pelvic organ prolapse is unique in each patient, and its thorough understanding is key to successful treatment.

M. Caretto • A. Giannini • E. Russo • P. Mannella
Division of Obstetrics and Gynecology, Department of Experimental and Clinical Medicine, University of Pisa, Pisa, PI, Italy

T. Simoncini (✉)
Division of Obstetrics and Gynecology, Department of Experimental and Clinical Medicine, University of Pisa, Pisa, PI, Italy

Division of Obstetrics and Gynecology, Department of Clinical and Experimental Medicine, University of Pisa, Pisa, PI, Italy
e-mail: tommaso.simoncini@med.unipi.it

M. Birkhaeuser, A.R. Genazzani (eds.), *Pre-Menopause, Menopause and Beyond*, ISGE Series, https://doi.org/10.1007/978-3-319-63540-8_27

27.2 Function and Dysfunction of the Pelvic Floor

Pelvic floor laxity depends on muscle injury and progressive pelvic floor weakening. These result from connective tissue degradation [1], pelvic denervation [2] and devascularization and anatomic modifications [3], all determining a decline in mechanical strength and dyssynergic pelvic floor function, predisposing to prolapse [4]. Pelvic floor consists of several muscles, all fundamental for the support and function of female pelvic structures. The levator ani constitutes the floor of the pelvis; it is composed of three different parts: the pubo-coccygeus, pubo-rectalis and ileo-coccygeus muscles. The pubo-coccygeus is the main part of the levator ani and it extends from the pubis toward the coccyx. The two parts (right and left) of the pubo-rectalis, behind the ano-rectal junction, arrange a muscular sling. The ileo-coccygeus is the smallest part of the levator ani. In women with normal pelvic statics, smooth muscle fibers in the anterior vaginal wall are organized in tight bundles orientated in circular and longitudinal order. In comparison, in women with POP the vaginal muscularis presents a decline of overall smooth muscle amount, fewer, smaller and disorganized bundles [5]. Levator ani injury has an established role in the pathophysiology of prolapse but does not explain all pelvic organ prolapses. Thirty percentage of women with prolapse show no sign of muscle injury on magnetic resonance imaging, underlining the fact that the disease process involves other factors as well. In this chain of events, failure of one of the functional and structural elements of the pelvic floor complex, e.g. the levator ani, results in increased mechanical load on other components (connective tissue and smooth muscle), which will eventually fail, as well [6]. On the other side, connective tissue abnormalities and smooth muscle alterations may represent the leading event in the development of prolapse [7]. Pelvic connective tissues are structured into a fascial sheet which covers the pelvic floor muscles and forms ligaments, connecting pelvic organs to the bony pelvis [8]. During evolution human female pelvis has undergone significant enlargement and architectural changes to allow for delivery of fetuses with increasing head diameters and upright standing and walking. Thus, connections of fascial structures to the pelvic sidewalls have progressively grown, suggesting a central role in the stabilization of the pelvic viscera of connective tissue [9]. Qualitative and quantitative alterations in collagen content and structure and in genes related to collagen remodeling in women with genital prolapse and stress urinary incontinence have been identified, which may represent individual predisposing factors for these conditions [10]. The vascular network has an important role in the pelvic floor, as well, and particularly for urinary continence [11].

27.3 Menopause and Aging: Impact on POP and UI

The lower urinary and female genital tracts are strictly related and both derive embryologically from the urogenital sinus. Half of postmenopausal women report urogenital symptoms [12]; these generally appear soon after the menopausal transition and worsen with time. Most of these symptoms such as dyspareunia, dysuria, frequency, nocturia, incontinence, and recurrent infections [13] are facilitated by declining levels of estrogens. Estrogen receptors (ER) are present in the epithelial tissues of the bladder, trigone, urethra, vaginal mucosa, and in the support structures of the utero-sacral ligaments, as well as in levator ani muscles and pubo-cervical fascia. Progesterone receptors are also expressed in the lower urinary tract, even if with less density than estrogen receptors. There is evidence that progesterone has adverse effects on female urinary tract function [14], since it is linked to an increase in the adrenergic tone, provoking a decreased tone in the ureters, bladder, and urethra. This may explain why urinary symptoms worsen during the secretory phase of the menstrual cycle, and progesterone may be responsible for the increase in urgency during pregnancy, although the precise mechanism is not fully figured out. The role of menopause on pelvic floor dysfunction is unclear. Nor menopausal status [15] nor the length of hormone deficiency [16] has been associated with the risk or severity of POP. In spite of the evidence indicating generally positive effects of estrogens on the urogenital tract, and the biological rationale supporting the potential to strengthen or preserve the pelvic fascial and muscle system, there is no evidence supporting the use of estrogen therapy for the prevention or treatment of POP or UI in climacteric women [17]. In particular, available evidence does not show a beneficial effect of the use of estrogen therapy, both local and systemic, on stress urinary incontinence. On the other hand, recent studies underline that local estrogen therapy is effective for the treatment of urge urinary incontinence, overactive bladder and it can reduce the recurrence of urinary tract infections. In women with overactive bladder symptoms, neuromodulatory effects of estrogens could be beneficial, as estradiol reduces the amplitude and frequency of spontaneous detrusor muscle contractions [18].

27.4 Aging and Constipation

Aging can induce changes in the structure and function of the gastrointestinal tract, especially in the colon and in the ano-rectal region, which can impair bowel habits and evacuation mechanisms. Aging is associated with loss of neurons in both the myenteric and submucosal plexus (cholinergic neurons and interstitial cells of Cajal). In agreement, initial observations suggested that delayed colon transit time may occur with aging. However, more recent publications point out that in healthy elder individuals, in the absence of comorbidities, there is no significant change in gut transit time [19]. However prolonged colonic transit time reported in small groups of elderly patients could be due to an increased absorption of water, which may lead to the production of harder stools, as well as difficulty in evacuation. Adequate perception of rectal, anal, and perianal region is of paramount importance in order to have a normal defecation. However, within aging, there could be a reduced rectal sensation and an increased rectal compliance: these alterations require larger stool volumes to induce the classical "call to stool," with a consequent difficult defecation, possibly of small feces. Thus, elderly people may need to have larger volumes of bowel content to stimulate rectal sensation and promote a normal defecation. Changes in the anatomy of the anal canal, internal anal sphincter degeneration and external anal sphincter atrophy have been associated with aging as much as tissue atrophy resulting in reduced distensibility. These observations, taken together, could further explain the reason why aging predisposes to alterations of the pelvic floor. Moreover, a pudendal nerve injury can also play a role in the onset of constipation (e.g., obstructed defecation) in the elderly, particularly in women, leading to an abnormal perineal descent and causing a prolapse of the anal canal or of the anterior rectal mucosa with a consequent alteration of rectal emptying [20]. A recent study [21] seems to confirm this concept. In a group of 334 women with obstructed defecation, after eliminating the confounding effect of vaginal delivery from the risk factors, the authors find that rectocele, intussusception, rectocele associated with intussusception, rectocele associated with mucosal prolapse, and grade III enterocele/sigmoidocele increase with age. Conversely, in women aged <50 years paradoxical contraction or lack of relaxation of the pelvic floor muscles seem to be the most frequent causes of obstructed defecation.

27.5 Personalizing Pelvic Floor Reconstructive Surgery in Aging Women

Urinary incontinence and pelvic organ prolapse have been considered for a long time a necessary compound of aging and their consequences have been accepted in spite of the enormous impact on quality of life. The use of aids such as diapers, sleepers for the night and pessaries has become widespread in elder women, and this has brought along significant direct costs to patients and to those health services covering for these tools. Access to surgical treatment has been traditionally limited in ageing women with pelvic floor dysfunction. Concurrence of chronic systemic diseases has often been a discouraging factor to candidate these women for surgery.

Tailoring surgical strategies is one of the most engaging parts of pelvic floor reconstruction. Surgery can be adapted to accomplish goals that can be very different based on the age and functional status of the patient. Reconstruction of a failed pelvic floor can be obtained through re-creation of an anatomical support that resembles as much as possible the original. But it can also be achieved through an attempt to solve specific complaints, even without correcting completely anatomy. This is often the case in elderly individuals, where a multitude of factors affect the final result of any reconstructive surgery. This is due to the possibility that aging-associated changes in the function of the bladder or of the rectum may be unveiled or decompensated by an untailored reconstruction. Thus a thorough understanding of the underlining functional status of pelvic organs is much more important in aging women than in younger ones before proceeding to surgery.

A simple evaluation of bladder function both during filling and during voiding is a critical step for pre-surgical assessment [22]. Urodynamic signs of overactive bladder are frequently found in aging individuals, even in the absence of clinical symptoms. This condition is more frequent in elder women because of multiple causes, often difficult to detect and to correct [23]. Atrophy of the uro-genital mucosae often increases the sensitivity of the bladder wall to filling and to bacterial contamination, enhancing muscarinic activity within the bladder. According to the integral theory of Papa Petros [24], intermediate or advanced prolapse of the bladder may per se induce bladder hyperactivity because of the stretching of the nerve fibers endowed in the elongated utero-sacral ligaments.

A correct understanding of the functional ability to empty the bladder is also key to surgical planning. Advanced bladder prolapse is frequently associated with clinical urinary outlet obstruction, with difficult and incomplete voiding. Post-void residual urine volume is directly linked to vesico-urethral reflux and to recurrent urinary infections. These are dangerous per se, but also represent the most common cause of urinary urgency. On the other side, bladder outlet obstruction due to advanced cystocele can mask a latent stress urinary incontinence that will develop upon surgical anatomic correction. Understanding these variables is important to provide correct information to patients, in addition to providing an adequate surgical plan.

An extremely important diagnostic item before considering any pelvic floor reconstructive treatment in an elderly individual is to identify the presence of a hypotonic bladder. This condition is common in this age range due to bladder muscle atrophy and to altered nerve control. It is not unusual that a woman with a partially denervated bladder presents with a leading symptom of urinary incontinence due to bladder sphincter insufficiency. If a concomitant bladder muscle weakness is not recognized the performance of anti-incontinence procedures such as retro-pubic or trans-obturator slings may solve incontinence, while creating obstruction. This may require later removal of the mesh but in frail women may eventually lead to irreversible bladder over-distension requiring self-catheterization for the rest of life [25].

Thus, urodynamic evaluation is particularly important in the pre-operative workup of aging women with pelvic floor dysfunction [26]. A cystometric test and a urinary flowmetry can provide valuable elements to tailor reconstructive surgery and to enhance its outcomes with appropriate medical treatments.

Vaginal atrophy is frequent in aging women. Besides being bothersome, it also carries a higher risk of complications for pelvic floor reconstruction, particularly when trans-vaginal prostheses are needed. Risk of mesh erosion is higher in the presence of vaginal atrophy, and shrinkage of the prosthetic material can lead to intractable dyspareunia in women with an atrophic vagina. Pelvic floor surgeons frequently use pre- and post-operative administration of local estrogen preparations to overcome such problems, but compliance is low, often for the difficulty to insert cream applicators or suppositories in the presence of prolapse or after surgery.

Another key point to correctly tailor reconstructive surgery is the assessment of rectal and anal sphincter function. A frequent mistake is to overlook bowel function in those patients that are surgically treated for anterior prolapse [27]. Constipation and obstructed defecation are very common in older people [28] and many drugs that are commonly used in this age range significantly worsen bowel function. It is also known that chronic constipation reduces the chances of success of surgical treatment, particularly in patients using drugs affecting bowel function. Altered defecation dynamics and slow intestinal transit are associated with steady increases in abdominal pressure. Strained or lengthy defecation represents a common reason for surgical failure, due to the progressive tearing of the reconstruction. In such instances, education of the patient to correct eating and drinking habits, and possibly the introduction of pharmacologic strategies to correct obstructed defecation, are mandatory [25].

On the opposite, some surgical procedures can lead to difficult or painful defecation. This is particularly common after suspension of the cervix or the vaginal cuff to the sacro-spinous ligaments with sutures or with meshes, because the suspended district pushes the rectum backwards to the sacrum. Some surgeons to reinforce fascial rectopexy use plication of the levator ani muscle. This procedure often determines painful intercourse and evacuation. The most troublesome condition is however when surgical reconstruction of a failed pelvic floor is performed in women with a deficient anal sphincter apparatus. These are patients that often present with impacted defecation, either because of a prominent rectocele that harbors the feces making expulsion difficult, or due to an obstructive enterocele squeezing the rectal ampule backwards. Such patients can be in a tight equilibrium, where the sphincter deficit compensates somewhat for the difficulty in defecation. However, if an effective correction of the obstructive component is achieved, these patients are more likely to develop gas or fecal incontinence, which is extremely invalidating and difficult to treat. A thorough understanding of fecal function through clinical assessment or appropriate diagnostic tools is thus important to provide correct information to patients on the possible risks of surgery and to tailor reconstruction.

The complex aspects of pelvic floor dysfunction should be addressed by physicians with a broader expertise that crosses disciplines, or in the context of multidisciplinary centers where urologists, gynecologists, and colo-rectal surgeons can interact to manage complex patients and to best cope with the multi-faceted aspects of pelvic floor dysfunction.

27.6 Tailoring Surgery for Urinary Incontinence in Elderly Individuals

Given the high incidence of urinary incontinence in the elderly population, much has been done in the recent years to develop adapted pelvic floor muscle training programs [29], more tolerable medical therapies [30] and less invasive and more effective targeted surgical approaches. Elder individuals should not be denied appropriate access to anti-incontinence surgery. Indeed, even at older ages, nonsurgical interventions are effective, but surgery is superior in terms of subjective and objective long-term success.

Table 27.1 Surgical strategies to correct urinary incontinence

Procedure	Indication
Sub-urethral slings	Stress urinary incontinence associated with urethral hypermobility
Retropubic tension-free vaginal tape (TVT)	SUI with ISD
Trans-obturator tape (TOT)	SUI
Tension-free vaginal tape—obturator (TVT-O)	SUI
Minislings	SUI
Bulking agents	Stress urinary incontinence with ISD or fixed urethra
Bulking agents	SUI with SUI or fixed urethra
Trans-abdominal procedures	Contraindications to slings
Retropubic colposuspension	SUI with ISD

The three main categories of anti-incontinence surgical procedures [31] are: (1) mid-urethral slings (2) urethral bulking agents, and (3) trans-abdominal retropubic urethropexies (Table 27.1).

Mid-urethral slings are the gold standard to treat stress urinary incontinence associated with urethral hypermobility. The rationale of these procedures stays in the restoration of a suburethral support that limits the movement of the mid-urethra during abdominal strain.

Different types of sub-urethral slings have been developed in the past 20 years, with the aim to obtain safer insertion. This has now led to an array of procedures that are also associated with slightly different functional effects, thereby permitting patient tailoring.

Retropubic placement of a sub-urethral sling (Tension-free Vaginal Tape—TVT) represents the first technique described. This procedure has high cure rates that have been shown to last up to 18 years after insertion. Due to the peculiar position of the sling, it also provides the best cure rate for women with urethral intrinsic sphincter deficiency. However, this technique is not devoid of risks, including, most importantly, bladder perforation, and de novo urge incontinence [32].

Trans-obturator placement of a sub-urethral sling (Trans-Obturator Tape—TOT) has been developed to avoid these complications and is nowadays considered by most urogynecologists a significant advancement over TVT in terms of intra-operatory risks. However, with this procedure the tape is left within the thigh abductor muscles and can occasionally retract the posterior branch of the obturator nerve resulting in a rare but troublesome development of groin and upper thigh pain. Thus caution should be taken when using this type of mesh in younger patients or in women that are active in sport, since pain may be more pronounced with increased muscle exercise.

Groin pain associated with TOT has pushed the development of devices that minimize placement of mesh through the obturator and adductor muscles, leading to the development of shorter meshes that are still inserted with the aid of trans-obturator needles, the so-called TVT Obturator (TVT-O), with the mesh entering the internal obturator fascia to a minimal extent [33]. Further evolution of this quest for minimizing the amount of mesh placement has led to the development of the so-called "minislings," or much shorter sub-urethral slings that present anchors allowing to fix them at the internal obturator fascia without penetrating the obturator muscle. These devices allow minimal surgical dissection, thereby making it possible their use in an ambulatory setting, and are not associated with pain. However, their long-term effectiveness needs to be demonstrated.

Currently, there is no data supporting the superiority of one of these procedures over the others in ageing women. Mastering all types of sub-urethral sling placement techniques is particularly important in the management of elder individuals, where the presence of intrinsic sphincter deficiency (ISD) and overactive bladder (OAB) are common. For instance, a TVT may be the best choice in a patient with ISD, while it could be the worst in the presence of OAB, where a TOT or a TVT-O may be preferred. Elder individuals may be better candidates for minislings, so to minimize surgical risks and hospital stay, since long-term efficacy may be less of a worry.

Bulking agents have been specifically developed for the treatment of elder women [34]. These agents are represented by a variety of non-resorbable or very-slowly resorbable dense preparations that can be injected in the peri-urethral space or under the urethral mucosa, at the level of the bladder neck. They result in the formation of a thickening of the urethral sphincter and in increased resistance to urine passage during abdominal stress. Placement of a bulking agent is a rather non-invasive procedure, since it can be administered on an outpatient basis. Plus, it is effective to address ISD and this is useful in elder women. However, the high costs and the limited duration of therapeutic success, which is about 8–12 months, significantly limit their widespread use. These agents are therefore often considered as the elective choice for those patients that, due to advanced age or co-morbidity, are best treated with a non-surgical procedure, so to avoid anesthesia.

Last, trans-abdominal retropubic urethral suspension procedures, such as the Burch or Marshall-Marchetti-Krantz procedures, can still be performed in selected cases. This is nowadays more acceptable than in the past, due to the standardization of these procedures through the use of mini-invasive techniques. The long-term cure rate for incontinence of retropubic suspension is lower than that of sub-urethral slings. Plus, these techniques provide a less reproducible elevation of the bladder neck, with the risk of over-correction with urinary outlet obstruction and de novo urgency. This is why most pelvic floor surgeons still prefer to insert a sub-urethral sling even when for other reasons a trans-abdominal procedure needs to be performed. However, with the widespread use of slings by non-expert surgeons, it becomes more frequent to see recurrent incontinence in women treated with more than one sling. In these patients a further trans-vaginal approach can be difficult and more likely to fail. In such conditions a retro-pubic approach remains a valid alternative and should be available at least in third-level centers [25].

27.7 Tailoring Surgery for Pelvic Organ Prolapse in Ageing Individuals

Pelvic organ prolapse (POP) is a common condition with an estimated incidence of up to 40% of women. The prevalence of POP is growing in Western countries due to increased life expectancy. In total, 30% of women aged 50–89 years require a consultation for pelvic floor dysfunction and the life-time risk of surgical repair is estimated at 11%, with almost one-third of the patients requiring repeat surgery.

A number of different surgical strategies to correct pelvic organ prolapse exist (Table 27.2). This field of surgery is nowadays undergoing a major technical and philosophical evolution.

The traditional approach used by urogynecologists to restore pelvic organ anatomy has been through the transvaginal route. Nearly 100 different techniques through the past 150 years have been described to repair POP trans-vaginally. The anatomical landmark and the surgical technique to perform trans-vaginal surgery are different compared with trans-abdominal procedures [35]. Trans-abdominal surgery to treat POP has not been widespread before the laparoscopic era, due to its invasiveness. Therefore most urogynecologists still hold to the cultural heritage of the trans-vaginal approach. However, the new generation of laparoscopic surgeons has recently pushed the number of abdominal procedures, showing that miniinvasive trans-abdominal POP correction is feasible and as effective as the traditional laparotomic technique.

Table 27.2 Surgical strategies to correct pelvic organ prolapse

Apical defect	Anterior defect	Posterior defect	Any prolapse
Trans-abdominal procedures			
Sacral colpo/cervicopexy	Abdominal paravaginal repair	Ventral rectopexy	
Abdominal lateral suspension			
Trans-vaginal/transrectal/transperineal procedures			
Iliococcygeus fascia fixation	Anterior colporraphy	Stapled transanal rectal resection (STARR) transtar	Colpocleisis
Levator myorrhaphy with apical fixation	Midline plication	Delorme procedure	
Mayo culdoplasty	Lahodny's procedure	Altemeier's procedure	
Utero-sacral ligament suspension	Vaginal paravaginal repair	Posterior colporraphy	
Sacrospinous ligament suspension	Anterior site-specific repair	Nichols' procedure	
		Richardson's procedure	
		Posterior site-specific repair	

When approaching an aging woman with pelvic organ prolapse, the three main alternative surgical strategies are fascial reconstruction of the defect, use of transvaginal augmentation or suspension with meshes, or abdominal suspension with meshes. In all cases total or supracervical hysterectomy can help achieve successful reconstruction, but its role is debated. The goals of any pelvic floor reconstructive surgery should be to achieve a durable result with the least invasive approach and a low rate of complications.

Fascial reconstructive techniques are performed transvaginally, and they are adequate to address intermediate prolapses, particularly if no or little apical descent is present. However, they fail to ensure a durable result in the presence of more advanced prolapses, with rates of recurrence that exceed 50% in most series in the mid-term. A specific challenge with this approach is the difficulty to ensure a stable apical attachment to the apical compartment and the need to remove the uterus to make this step more achievable. On the other side, fascial procedures are extremely safe and the least invasive approach, allowing for loco-regional anesthesia and for prompt return to normal activities. In the attempt to achieve more solid reconstruction while maintaining the advantages of vaginal surgery, mesh augmentation techniques have become popular. A number of shapes and materials have been developed, and kits have been designed by the industry to allow for more effective and easy application. Nowadays most kits allow for combined correction of anterior or posterior defects, combined with apical suspension. These devices have been developed to allow for uterine-sparing surgery and to overcome the surgical challenge of apical suspension with traditional fascial techniques. While being effective, these meshes have reached the news due to the incidence of complications, mostly due to erosion of the organs around the mesh, or to shrinkage or migration of the mesh. Such complications are often associated with bleeding, infections, pain, and troublesome intercourse, therefore requiring surgery for mesh removal. The use of "lighter" materials and a more careful selection of the correct candidates for this surgery have in part overcome these problems, yet it is more and more appreciated how placement of these meshes should be performed only by experienced surgeons.

Aging women may specifically benefit from the more solid restoration of anatomy combined with the remarkably little invasiveness of these procedures. Aging per se may also make less relevant possible complications that may turn into reduced caliber of the vagina, which may instead be a strong disincentive for younger, sexually active, women. However, the high prevalence of urogenital atrophy and of conditions that facilitate mesh infection, such as type 2 diabetes mellitus, sometimes warrants against the use of meshes in elderly individuals.

The last Cochrane revision on pelvic floor reconstructive surgery published in 2013 [35] outlines how abdominal procedures (sacral colpo/cervicopexy) have superior outcomes in terms of anatomic and subjective and objective cure rates when compared to vaginal procedures, including trans-vaginal sacro-spinous ligament suspension, utero-sacral ligament suspension and transvaginal meshes, particularly in elder women. As previously said, more widespread availability of skills in laparoscopic pelvic floor reconstruction has led to a revival of this excellent surgical technique. However, sacral colpopexy is a highly challenging procedure, requiring extensive dissections deep in the pelvis, the position of a high number of sutures, often in areas where triangulation of laparoscopic instruments is not effective.

Furthermore, the sacrum is a dangerous area, where potentially life-threatening bleeding complications may ensue. These issues still limit the performance of sacral colpopexy only to a handful of experienced surgeons, therefore limiting patient access to this procedure. If available, sacral colpo/cervicopexy is an excellent procedure for aging individuals. Indeed, notwithstanding the long operating time, if performed with mini-invasive surgery it is not a painful procedure and return to daily activities is as speedy as with vaginal procedures.

Similar to anti-incontinence surgery, there is no specific guideline supporting one type of POP repair vs. the others. Experience of each surgeon is an important factor influencing the choice of the technique. Based on available evidence, in the presence of an advanced apical defect or with recurrent POP an abdominal approach is the best option for an elder woman, so to limit the risk of complications and of further surgeries due to failures. A fascial vaginal approach is warranted because of its low morbidity in those patients with intermediate bladder or rectal prolapse. Mesh augmentation should be limited to selected patients where the risk/benefit ratio may be particularly favorable [35].

27.8 Future Trends in Pelvic Floor Surgery in Aging Women

Robotic surgery is the new emerging trend in many areas of medicine. Although this emerging technique is still in its infancy, it already offers tangible advantages over traditional laparoscopy. Enhanced vision and precision in instrument movement make it easier to perform difficult dissections. The 7 degrees of freedom in the movement of the instrument tips allow for gentle grasping of tissues and for the placement of precise and effective intracorporeal sutures. These advantages are exploited at their maximum in pelvic floor reconstructive surgery, where the dissection of the vescico-vaginal septum and of the recto-vaginal septum can be particularly complex. Better identification of the pre-sacral ligament and precision in managing the pre-sacral vessels also comes handy with robotic assistance.

Finally, the placement of stitches in narrow areas is much more precise and effective using robotic instruments. For these reasons, the potential advantages of robotic assistance for pelvic floor reconstruction have been explored. Robotic surgeons fiercely support the idea that the technical advantages of robotics do not simply make this complex surgery easier, but that it mostly improve its execution, thus possibly leading to better pelvic floor reconstruction [36]. Whether this is true or not is yet to be shown by appropriate trials. It is also likely that the ongoing evolution of the robotic platform, and the emergence of other types of medical robots will lead to even less invasive surgery and to a reduction in costs, thus making this surgery the best option available to treat complex and advanced POP in aging individuals.

An additional trend is the ongoing implementation of newer surgical strategies to better exploit the abdominal access for pelvic floor reconstruction. While so far the only standardized abdominal procedure for POP has been sacral colpopexy, new techniques are emerging. Ventral rectopexy [37] has been developed by colo-rectal surgeons to treat rectal prolapse and obstructed defecation syndrome, and shares a number of features with sacral colpopexy, including the anchoring of a biocompatible mesh to the sacral promontory.

Alternative strategies to suspend the apical compartment that avoid the risks of sacral fixation are also gaining momentum. Lateral mesh suspension of the apex to the abdominal wall has been described, with seemingly effective results [38]. Such new approaches will soon broaden the surgical armamentarium needed to tailor pelvic floor reconstruction.

Conclusions

Tailoring reconstructive surgery for incontinence or POP is particularly important in aging women. Thorough assessment of the functional status of the patient and of the pelvic organs is more important than in younger patients for decision-making regarding surgery. Careful discussion of the benefits and risks of every available procedure is of paramount importance, as much as a correct explanation of the expected functional results of surgery. This vibrant area of surgery is steadily evolving with the introduction of newer techniques and with technological advancements such safer prosthetic materials, anatomically designed mesh augmentation kits or the new robotic approach. The expected increase in prevalence of pelvic floor dysfunction as Western populations age more calls for more research in this area, so to offer to aging women better and more tailored solutions for their complaints, and to provide them with significant improvements in quality of life.

References

1. Soderberg MW, Johansson B, Masironi B, Bystrom B, Falconer C, Sahlin L et al (2007) Pelvic floor sex steroid hormone receptors, distribution and expression in pre- and postmenopausal stress urinary incontinent women. Acta Obstet Gynecol Scand 86(11):1377–1384
2. Dietz HP, Tekle H, Williams G (2012) Pelvic floor structure and function in womenwith vesicovaginal fistula. J Urol 188(5):1772–1777
3. Goepel C (2008) Differential elastin and tenascin immunolabeling in the uterosacralligaments in postmenopausal women with and without pelvic organ prolapse. Acta Histochem 110(3):204–209
4. Fitzpatrick CC, Elkins TE, DeLancey JO (1996) The surgical anatomy of needle bladderneck suspension. Obstet Gynecol 87(1):44–49
5. Badiou W, Granier G, Bousquet PJ, Monrozies X, Mares P, de Tayrac R (2008) Comparative histological analysis of anterior vaginal wall in women with pelvicorgan prolapse or control subjects. A pilot study. Int Urogynecol J Pelvic Floor Dysfunct 19(5):723–729
6. Chen BH, Wen Y, Li H, Polan ML (2002) Collagen metabolism and turnover in womenwith stress urinary incontinence and pelvic prolapse. Int Urogynecol J Pelvic Floor Dysfunct 13(2):80–87
7. DeLancey JO, Morgan DM, Fenner DE, Kearney R, Guire K, Miller JM et al (2007) Comparison of levator ani muscle defects and function in women with andwithout pelvic organ prolapse. Obstet Gynecol 109(2 (Pt 1)):295–302

8. De Blok S (1982) The connective tissue of the adult female pelvic region. A dissectionalanalysis. Acta Morphol Neerl Scand 20(2):191–212
9. Pinkerton JH (1973) Some aspects of the evolution and comparative anatomy ofthe human pelvis. J Obstet Gynaecol Br Common 80(2):97–102
10. Jackson SR, Avery NC, Tarlton JF, Eckford SD, Abrams P, Bailey AJ (1996) Changes in metabolism of collagen in genitourinary prolapse. Lancet 347(9016):1658–1661
11. Enhorning GE (1976) A concept of urinary continence. Urol Int 31(1/2):3–5
12. Bruce D, Rymer J (2009) Symptoms of the menopause. Best Pract Res Clin Obstet Gynaecol 23(1):25–32
13. Bygdeman M, Swahn ML (1996) Replens versus dienoestrol cream in the symp-tomatic treatment of vaginal atrophy in postmenopausal women. Maturitas 23(3):259–263
14. Hextall A, Bidmead J, Cardozo L, Hooper R (2001) The impact of the menstrualcycle on urinary symptoms and the results of urodynamic investigation. BJOG 108(11):1193–1196
15. Lawrence JM, Lukacz ES, Nager CW, Hsu JW, Luber KM (2008) Prevalence and co-occurrence of pelvic floor disorders in community-dwelling women. Obstet Gynecol 111(3):678–685
16. Versi E, Harvey MA, Cardozo L, Brincat M, Studd JW (2001) Urogenital prolapse andatrophy at menopause: a prevalence study. Int Urogynecol J Pelvic Floor Dysfunct 12(2):107–110
17. Ismail SI, Bain C, Hagen S (2010) Oestrogens for treatment or prevention of pelvicorgan prolapse in postmenopausal women. Cochrane Database Syst Rev 2010(9):CD007063
18. Nappi RE, Davis SR (2012) The use of hormone therapy for the maintenance of urogynecological and sexual health post WHI. Climacteric 15(3):267–274
19. Bitar K, Greenwood-Van Meerveld B, Saad R, Wiley JW (2011) Aging and gastroin-testinal neuromuscular function: insights from within and outside the gut. Neurogastroenterol Motil 23(6):490–501
20. McFarland LV, Dublin S (2008) Meta-analysis of probiotics for the treatment of irritable bowel syndrome. World J Gastroenterol: WJG 14(17):2650–2661
21. Murad-Regadas SM, Rodrigues LV, Furtado DC, Regadas FS, Olivia da SFG, Regadas Filho FS et al (2012) The influence of age on posterior pelvic floor dys-function in women with obstructed defecation syndrome. Tech Coloproctol 16(3):227–232
22. Collins CW, Winters JC (2014) AUA/SUFU adult urodynamics guideline: a clinical review. Urol Clinics North Am 41:353–362
23. Mannella P, Palla G, Bellini M, Simoncini T (2013) The female pelvic floor through midlife and aging. Maturitas 76:230–234
24. Petros PE, Ulmsten UI (1990) Cure of urge incontinence by the combined intravaginal sling and tuck operation. Acta Obstet Gynecol Scand Suppl 153:61–62
25. Mannella P, Giannini A, Russo E, Naldini G, Simoncini T (2015) Personalizing pelvic floor reconstructive surgery in aging women. Maturitas 82(1):109–115
26. Rosier PF, Giarenis I, Valentini FA, Wein A, Cardozo L (2014) Do patients with symptoms and signs of lower urinary tract dysfunction need a urodynamic diagnosis? Neurourol Urodyn 33(5):581–586
27. Davis K, Kumar D (2005) Posterior pelvic floor compartment disorders. Best Pract Res Clin Obstet Gynaecol 19:941–958
28. Gallegos-Orozco JF, Foxx-Orenstein AE, Sterler SM, Stoa JM (2012) Chronic constipation in the elderly. Am J Gastroenterol 107:18–25
29. Bo K, Hilde G (2013) Does it work in the long term? A systematic review on pelvic floor muscle training for female stress urinary incontinence. Neurourol Urodyn 32(3):215–223
30. Rahn DD, Carberry C, Sanses TV, Mamik MM, Ward RM, Meriwether KV et al (2014) Vaginal estrogen for genitourinary syndrome of menopause: a systematic review. Obstet Gynecol 124:1147–1156
31. Holroyd-Leduc JM, Straus SE (2004) Management of urinary incontinence in women: scientific review. JAMA 291:986–995
32. Lee JK, Dwyer PL, Rosamilia A, Lim YN, Polyakov A, Stav K (2011) Persistence of urgency and urge urinary incontinence in women with mixed urinary symptoms after midurethral slings: a multivariate analysis. BJOG 118:798–805

33. Waltregny D, de Leval J (2009) The TVT-obturator surgical procedure for the treatment of female stress urinary incontinence: a clinical update. Int Urogynecol J Pelvic Floor Dysfunct 20(3):337–348
34. Cox A, Herschorn S, Lee L (2013) Surgical management of female SUI: is there a gold standard? Nat Rev. Urol 10:78–89
35. Maher C, Feiner B, Baessler K, Schmid C (2013) Surgical management of pelvic organ prolapse in women. Cochrane Database Syst Rev 4:CD004014
36. Sajadi KP, Goldman HB (2015) Robotic pelvic organ prolapse surgery. Nat Rev Urol 12(4):216–224
37. Mercer-Jones MA, D'Hoore A, Dixon AR, Lehur P, Lindsey I, Mellgren A et al (2014) Consensus on ventral rectopexy: report of a panel of experts. Color Dis 16:82–88
38. Dubuisson J, Eperon I, Dallenbach P, Dubuisson JB (2013) Laparoscopic repair of vaginal vault prolapse by lateral suspension with mesh. Arch Gynecol Obstet 287:307–312

Index

M. Birkhaeuser, A.R. Genazzani (eds.), *Pre-Menopause, Menopause and Beyond*, ISGE Series, https://doi.org/10.1007/978-3-319-63540-8

I

K

L

M

Printed by Printforce, the Netherlands